2015-2016

# Managing Contraception
for your pocket

AF856185

Mimi Zieman
Robert A. Hatcher
Ariel Z. Allen



February 2015

## COPYRIGHT INFORMATION



**Suggested formal citation:**
Zieman M, Hatcher RA., Allen A. Z. *Managing Contraception 2015-2016*. Tiger, Georgia: Bridging the Gap Foundation, 2015.

## IMPORTANT DISCLAIMER

The authors remind readers that this book is intended to educate health care providers, not guide individual therapy. The authors advise a person with a particular problem to consult a primary-care clinician or a specialist in obstetrics, gynecology, or urology (depending on the problem or the contraceptive) as well as the product package insert and other references before diagnosing, managing, or treating the problem. **Under no circumstances should the reader use this handbook in lieu of or to override the judgment of the treating clinician.** The order in which diagnostic or therapeutic measures appear in this text is not necessarily the order that clinicians *should* follow in each case. The authors and staff are not liable for errors or omissions.

Twelth Edition, 2015-2016
ISBN 978-0-578-15378-0
Printed in the United States of America
Bridging the Gap Foundation

On 200 pages, we cannot possibly provide you with all the information you might want or need about contraception. Many of the questions clinicians ask are answered in the textbook ***Contraceptive Technology*** or in detail on our website. Visit us regularly at: **www.managingcontraception.com**

➔ **Since the most lethal forms of ovarian cancer start in a women's fallopian tubes and then spread to her ovaries, how should tubal sterilization procedures, the most commonly utilized method of contraception, both in the United States and worldwide be performed? READ ON.**

2015-2016

# Managing Contraception
*for your pocket*

**Mimi Zieman, MD**
Adjunct Associate Professor of Gynecology and Obstetrics
Emory University School of Medicine

**Robert A. Hatcher, MD, MPH**
Professor Emeritus of Gynecology and Obstetrics
Emory University School of Medicine

**Ariel Z. Allen**
Student
Washington University in St. Louis

We want to thank the following individuals who contributed mightily as authors of previous editions of ***Managing Contraception:***

**Rachel Blankstein**

**Carrie Cwiak, MD, MPH**

**Philip D. Darney, MD, MSc**

**Mitchell D. Creinin, MD**

**Harriet R. Stosur, MD**

**Anita Nelson, MD**

**Erika Pluhar, PHD**

**Alston Watt, MsH**

**Technical and Computer Support:**
**DID Media, LLC., Cornelia, Georgia**
**Jason Blackburn**

Previous editions of this book enjoyed the support of both the Packard Foundation and an anonymous foundation.

*Bridging the Gap Foundation • Tiger, Georgia*
Please consider making a contribution to this 501-C3 organization.
The extent to which we can make this 2014-2015 edition of *Managing Contraception* available to medical students, residents and family planning programs internationally depends on contributions from people like you. Since the first edition of *Managing Contraception*, over **800,000 of the 1,075,000** copies of this book have been **given away at no cost** to medical students, residents, nursing and nurse midwifery students and family planning nurse practioners.

## OUR MISSION

The mission of *Bridging The Gap Foundation* is to improve reproductive health and contraceptive decision-making of women and men by providing up-to-date educational resources to the physicians, nurses and public health leaders of tomorrow.

## OUR VISION

Our vision is to provide educational resources to the health care providers of tomorrow to help ensure informed choices, better service, better access to service, happier and more successful contraceptors, competent clinicians, fewer unintended pregnancies and disease prevention.

We hope this e-book will make important information accessible to more people.

## *www.managingcontraception.com*

### Examples of questions answered on this website:

***I received a Mirena IUD on the 13th of October. My question is: From October 28th through November 4th I have been having a period. It's been 8 days. Is that normal*?**

**Reply on November 4th:**
Bleeding days exceed days with no blood for the first month using Mirena (not for everyone, but this is on average). You may continue to have more days of spotting or bleeding in the days or weeks or even months ahead. I hope the ➔ bleeding is becoming less over time. In time, women using Mirena have 90% LESS blood loss, less pain, less cramping and less symptoms for endometriosis than women of the same age using no hormonal method of contraception.

➔ Close to 30% of all women consider their menstrual beeding to be heavy. Because of missed work women with heavy menstrual bleeding earn an average of $1692 ➔ less annually than women with normal menses. Which hormonal medication was found by Gupta in 2013 to be most effective in decreasing heavy menstraul bleeding and accompanying symptons? See page XXX for the answer and references.

Robert A. Hatcher, MD, MPH
Emeritus Professor of Gynecology and Obstetrics
Emory University School of Medicine, Atlanta, GA

# HOW TO USE MANAGING CONTRACEPTION

This guide is designed to give up-to-date, immediate clinical information that is evidence-based. For more comprehensive information, we refer you to ***Contraceptive Technology***, an in-depth textbook, which is available through the website (www.managingcontraception.com) or in CD-ROM format.

***Managing Contraception*** is also be used extensively as a teaching tool.

Medical, nursing or public health students OR residents can be taught using ***Managing Contraception.***

Have fun with it! Bring examples of different birth control methods to show, props, etc.

One long-time user of past editions of Managing Contraception told attendees at the 2014 Contraceptive Technology conference in Atlanta:

> ***"I carry the little book, Managing Contraception, with me at all times. I have a copy on my desk at home, in my office at work, and on the exam tables where I see patients. I have a copy in my car, in each of my lab coats, and the suitcase I take on trips."*** ←

Thanks for your enthusiasm for this little book, **Dr. Eva Lathrop**. We authors also carry *Managing Contraception* with us at all times because we cannot possible remember all the details. ←

# DEDICATION

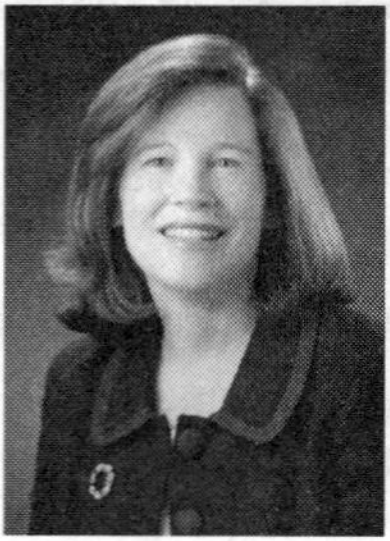

The 2015-2016 edition of Managing Contraception is dedicated to a person who has spent much of the last 30 years helping family planners across the globe improve the way we provide the remarkable contraceptives at our disposal.

After graduating from Middlebury College in Vermont as a biology major, Kate Curtis received an MSPH from the University of North Carolina in Chapel Hill with a concentration in Reproductive Health Epidemiology. She received her PhD from the Epidemiology Department at the School of Public Health at UNC Chapel Hill.

She then went to the Centers for Disease Control in Atlanta where she has been since 1998. She has worked primarily on two important questions for the past 16 years.

1) **Who Can Use Each of The Modern Contraceptives?**

2) **How to Provide These Methods?**

The first of these questions was answered by reviewing all of the relevant literature published on use of contraceptives in women with various medical conditions and convening a panel of experts to make recommendations which became the World Health Organization (WHO) Medical Eligibility Criteria. Later, with the leadership of Kate Curtis and Bert Peterson, this document was revised and updated for a U.S. audience creating the US Medical Eligibility Criteria. Thank you Kate Curtis for helping us answer important clinically relevant questions related to **WHO** can use particular methods such as:

**Can a woman who has had a blood clot use a levonorgestrel intrauterine device (Mirena)?**

**If a woman smokes can she use birth control pills?**

**Can a woman with endometrial hyperplasia use a Nexplanon implant?**

Katie Curtis next brought her competence and caring to the development of international and then U.S. documents that describe HOW the various methods are to be used: The Selected Practice Recommendations (SPR) for Contraceptive Use answer questions like:

**For how long is backup contraception required when starting pills, IUDs or implant?**

**When can postpartum women start using combined hormonal methods?**

**Are prophylactic antibiotics indicated for women receiving an IUD?**

**If a woman has had a pelvic infection, can she use an IUD?**

Dr. Jeffrey Peipert of Washington University in St. Louis and the St. Louis Contraceptive CHOICE Project suggested that "Dr. Kate Curtis has done the very important work which benefits all of us each day as we try to best serve our patients. Her work is incredibly important."

Kathryn M. Curtis has a remarkable toolkit that she has brought to the table consistently over the past two decades.

She brings together hardworking, dedicated groups of 5, 20 or 40 individuals willing to spend prodigious amounts of time on developing recommendations that have opened the door for providing contraceptives to a wider group of women. She carries to each meeting three or four huge books (three hole binders) each containing the scientific studies that could inform her panel of experts so that their conclusions could be as evidence based as possible.

Kate has a quiet energy and strength that never seem to become used up. She is kind and builds friendships along the way.

Robert Frost said that **"the best way out is always through."** Kate is a person who works through each challenge slowly and carefully. And all of us in family planning benefit daily from her attention to detail, patience, wisdom and hard work.

**Bob Hatcher and Mimi Zieman**

Atlanta, Georgia
January 2015

## IMPORTANT CONTACTS

| TOPIC | ORGANIZATION | PHONE NUMBER | WEBSITE |
|---|---|---|---|
| Abortion | Abortion Hotline (NAF) | (202) 667-5881 | www.prochoice.org |
| Abuse/Rape | National Domestic Violence Hotline | (312) 663-3520 | |
| | | 800-799-SAFE | www.ndvh.org |
| Adoption | Adopt a Special Kid-America | 888-680-7349 | www.adoptaspecialkid.org |
| | Adoptive Families of America | 800-372-3300 | www.adoptivefamilies.org |
| Breastfeeding | La Leche League | 800-LA-LECHE | www.lalecheleague.org |
| Contraception | Managing Contraception/ Bridging the Gap Communications | (770) 887-8383 | www.managingcontraception.com |
| | Planned Parenthood Federation of America | 800-230-PLAN | www.ppfa.org |
| | Family Health International | (919) 544-7040 | www.fhi.org |
| | World Health Organization | 011-41-22-791-21-11 | www.who.int |
| | Assoc. of Reproductive Health Professionals (ARHP) | (202) 466-3825 | www.arhp.org |
| Counseling | Depression and Bipolar Support Alliance | 800-826-3632 | www.ndmda.org |
| Emergency contraception | Emergency Contraception Information | 888-NOT-2-LATE | not-2-late.com |
| HIV/AIDS | Ntl. HIV/AIDS Clinicians' Consultation Center | | www.ucsf.edu/hivcntr |
| | Post-Exposure Prophylaxic Hotline (PEP) | 888-HIV-4911 | |
| Pregnancy | Lamaze International | 800-368-4404 | www.lamaze.org |
| | Depression After Delivery | 800-944-4773 | depressionafterdelivery.com |
| STIs | CDC Sexually Transmitted Disease Hotline | 800-342-AIDS | cdc.gov/nchstp/dstd/dstdp.html |

## HOW TO USE THIS BOOK

1. Chapter 29 is taken directly from the most recent CDC recommended guidelines for the treatment of STIs. STIs alphabetized on Page 166.
2. Color photos of pills help you to determine the pill your patient is/was on (A22 - A33)
3. The pages on the menstrual cycle concisely explain a very complicated series of events. Study pages 1-4 over and over again. Favorite subjects for exams!
4. Important: Sprintec (A27) and Tri-Sprintec (A31) are available for $10 per single cycle and $24 for three cycle ($8 per cycle) at Wal-Mart and other big box stores.
5. Algorithms throughout book; several that might help you are on the following pages:
   - Page 121: Choosing a pill
   - Page 122: What to do about breakthrough bleeding or spotting on pills
   - Page 146: Late for Depo-Provera injection
6. New algorithyms in this edition
   - → Late or missed pills (page 126)
   - → Recommended steps after vomiting or diarrhea on pills (page 127)
   - → Late or detached patch (page 130)
   - → Late placement of vaginal ring (page 134)

# ABBREVIATIONS USED IN THIS BOOK

**ACOG** American College of Obstetricians & Gynecologists
**AIDS** Acquired immunodeficiency syndrome
**AMA** American Medical Association
**ASAP** As soon as possible
**BBT** Basal body temperature
**BCA** Bichloroacetic acid
**BID** Twice daily
**BMI** Body Mass Index
**BP** Blood pressure
**BTB** Breakthrough bleeding
**BTL** Bilateral tubal ligation
**BV** Bacterial vaginosis
**CA** Cancer (if not California)
**CDC** Centers for Disease Control and Prevention
**COCs** Combined oral contraceptives (estrogen & progestin)
**CMV** Cytomegalovirus
**CT** Chlamydia trachomatis
**CVD** Cardiovascular disease
**D & C** Dilation and curettage
**D & E** Dilation and evacuation
**DCBE** Double contrast barium enema
**DMPA** Depot-medroxyprogesterone acetate (Depo-Provera)
**DUB** Dysfunctional uterine bleeding
**DVT** Deep vein thrombosis
**E** Estrogen
**EC** Emergency contraception
**ECPs** Emergency contraceptive pills ("morning-after pills")
**ED** Erectile dysfunction
**$E_2$** Estradiol
**EE** Ethinyl estradiol
**ENG** Etonorgestrel
**EPA** Environmental Protection Agency
**EPT** Estrogen-progestin therapy
**ET** Estrogen therapy
**EVA** Ethylene vinyl acetate
**FAM** Fertility awareness methods
**FDA** Food and Drug Administration
**FH** Family History
**FSH** Follicle stimulating hormone
**GAPS** Guidelines for Adolescent Preventive Services
**GC** Gonococcus/gonorrhea
**GI** Gastrointestinal
**GnRH** Gonadotrophin-releasing hormone
**HBsAg** Hepatitis B surface antigen
**HAV** Hepatitis A virus
**HBV** Hepatitis B virus
**HCG** Human chorionic gonadotrophin
**HCV** Hepatitis C virus
**HDL** High density lipoprotein
**HIV** Human immunodeficiency virus
**HMB** Heavy menstrual bleeding
**HPV** Human papillomavirus
**HSV** Herpes simplex virus (I or II)
**H(R)T** Hormone (replacement) therapy
**IM** Intramuscular
**IPPF** International Planned Parenthood Federation
**IUC** Intrauterine contraceptive
**IUD** Intrauterine device
**IUP** Intrauterine pregnancy
**IUS** Intrauterine system
**IV** Intravenous
**KOH** Potassium hydroxide
**LARC** Long acting reversible contraception
**LAM** Lactational amenorrhea method

| | |
|---|---|
| LARC | Long acting reversible contraceptives |
| LDL | Low-density lipoprotein |
| LGV | Lymphogranuloma venereum |
| LH | Luteinizing hormone |
| LMP | Last menstrual period |
| LNG | Levonorgestrel |
| MI | Myocardial infarction |
| MIS | Misoprostol |
| MMG | Mammogram |
| MMPI | Minnesota Multiphasic Personality Inventory |
| MMR | Mumps Measles Rubella |
| MMWR | Mortality and Morbidity Weekly Report |
| MPA | Medroxyprogesterone acetate |
| MRI | Magnetic resonance imaging |
| MSM | Men who have sex with men |
| MTX | Methotrexate |
| MVA | Manual vacuum aspiration |
| N-9 | Nonoxynol-9 |
| NFP | Natural family planning |
| NSAID | Nonsteroidal anti-inflammatory drug |
| OA | Overeaters Anonymous |
| OB/GYN | Obstetrics & Gynecology |
| OC | Oral contraceptive |
| OR | Operating Room |
| OTC | Over the counter |
| P | Progesterone or progestin |
| Pap | Papanicolaou |
| PCOS | Polycystic ovarian syndrome |
| PE | Pulmonary embolism |
| PET | Polyesther (fibers) |
| PG | Prostaglandin |
| pH | Hydrogen ion concentration |
| PID | Pelvic inflammatory disease |
| PLISSIT | Permission giving<br>Limited information<br>Simple suggestions<br>Intensive<br>Therapy |
| PMDD | Premenstrual dysphoric disorder |
| PMS | Premenstrual syndrome |
| po | Latin: "per os"; orally, by mouth |
| POCs | Progestin-only contraceptives |
| POP | Progestin-only pill (minipill) |
| PP | Postpartum |
| PPFA | Planned Parenthood Federation of America |
| PRN | As needed |
| qd | Once daily |
| qid | Four times a day |
| RR | Relative risk |
| Rx | Prescription |
| SAB | Spontaneous abortion |
| SHBG | Sex hormone binding globulin |
| SPT | Spotting |
| SSRI | Selective Serotonin Reuptake Inhibitors |
| STD | Sexually transmitted disease |
| STI | Sexually transmitted infection |
| Sx | Symptoms |
| TAB | Therapeutic abortion/elective abortion |
| TB | Tuberculosis |
| TCA | Trichloroacetic acid |
| tid | Three times a day |
| TSS | Toxic shock syndrome |
| URI | Upper respiratory infection |
| US MEC | US Medical Eligibility Criteria |
| UTI | Urinary tract infection |
| VTE | Venous thromboembolism |
| VVC | Vulvovaginal candidiasis |
| WHO | World Health Organization |
| ZDV | Zidovudine |

# CHAPTER 1
# The Menstrual Cycle

www.noperiod.com

## SEVERAL KEY POINTS ON MENSTRUAL PHYSIOLOGY:

- ***What initiates menses (and the next cycle)*** is atrophy of the corpus luteum on or about day 25 of a typical 28 day cycle. This atrophy is initiated by a decline in LH release from the anterior pituitary gland and results in a fall in serum estrogen (E) and progesterone (P) levels. Without hormonal support, the endometrium sloughs. This drop in hormonal levels is also detected by the hypothalamus and pituitary, and FSH levels increase to stimulate follicles for the next cycle (Fig. 1.1 and 1.2).
- ***Anovulation in women NOT on hormonal contraception leads to prolonged cycles, oligomenorrhea, amenorrhea or irregular bleeding.*** It contributes to difficulty becoming pregnant for some women. The absence of progesterone in anovulatory women *not* on hormones or a contraceptive that provides a progestin places these women at risk for endometrial hyperplasia and endometrial cancer. The uterus of these women is being exposed over and over again to unopposed estrogen. Recovery of ovarian function and return of ovulation has been demonstrated in women with functional hypothalamic amenorrhea who have been treated with cognitive behaviorial therapy designed to improve coping skills for circumstances and moods that exacerbate stress *[Berga-2003]*. Similar results have also been achieved in women treated with hypnotherapy *[Tschugguel-2003]*
- ***The two-cell, two gonadotrophin theory:*** At the very beginning of the cycle, the outer theca cells can only be stimulated by LH and produce androgens (testosterone and androstenedione) and the inner granulosa cells can only be stimulated by FSH. Androgens diffuse toward the inner layer *granulosa* cells where they are converted into estradiol ($E_2$) by FSH-stimulated aromatase.
- In a developing follicle, ***low androgen levels*** not only serve as the substrate for FSH-induced aromatization, but also stimulate aromatase activity. On the other hand, ***high levels of androgens*** (an "androgen-rich" environment as in some women with polycystic ovaries) lead to inhibition of aromatase activity and to follicular atresia.
- The female infant is born with 1-2 million follicles, most of which undergo atresia before puberty. Only about 10-20 follicles each month are recruited by rising FSH levels. The recruitment actually occurs during the late luteal phase of the preceeding cycle. Of those 10-20 follicles, usually only one dominant follicle ovulates. The number of follicles stimulated each month depends on the number of follicles left in the residual pool.
- FSH levels are low before ovulation as a result of negative feedback on FSH of $E_2$ and inhibin B. The dominant follicle "escapes" the effects of falling FSH levels before ovulation, because it has more granulosa cells, more FSH receptors on each of its granulosa cells, and increased blood flow. Cut off from adequate FSH stimulation, the other nondominant follicles undergo atresia.
- When $E_2$ production is sustained at sufficient levels (about 200 pg/ml) for more than 50 hours, negative feedback of $E_2$ on LH reverses to positive feedback. The LH surge occurs, and about 12 hours later an oocyte is extruded.
- About 50,000 granulosa cells form the corpus luteum. Some granulosa cells continue to produce $E_2$ and inhibins but many join the outer layers of theca cells to produce progesterone (P). Inhibin selectively suppresses FSH, not LH. The highest levels of inhibin are during the mid-luteal phase (primarily inhibin A now), causing FSH levels to be the lowest in the mid-luteal phase. At the end of the cycle (10-14 days after ovulation) if the corpus luteum is not rescued by HCG produced by the implanted trophoblast (pregnancy), the corpus luteum will undergo programmed atresia. Falling $E_2$, P, and inhibin levels induce the release of FSH to initiate another cycle.

**Figure 1.1 Menstrual cycle events - Idealized 28 Day Cycle**

[Hatcher RA, et al. *Contraceptive Technology*. 20th ed. New York: Irvington, 2011:37]

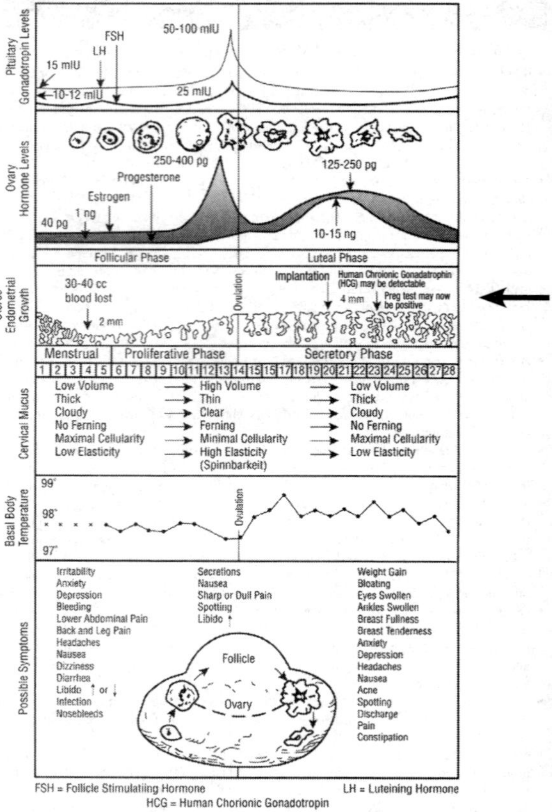

## Figure 1.2 Regulation of the menstrual cycle

[Hatcher RA, et al. *Contraceptive Technology*. 20th ed. New York: Irvington, 2011:32]

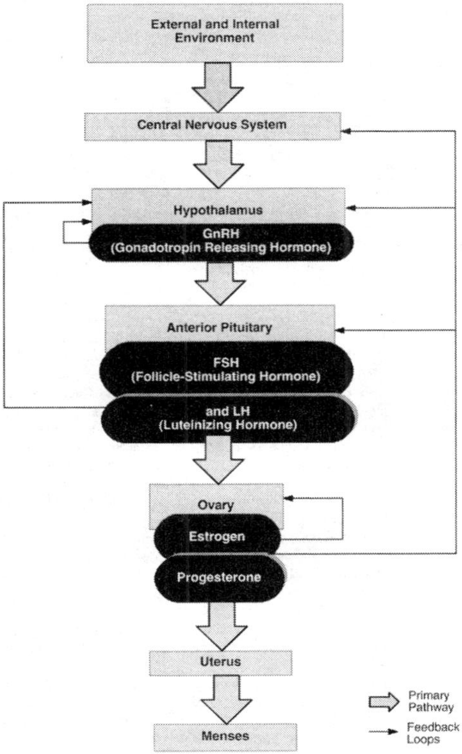


Primary hormone pathways (⇨) in the reproductive system are modulated by both negative and positive feedback loops (→). Prostaglandins, secreted by the ovary and by uterine endometrial cells, also play a role in ovulation, and may modulate hypothalamic function as well.

## *Is Menstruation Obsolete? Who Needs a Period?*

The extended or continuous use of pills causes women to have fewer "pill periods". Most, but not all, women like this *[Ropes-2002]*. Decreased periods or no periods at all is important to discuss with women considering use of continuous pills, Depo-Provera injections, the Mirena IUD or the implant. A 2003 Gallop poll found that 99% of female gynecologists consider menstrual suppression safe.

**Very Important Counseling Mesage:**
Educate women that a "pill period" is, by definition, arbitrary, which is why the timing of the pill period can be manipulated.

***What is "natural" — 50, 150, or 450 menstrual periods in a woman's lifetime?*** In **prehistoric times** women had **50** menstrual cycles or fewer. In **Colonial America**, when women were having an average of 8 babies and nursing each baby for 2-3 years, women averaged **150** menstrual periods per lifetime. **Currently** in America women who are not on contraceptives that markedly decrease the number of periods have on average **450-480** menstrual cycles per lifetime. *[Segal, 2001]*

Some women find regular menses reassuring, positive, "natural" or important evidence that they are still capable of reproducing. Many women regularly experience inconvenience, messiness, blood loss, painful menses, cyclic migraines, depression, ovarian cysts, and/or breast tenderness, would be happier having periods less often, or not at all (also see discussion of extended use of COCs on page 100).

Many women feel both positively and negatively about their periods. Close to half of all GYN visits are for difficulties women experience at the time of their menses. *[Segal, 2001]* Women experiencing symptoms associated with their menses may benefit from contraceptives that alter the likelihood of ovulation, the amount of blood lost each month, or the extent of menstrual cramping and pain. In some instances, women may benefit from contraceptives that completely eliminate monthly periods. This is particularly likely to be true for women with any of the following cyclic symptoms: PMS, endometriosis, dysmenorrhea, depression, headaches, seizures, nausea, vomiting, breast enlargement or tenderness or very heavy bleeding. Unfortunately, few women are aware of the noncontraceptive benefits of contraceptives *[Peipert, 1993]* or of basic contraceptive knowledge *[Davis, 2006]*.

**Clearly some women choose contraceptives to gain relief from symptoms related to their menstrual cycles. Others discontinue contraceptives due to undesirable effects on the patterns of their menses.** In the pages ahead, the advantages and disadvantages of each contraceptive related to the menstrual cycle are described.

A provocative book by Coutinho and Segal raises the question: ***Is Menstruation Obsolete?*** *[Coutinho, 1999]* These two individuals played pivotal roles in the research leading to the approval of a number of our current contraceptives. Here is a comment on their book:

Kate Miller, MPH, of the University of Pennsylvania states: ***One of the difficulties of regular menstruation is the usual assembly of monthly symptoms - cramps, headache, fatigue, irritability - which are often dismissed as part of "the curse" that women must simply endure. Since women tolerate these symptoms so regularly, they may not automatically include them in the "risks" of monthly menstruation. The reader is encouraged to recognize what may have previously gone unnoticed: that this monthly discomfort is simply not obligatory. In fact, it can be a startling exercise for a woman to imagine her life without the hassles and ailments of regular menstruation. This is a message whose time has come.***

It is a leading theory that ovarian cancers usually originate in the fimbria of the fallopian tubes. At the time of tubal sterilization, removal of the tubes (salpingectomy) should be considered.

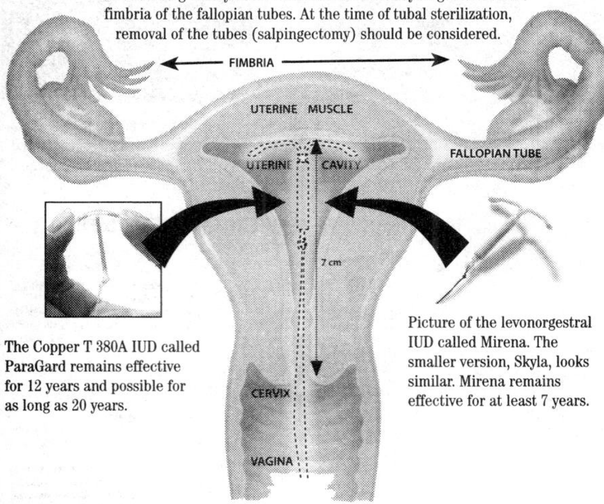


The Copper T 380A IUD called ParaGard remains effective for 12 years and possible for as long as 20 years.

Picture of the levonorgestral IUD called Mirena. The smaller version, Skyla, looks similar. Mirena remains effective for at least 7 years.

**In this diagram, the distance from the opening of the cervix up to the top of the uterine cavity measures 7.0 centimeters (just less than 3 inches). Before having a baby, 70% of women 15-25 years of age have a uterus this size or larger. A uterus this size has adequate room for a Mirena or ParaGard IUD in over 90% of women.**

## WHAT ARE THE ADVANTAGES OF THE HORMONAL IUD? (more on page 89)

- Mirena decreases menstrual cramping and dramatically decreases menstrual blood loss. In fact, the Mirena IUD is the most effective medical therapy for heavy menstrual bleeding. [Gupta 2013, NEJM]
- About 20% of women experience an absence of menstrual bleeding after one year of using the Mirena IUD. happens in just 4% after one year in users of the Skyla levonorgestrel IUD [Skyla package insert]
- Mirena appears to have a 50% protective effect against pelvic infections.
- Endometrial cancer is one of the most common reproductive cancers in women. It can be prevented if postmenopausal women on estrogen therapy use Mirena.
- Mirena IUDs are often prescribed for women with:
  - Heavy menstrual bleeding
  - Endometriosis
  - Anemia
  - Fibroids
  - Cramping or pain with periods
  - Adenomyosis
  - Dysfunctional uterine bleeding (DUB)
  - Endometrial hyperplasia (and occasionally for stage 1 endometrialca)

# CHAPTER 2

## Counseling Guidelines

www.gmhc.org, www.plannedparenthood.org, www.bedsider.org, www.choiceprojectwustl.edu

One of the main paradigm shifts we would like to emphasize is that women should be encouraged to consider a LARC (long-acting reversible contraceptive) method as a first-line option when wanting to prevent pregnancy. These methods, IUDs and implants, are among the most effective methods, and therefore, should be considered first.

### COMPARING TYPICAL EFFECTIVENESS OF CONTRACEPTIVE METHODS

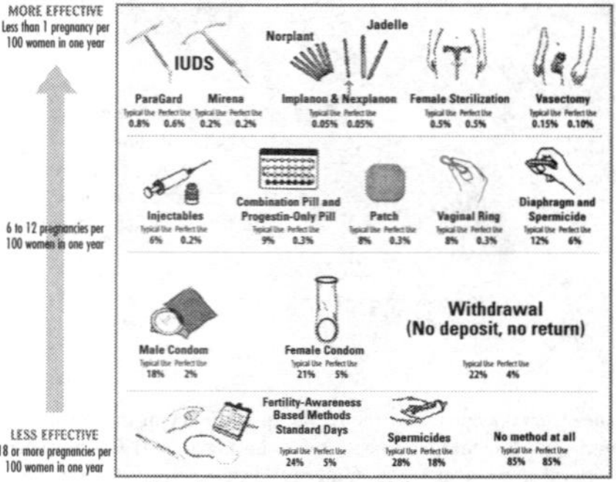


**Thank you James Trussell for these numbers!**

**How to make your method most effective**

**After procedure, little or nothing to do or remember.**
Vasectomy: **Use another method for first 3 months and until there are no motile sperm on 2 semen analyses.**
Injections: **Get repeat injections on time**
Pills: **Take a pill each day**
Patch, Ring: **Keep in place, change on time**
Condom, Diaphragm: **Use correctly every single time you have sex**
Fertility-awareness based methods: **Abstain or use condoms on fertile days. Newest methods (Standard Days Method and Two Day Method) may be easier to use and consequently more effective.**
Withdrawal, spermicide: **Use correctly every time you have sex.**

***Adapted from WHO 2007 and Contraceptive Technology, 20th Edition, 2011***

***Advantages of counseling:***

- Repeatedly encourage use of most effective, least complicated methods
- Goal is reducing unintended pregnancies, now 50% of U.S. pregnancies
- Involves patient in his/her own care and dispels misconceptions, myths and rumors
- Improves success with complicated regimens
- Advises change of risky behaviors
- Facilitates the decision-making process regarding contraception and STI prevention
- Explains possible side effects, which reduces anxiety, increases success with method and encourages clients to contact if problems occur, reducing severity of complications
- Strengthens the provider/patient relationship
- Encourages patient responsibility for his/her health decisions
- Ensures and maintains *confidentiality*

Each night, 700,000 to 1 million women in the US who do not want to become pregnant have sex with no protection. One of the most important questions is: *Are you repeatedly having unprotected sex? If yes, what is your plan for birth control?*
"If preventing an unwanted pregnancy is important to you, and you are repeatedly having unprotected intercourse, strongly consider using one of the two IUDs or the implant."

***Principles of good counseling: Allow plenty of time***

- Know what you are talking about!
- *Listen*, look at your patients, allow them to speak freely, paraphrase what you hear
- *Respect,* recognize and accept each individual's unique situation
- Accept and anticipate that behavior change occurs slowly and incrementally.
- Remain *sensitive*; acknowledge that sex/sexuality are very personal
- Be *nonjudgmental* and encourage *self-determination;* avoid *false reassurance*
- ***Urge all your patients to know their HIV status;*** each encounter offers opportunity to counsel about STI/HIV prevention and contraception
- Inquire about problems patients may have had with previous medical recommendations
- Realize your patient will remember only 1-4 points from each visit. Avoid information overload and provide written information at appropriate reading level for later reference

***Reproductive/Contraceptive Goals:***

| GOAL: | MAIN CONTRACEPTIVE CONCERNS MAY BE: |
|---|---|
| Delaying birth of first child | Effectiveness of method, future fertility and STIs; explain EC |
| Avoiding abortion | Need for maximal effectiveness; Tell about ECs;<br>May want to use 2 methods consistently |
| Spacing births | Balance of efficacy & convenience; explain EC; safety with breastfeeding |
| Completed childbearing | Needs effective method for long term |

Also see "Increasing Contraceptive Effectiveness" -Seven Suggestions, page 39.

**In providing each contraception, keep your antennea up for the myths that are discouraging women and men, boys and girls from using this method. Seven myths:**

1. **IUDs cause abortion.** No, both Mirena and Paragard IUDs prevent fertilization, thus preventing both spontaneous abortions (miscarriages) and the need for induced abortions due to unintended pregnancies.
2. **Condoms are not effective at preventing sexually transmitted infections.** WRONG: According to the CDC, condoms are highly effective vs. STIs, providing an essentially impermeable barrier to particles the size of STI pathogens. Women using IUDs, impants, pills, rings, patches, or injections should use condioms, too!
3. **Hormonal contraceptives cause cancer.** DEFINITELY WRONG! Pills prevent colon, ovary and endometrial cancer. Pills do not increase a woman's risk for breast cancer. Mirena IUDs prevent endometrial hyperplasia and endometrial cancer. *[Speroff 2001]*
4. **Women with fibroids cannot use a Mirena IUD.** WRONG: In fact, Mirena IUDs decrease fibroid bleeding and, perhaps, fibroid size.
5. **Women cannot use an IUD until they have had a baby.** NO, both the World Health Organization and the Centers for Disease Control (CDC) consider the IUD an acceptable choice for women who have not had a baby. IUDs do not cause pelvic infections or ectopic pregnancies. Mirena appears to prevent pelvic imflammatory disease (Toivin 1991).
6. **IUDs are just too expensive.** Well, they may have a high up-front cost, over time, IUDs are definitely the most cost effective reversible contraceptives. 100% cost $0 if a woman is covered by the Affordable Care Act.
7. **IUDs increase an adolescent's risk of PID, STDs, and infertility.** A 2007 Committee Opinion of ACOG concluded that the IUD does not increase an adolescent's risk of PID, STDs or infertility and that the levonogestrel IUD may lower the risk of PID.

## WHAT DOES STRUCTURED COUNSELING MEAN?

***Carefully planned structured counseling may include:***

- Repetition of a specific message at the time of the initial visit
- Having the patient repeat back her understanding of a message
- Use of a clear, concise videotape
- Asking the patient if she has questions about the videotape
- Written information and instructions that highlight key messages
- Repetition at each follow-up visit
- Checklist for patient to fill out at ***each*** follow up visit

*Example: Structured counseing for Depo-Provera**

- **The message: Depo-Provera will change your periods.** No woman's periods stay the same as they were before starting Depo-Provera. Ask: ***"Will you find it acceptable if there are major changes in your periods?"*** If no, steer clear of DMPA (as well as progestin-only pills, Implanon, Nexplanon, Mirena)
- Have the patient repeat back her understanding of the message, particularly that **over time women stop having periods most months.** Women tend to have very irregular menses almost immediately
- Use of a clear, concise videotape
- Asking the patient if she has questions about the videotape
- Written instructions that clearly highlight the key messages
- Asking at each 3-month visit what has happened to a woman's pattern of bleeding, whether amenorrhea has begun and how she feels about her pattern of bleeding

***Checklist for Depo-Provera patient to fill out <u>at each follow up visit</u>. Please check yes or no. Tell us if you have/are:***

| | | |
|---|---|---|
| Spotting or irregular vaginal bleeding | ☐ Yes | ☐ No |
| Missed periods or very, very light periods | ☐ Yes | ☐ No |
| Concern over your pattern of vaginal bleeding | ☐ Yes | ☐ No |
| Depression, severe anxiety or mood changes | ☐ Yes | ☐ No |
| Gained 5 pounds or more | ☐ Yes | ☐ No |
| Questions you want to ask us about Depo-Provera injections | ☐ Yes | ☐ No |
| Any wrist, hip or other fractures | ☐ Yes | ☐ No |
| Using calcium supplements | ☐ Yes | ☐ No |
| Regular exercise | ☐ Yes | ☐ No |

* Continuation rates for women started on Depo-Provera are only 40-60% at one year. Structured counseling has been shown to improve these rates. See Page 144 for more details that include the results of a randomized study in Mexico.
Structured counseling is important for women starting any method of contraception, including barrier methods.

# CHAPTER 3

## Providing Quality Family Planning Services (QFP)

**Screening Recommendations for Women of Reproductive Age Related to Family Planning Services**

### Recommendations from CDC and the U.S Office of Population Affairs

http://www.cdc.gov/mmwr/preview/mmwrhtml/rr6304a1.htm?s_cid=rr6304a1_w

**The full CDC document outlines how to determine need for services e.g., assessing reason for visit, whether she has another source for primary care, need for STD services etc.**

➢ *Document is organized by different types of visits made, or need for, contraceptive services, pregnancy test visit, infertility visit, preconception health visit, STD services, and related preventive health services*

➢ *The screening recommendations in this chapter are detailed mostly under preconception health services but apply regardless of a woman's childbearing intentions*

➢ *These recommendations do not include all preventive health services that women of reproductive age may need e.g. screening for lipid disorders or skin cancer. Although imp't for primary care, they are not related to Family Planning Services*

➢ *Full recommendations at: http://www.cdc.gov/mmwr/preview/mmwrhtml/rr6304a1.htm?s_cid=rr6304a1_w*

- **Intimate partner violence:** screen and refer to intervention services
- **Alcohol, smoking and drug use:** screen and refer to intervention services
- **Immunization:** screen for status and provide or refer including influenza, Tdap, MMR, Varicella, Pneumococcal and meningococcal.
  - ACOG recommends rubella titers in women unsure of MMR status
- **Depression:** screen when staff-assisted depression care supports are in place
  - if patient experiencing depression, assess risk for suicide
- **Obesity:** screen with height, weight, BMI and if obese refer for intensive counseling and behavioral interventions
- **Blood pressure:** measure routinely
  - If less than 120/80 screen every 2 years
  - If 120-139/80-89 screen yearly
- **Diabetes:** screen in all adults with sustained BP (treated or untreated) more than 135/80
- **Chlamydia:** all sexually active women ≤ 25 annually and > 25 with risk factors for CT

| RISK FACTORS FOR CT | |
|---|---|
| • New partners | • >1 partner |
| • Partners with other partners | |

  - If treating for CT, rescreen at 3 months for re-infection
  - Screen pregnant women at time of their pregnancy test if care may be delayed
- **Gonorrhea:** screen all sexually active women at risk annually

| RISK FACTORS FOR GC | |
|---|---|
| • Age <25 | • previous GC infection, |
| • presence of other STDs | • new or multiple partners |
| • inconsistent condom use | • commercial sex work, drug use |

  - If treating for GC, rescreen at 3 months for re-infection
  - Screen pregnant women at time of their pregnancy test if care may be delayed

- **Syphilis:** screen those at risk:

| RISK FACTORS FOR SYPHILIS | |
|---|---|
| • MSM | • sex workers |
| • those who exchange sex for drugs | • in adult correctional facilities |
| • high prevalence areas | |

  - Screen pregnant women at time of pregnancy test if care may be delayed
- **HIV:** screen ages 13-64 routinely and high risk annually

| RISK FACTORS FOR HIV |
|---|
| • injection drug users and their partners |
| • those who exchange sex for money or drugs and their partners, |
| • partners of HIV infected |
| • MSM |
| • people with more than 1 partner since last HIV test |

- **Hepatitis C:** one time testing for people born between 1945-1965 (account for 75% of chronic HCV infections) as well as those at high risk.

| RISK FACTORS FOR HCV | |
|---|---|
| • Born between 1945-1965 | • Ever injected illegal drugs |
| • Received clotting factors before 1987 | • Ever on chronic hemodialysis |
| • Received organ transplant | • Blood transfusion before 1992 |
| • Persistently abnormal alanine aminotransferase | |
| • Needles stick by someone HCV positive | |
| • Child born to HCV positive woman | |

- **HPV vaccine:** offer to ages 11-26
- **Hepatitis B vaccine:** offer to all unvaccinated under 19 years and all adults who are unvaccinated and do not have documented hx of Hepatitis B infection
- **Cervical cytology:** pap smears age 21-65 every 3 years, ages 30-65 screen with combination of cytology and HPV testing every 5 years

  **The need for cervical cytology should not delay initiation or hinder continuation of contraception**

- **Clinical Breast Exam:** can be recommended. USPSTF says there is insufficient evidence to assess balance of benefits vs. harms. ACOG recommends screening Q3yrs ages 20-39 and yearly after 40
- **Mammography:** ages less than 50 screen based on individual patient's risk, 50-74 screen biennially, ACOG-recommends annual screening more than 40 yrs

## STD RECOMMENDATIONS:

- Provide high-intensity behavioral counseling for those at risk including: all sexually active adolescents, adults with current STD or in past year, adults with multiple partners, or live in high prevalence communities
- When treating for an STD, counsel about need for partner treatment
  - partners in the past 60 days for CT and GC
  - 3 months for primary syphilis and 6 months for secondary syphilis PLUS the duration of lesions or signs
  - if partners cannot be examined, expedited partner therapy (giving prescription to treat partner for GC or CT) can be offered if permissible by state laws.
- Advise to refrain from unprotected sexual intercourse during Rx
- Return for retesting in 3 months
- Encourage condom use

# CHAPTER 4
# Taking a Sexual History
www.siecus.org

***Taking Sexual Histories***
Explain to the patient that obtaining sexual information is necessary to provide complete care, but reassure her/him that she/he has the right to discuss only what she/he is comfortable divulging. Ask patients less direct questions in the beginning to build trust, then ask the questions that explicitly address sexual issues once you have their confidence. **Be cautious about what information you place on the chart.** Medical records are not necessarily confidential and can be reviewed by insurance companies **(may also be subpoenaed in legal proceedings)**

***Suggestions for Initiating the Sexual History***
- I will be asking some personal questions about your sexual activity to help me make more accurate diagnoses. This is a normal part of the exam I do with all patients
- **To help keep accurate medical records, I will be writing down some of your responses. If there are things you do not want me to record, please tell me**
- Some patients have shared concerns with me related to their risks of infections or concerns about particular sexual activities. If you have any concerns, I would be happy to discuss them with you

***Sexual History Questions***
*Beware! People may have great difficulty giving honest answers to the following intimate questions.*
- **What are you doing to protect yourself from HIV and other infections? OR What are you doing that puts you at risk for HIV?**
- Do you have questions regarding sex or sexual activity?
- How old were you when you had your first sexual experience? What Happened?
- Do you have sex with men, women or both?
- Do you need contraception? How are you protecting yourself from unwanted pregnancy?
- How many sex partners have you had in the last 3 months? in the last 6 months? in your lifetime?
- How many sex partners does your partner have? Can you discuss this together?
- Do you have penis in vagina sex? penis in mouth sex? penis in rectum sex?
- Do you drink alcohol or take drugs in association with sexual activity?
- Have you ever been forced or coerced to have sex? What kind of force was used?
- Are you now in a relationship where you feel physically, sexually, or emotionally threatened or abused?
- When you were younger, did anyone touch your private body parts or ask you to touch theirs?
- Have you ever had sex for money, food, protection, drugs or shelter?
- Do you enjoy sex? Do you usually have orgasms? Do you ever have pain with sex?
- Do you or your partner(s) have any sexual concerns?
- Do you awaken from sleep and you are having intercourse? (If this happens often, condoms and other barrier methods may not be the best method for you.)

***Avoid Assumptions***: Making assumptions about a patient's sexual behavior and orientation can leave out important information, undermine patient trust and make the patient feel judged or alienated, causing her to withhold information. This can result in diagnostic and treatment errors. Do not assume that patients:
- ARE sexually active and need contraception
- Are NOT sexually active (e.g., older patients, young adolescents)
- Are heterosexual, homosexual or bisexual OR know if their partners have other partners
- Have power (within a relationship) to make or implement their own contraceptive decisions

# CHAPTER 5

## Sexual Dysfunction

www.herhealth.com, www.newshe.com or www.assect.org

### FEMALE

***Dyspareunia***

- *Definition:* Pain during vaginal intercourse or vaginal penetration
- *Key questions:* Do you have pain with vaginal penetration? Do you have pain with early entry or in the mid vaginal area? Is there pain with deep thrusting? Is pain occasional or consistent? With every partner? Does the pain change with different sexual positions? Are you aroused and lubricated before penetration?
- *Causes:* Organic - vestibulitis, urethritis/UTI, vaginitis, cervicitis, vulvodynia, vulvar dystrophy, interstitial cystitis, traumatic deliveries (forcep or vacuum extractions), hypoestrogenism, PID, endometriosis, surgical scars or adhesions, pelvic injuries, tumors, hip joint or disc pain, female circumcision, orgasmic spasm, lack of foreplay, lubrication
  Psychological - current or previous abuse, relationship stress, depression, anxiety, fear of sex or fear of pregnancy
- *Treatment:* Directed to underlying pathology including depression. If dyspareunia is chronic, consider supplementing medical management with supportive counseling and sex therapy

***Vaginismus (special case of dyspareunia)***

- *Definition:* Painful involuntary spastic contraction of introital and pelvic floor muscles
- *Causes:* Organic - may be secondary to current or previous dyspareunia and its causes. Psychological - sexual abuse, fears of abnormal anatomy (e.g. terror that vagina will rip with penile or speculum introduction), negative attitudes about sexuality
- *Treatment:* Education is critical. Insight into underlying causes helps. After source is recognized, start progressive desensitization exercises, which may include self manipulation, dilators and/or biofeedback and pelvic floor physical therapy. Sex therapist/psychologist intervention may be needed to deal with unconscious fears unresponsive to education

***Decreased Libido (Hypoactive Sexual Desire)***

- *Definition:* Relative lack of sexual desire defined by individual as troublesome to her sexual relationship (there is no absolute "normal" level)
- *Causes:* **Organic** - may be due to acute or chronic debilitating medical condition (e.g., diabetes, stroke, spinal cord injury, arthritis, pain, cancer, chronic obstructive pulmonary disease, coronary artery disease, etc.), medications (e.g. sedatives, narcotics, hypnotics, anticonvulsants, centrally-acting antihypertensives, tranquilizers, anorectics, oral contraceptives, Depo-Provera, and some antidepressants), dyspareunia, incontinence, alcohol, hormonal imbalance, or healing episiotomy or other surgical scars; Sexual practices - inadequate sexual stimulation or time for arousal. Sexual desires discordant with partner's desires
  **Psychological** - depression, anxiety, exhaustion, life stress (finances, relationship problems, etc.), poor partner communication, lack of understanding about impacts of aging. Change in body image (breast-feeding, postpartum, weight gain, cancer, or post mastectomy or hysterectomy)
- *Treatment:* Treat underlying causes where possible. Rule out hyperactive sexual desire disorder of partner. Reassure about normalcy, if appropriate. Help patient create time and special space for sexual expression - no distractions from children, telephone, household chores. Suggest variety in sexual practices perhaps with aid of fantasies (romantic novels, films, etc). Exogenous testosterone therapy has yielded mixed results in studies and is not FDA approved. New drugs and creams, causing increased blood flow to the clitoris, may increase sexual arousal for those women whose problems started after developing a

medical disorder and had normal function previously. Consider referral to sex therapist. Read *For Each Other* by Lonnie Barbach and *Women, Sex & Desire* by Elizabeth Davis or *Our Bodies, Ourselves* by the Boston Women's Health Collective

***Excessive Sexual Desire (Hyperactive Sexual Desire)***
- *Definition:* Excessive sexual activity resulting in social, psychological and physical problems. See Diagnostic and Statistical Manual of Mental Disorders, Fourth Edition (DSM-IV)
- *Cause:* Low self esteem; abuse; attention seeking; acting out; mania; bipolar disease
- *Treatment:* Refer for psychological counseling and therapy and Sex Addicts Anonymous

***Orgasmic Disorders: Anorgasmia or Primary Anorgasmia***
- *Definitions:*
  - *Preorgasmia or Primary Anorgasmia:* Never experienced orgasms and desires to be orgasmic
  - *Secondary Anorgasmia:* Orgasmic in past, no orgasms currently, desirous of orgasm
- *Cause:* Organic - may be secondary to dyspareunia, neurological, vascular disease, medications (e.g. sedatives, narcotics, hypnotics, anticonvulsants, centrally-acting antihypertensives, tranquilizers, anorectics, and some antidepressants - particularly SSRI class antidepressants), or poor sexual techniques of partner (painful, rapid ejaculation) Psychological - negative attitude about sexuality, chronic relationship stress; lack of knowledge about body and sexual response, depression, life stress
- *Treatment:* Treat underlying organic causes, if possible. Explain sexual response (suggest reading ***Our Bodies, Ourselves*** or ***For Yourself***). Add behavioral/psychological approach using PLISSIT model (see Abbreviations, Page ix), and sensate focusing exercises. Help couple set alternative pleasuring goals. Refer to sex therapist if initial interventions not successful. Have woman learn how to have an orgasm on her own in comfortable environment and then she can teach her partner how to pleasure her. Recommend use of lubricants, vibrators and sex toys.

## MALE

***Decreased Libido (Hypoactive sexual desire disorder)***
- No absolute level is "normal"; "decreased libido" is usually related to previous experience, partner's expectations, or perceived societal norms
- Evaluation and treatment similar to female's (see above)

***Excessive Sexual Desire (Hyperactive Sexual Desire)***
- *Definition:* Excessive sexual activity resulting in social, psychological and physical problems.
- *Cause:* Abuse at young age; attention seeking; acting out; mania; other such as bipolar disease
- *Treatment:* Refer for psychological counseling and therapy, Sex Addicts Anonymous after therapy

***Premature (Rapid) Ejaculation***
- *Definition:* Recurrent ejaculation before or shortly after vaginal penetration or ejaculation occurs earlier than patient or partner desires. Average time from entry to ejaculation in "normal" couples is 2 minutes; shorter interval is consistent with diagnosis.
- *Causes:* Organic - urethritis, prostatitis, neurological disease (e.g. multiple sclerosis). Psychological - learned behavior, anxiety (especially among teens)
- *Treatment:* Education and reassurance is important. If goal is pleasuring of partner, teach other techniques to arouse her or him prior to intercourse and/or to achieve orgasm. "Start and stop" technique can be used to prolong erection; man stops stimulation for at least 30 seconds when he feels ejaculation imminent. "Squeeze" technique helpful; when man feels impending ejaculation, partner firmly squeezes the head of the penis beneath the glans for 4-5 seconds to decrease erection. Selective serotonin reuptake inhibitors (SSRIs) in low doses may be helpful if these other techniques are not adequate. Refer to sex therapist (or urologist if cause organic) for additional treatment if needed. Condoms are available with benzocaine to decrease sensation and reduce premature ejaculation

***Delayed (Retarded) Ejaculation/Anorgasmia***

- *Definition:* Inability to or difficulty in experiencing orgasm and ejaculation with a partner
- *Cause:* usually psychological; learned behavior; may occur when a man has masturbatory patterns that cannot be duplicated with partner; overemphasis on sexual performance; medications such as SSRI's. Rule out organic problems carefully
- *Treatment:* referral to sex therapist recommended

***Erectile Dysfunction/Disorders (ED) (Impotence)***

- *Definition:* Inability to attain or sustain an erection that is satisfactory for coitus
- *Primary:* never achieved erection
- *Causes:* Organic - low testosterone levels due to hypothalamic-pituitary-testicular disorder; severe vascular compromise. Psychological - usual cause
- *Secondary:* current inability to attain or maintain erection (may be situational)
- *Causes:* Organic - diabetes mellitus, alcohol abuse, hypothyroidism, drug dependency, medications (e.g. sedatives, narcotics, hypnotics, anticonvulsants, centrally-acting antihypertensives, tranquilizers, anorectics, illegal drugs, and some antidepressants), hypopituitarism, penile infections, atherosclerosis, aortic aneurysm, multiple sclerosis, spinal cord lesions, orchiectomy or prostatectomy
  Psychological - depression, relationship stress, prior abuse, etc. Suspect when patient has morning erection or is able to masturbate to ejaculation
- *Treatment:* Treat underlying cause. Switch medications if possible. Same measures that help women's sexual desire may be useful. Medical or mechanical treatments available:
  1. *Testosterone.* Shown to be useful in wasting diseases (AIDS) and other low testosterone conditions. Available in patches for ease of use
  2. *Phosphodiesterase inhibitors:* Viagra, Cialis, Levitra. Use caution in patients with cardiovascular disease. Not to be used when taking nitrates because it can drop blood pressure.
  3. *Alprostadil injections (Edex or Caverject)* prostaglandin E1 ~ 1 cc injected into corpus cavernosa (strengths 125 µg - 1000 µg). Excessive injection may cause priapism. Erection achieved with stimulation lasts 30-60 minutes. Avoid in anticoagulated patients and with vasoactive medications.
  4. *Alprostadil suppository (Muse)* prostaglandin pellet E1 (125-1000 µg) placed inside urethra. Erection occurs as drug absorbed. 70% successful. Contraindications - anatomical penile abnormalities (strictures, hypospadias, etc.), and thrombosis risk factors. Limit 2/day
  5. *Yohimbine hydrochloride.* Prescription pill composed of indole alkaloid. Modestly successful. Avoid in psychiatric patients.
  6. *Vacuum Erection Device (VED).* Use of a vacuum pump and different size rubber bands maintains an erection for 30 minutes. Safe and effective (90% success rate).
  7. *Penile implants (prostheses).* Permanent bendable rods or inflatable reservoirs implanted surgically into penis. Activated/inflated for intercourse. Success rate high, but associated with surgical risks and the risk that natural erections disappear
  8. *Microsurgery.* Used in men with atherosclerosis of penile arteries or venous pathology; over 50% success rate

# CHAPTER 6

## Adolescent Issues

**advocatesforyouth.org, youngwomenshealth.org, teenwire.com, arhp.org/arhpframepated.htm, www.askdurex.com**

**To improve contraceptive effectiveness, prevent sexually transmitted infections, and prevent infertility due to tubal occlusion, CONDOMS should be used by most adolescents using ANY contraceptive, including, of course, the extremely effective "forgettable" methods - IUDs and implants.**

Talking to adolescent patients about the benefits of delaying sexual activity, the correct use of contraceptives, and the need for protection for STI's and HIV is important:

- The teen pregnancy rate among all teens has decreased since 1990 due to more teens delaying sex and sexually active teens using contraception more consistently *[Santelli-2004]*
- However, the pregnancy rate remains very high among sexually experienced teen girls (31%), especially among teens who start having sex before age 15 (46%), Hispanic teens (52%), and teens who have more than 1 partner (37%) *[National Survey of Family Growth-2002]*
- Teens who used a method of contraception the first time they had sex are less likely to have been involved in a pregnancy than those who did not *[NSFG-2002]*
- Recent study showed a decline in condom use after starting OCs. Subjects who were advised to ALWAYS use a condom, had a 50% increase in consistent condom use. *[Morroni et al 2014]*

### COUNSELING CHALLENGES POSED BY ADOLESCENTS

***Teens are not "young adults."*** Developmentally appropriate approaches are needed.

- Age 11-14 – teens are very concrete, egocentric (self-focused) and concerned with personal appearance and acceptance, and have a short attention span. They will start sexual maturation and abstract thinking in this period
- Age 14-15 – teens are peer oriented and authority resistant (challenge boundaries), and have very limited images of the future
- Age 16-17 – teens are developing logical thought processes and goals for the future. Develop a stronger sense of identity. Thinking becomes more reflective
- Age 18 and above – development of distinct identity and more settled ideas and opinions

***Nonjudgmental, open-ended and reflective questions*** are better than direct yes-no inquiries. Try reflective questions such as "What would you want to tell a friend who was thinking about having sex?" instead of "You're not having sex, are you?"

**CONFIDENTIALITY:** Adolescents are often afraid to obtain medical care for contraception, pregnancy testing or STI treatment because they fear parental reaction. Over two-thirds of teens never discuss sexual matters with their parents; over one-half feel that their parents could not handle it. All teens should be entitled to confidential services and counseling, but billing systems and/or laws in some states affect their confidential access to family planning services. Know your local laws and refer to sites that may be able to meet all the teen's needs if your practice can not.

**Long Acting Reversible Contraceptives, also called LARC methods or forgettable methods (IUDs, implants), are the most effective methods of preventing teen pregnancy.**

**ADOLESCENTS AND THE LAW:** This table provides information on an adolescent's right to consent to reproductive health, contraception, and abortion services.

***Table 6.1 Adolescents and the Law - www.guttmacher.org/statecenter/spids/spib_OMCL.pdf***

| | | | | | | |
|---|---|---|---|---|---|---|
| AL ✳□★ | DE ●■□✦ | IN ✳■★ | MA ●■★ | NV ■★ | OH ○■★ | TX ■□★✦ |
| AK ●■✦ | DC ●■✚ | IA ●■✦ | MI ■□★ | NH ■✚★ | OK ■□✦★ | UT ■★✦ |
| AZ ●■★ | FL ✳■✦ | KS ✳■□★ | MN ●■□✦ | NJ ■□✧ | OR ●■□✚ | VT ■✚ |
| AR ●■□★ | GA ●■□✦ | KY ●■□★ | MS ✳■★ | NM ●■☆ | PA ✳■★ | VA ●■★ |
| CA ●■☆ | HI ✳■□✚ | LA ✳■□★ | MO ■□★ | NY ●■✚ | RI ○■★ | WA ●■✚ |
| CO ●■✦ | ID ●■★ | ME ✳■□✚ | MT ●■□ | NC ●■★ | SC ■★ | WV ■✦ |
| CT ✳■✚ | IL ✳■□✧ | MD ●■□✦ | NE ■★ | ND ○■□★ | SD ■✦ | WI ○■★ |
| | | | | | TN ●■★ | WY ●■★✦ |

● = All minors may consent to contraceptive service
✳ = Some minors may consent (e.g. married, pregnant, age)
○ = No explicit policy related to minors' access to contraceptive services
■ = Minor may consent to testing and treatment for STDs. Some states specify age (e.g. 12 or 14)
□ = Physician may inform parents but is not required to
★ = Parental consent required before a minor may obtain an abortion
☆ = Parental consent law exists but not in effect (e.g., declared unenforceable by courts)
✦ = Parental notification required before a minor may obtain an abortion. In some states, parental notification is not necessary if a risk for the minor is perceived (i.e. telling parents may result in harm to minor) For DE females <16, OR <15, SC <17
✧ = Parental notification law exists but not in effect (e.g., declared unenforceable by courts)
✚ = Does not require parental involvement before a minor may obtain an abortion

*Sources: State Policies in Brief: An Overview of Minors' Consent Law. As of June 2012 Guttmacher Institute.*

***Note**: Many of the laws contain specific clauses that affect their meaning and application. The authors encourage readers to consult the above documents (updated monthly) for more details: www.agi-usa.org.*

## TEENS AND CONTRACEPTION

The pelvic exam may be a barrier to initiating contraceptive use. It is not necessary to perform a pelvic exam prior to prescribing any contraceptive other than an IUD *[Stewart-2001]*

## ADOLESCENTS AS RISK TAKERS

- Full evaluation of behaviors is important to personalize counseling. Teens must move away from parental authority figures to become independent adult individuals, but, along the way, they may take excessive risks in many areas, including sexuality
- HEADSS interview technique helpful as an organized approach. Ask each teen about Home, Education, Activities, Drugs, Sexuality (activity, orientation and abuse) and Suicide
- Look for the female athletic triad: eating disorders, amenorrhea and osteoporosis. This triad of symptoms may also occur in women who do not exercise excessively
- Discuss keeping emergency contraceptive pills at home and provide a prescription if needed or desired
- The single-rod implant is a highly effective method for use in this age group
- Both copper and levonorgestrel IUDs are safe and effective methods for nulliparous and parous adolescents (US MEC category 2)
- As in adults, bone mineral density quickly recovers after discontinuation of DMPA use to levels as high as non-users by 12 months *[Curtis-2006]*. DEXA scans are NOT indicated in this age group as the scores cannot predict fracture risk in adolescents

## HEALTH CARE SCREENING FOR ADOLESCENTS

- Initiate pap smear screening beginning at age 21, unless immune deficient or other special circumstances warrant earlier screening
- HPV typing is not indicated in this age group since low-risk HPV infections are so common and resolve spontaneously (ASCCP, ACOG Guidelines)
- Teaching self breast examination is not recommended in women younger than 19 years old as it leads to many false positives and takes time from higher priority counseling issues

## SEX EDUCATION

Abstinence-only sex ed programs have been found ineffective in preventing or delaying teenagers from having sexual intercourse, and have no impact on likelihood that if they do have sex, they will use a condom. Moreover, sex education, contraception and STIs curricula offered in many schools are not medically correct. The information teens obtain from peers is also often inaccurate. Common **MYTHS** are:

- *You cannot get pregnant the first time you have intercourse*
- *You cannot get pregnant if you douche after sex*
- *Having sex or having a baby makes you a woman, makes your boyfriend love you, and gets you the attention you deserve*
- *Making a girl pregnant means that you are a man*

***Adolescents need very concrete information and opportunities to role play and practice:***

- How to open and place a condom and where to carry it
- How to negotiate NOT having sex and, in other cases, condom use
- How to punch out the pills, where to keep the pack, and how to remember them
- The remarkable advantages of continuous and extended use of pills to decrease the very high (9%) typical use failure rate of combined pills.
- Dual protection: condoms and another contraceptive
- How to access and use emergency contraceptive pills and IUDs

## TEENS AND SEXUALLY TRANSMITTED INFECTIONS

- Although adolescents and young adults 15-24 years old account for 25% of the sexually active population, they experience almost half of the newly acquired cases of STIs annually *[Guttmacher-2008]*
- HPV infections account for half of the newly acquired STIs in this age group. The HPV vaccine, Gardasil, provides immunity against types 6, 11, 16 and 18, and is recommended for all girls and young women aged 9-26 *[CDC-2007]*
- Gardasil is also now approved for use in boys and men ages 9-26 for the prevention of warts
- Cervarix, another HPV vaccine for females ages 10-25 approved. Targets HPV types 16 and 18. Also given as series of 3 injections
- Annual screening for gonorrhea, Chlamydia, and HIV is recommended for all sexually active people in this age group. Treatment for gc and ct should be followed by a rescreening test for reinfection in 3 months.
- Infertility due to tubal occlusion has led to increasing need for expensive in vitro fertilization in the United States

## TEEN BIRTH RATES AND ABORTION RATES

In 2002, 75 out of 1000 U.S. women ages 15-19 got pregnant— a rate 11 times greater than in the Netherlands and four times higher than in Germany. But, in 2010, teen birth rate hit lowest rate in 70 years: 34.3 births per 1,000 girls 15-19 y/o. *[CDC National Center for Health Statistics]*. During the 2008-2013 period, the mean annual rates of pregnancy, birth and abortion among CHOICE participants were 34.0, 19.4, and 9.7 per 1000 teens, respectively. In comparison, rates of pregnancy, birth, and abortion among sexually experienced U.S. teens in 2008 were 158.5, 94.0, and 41.5 per 1000,respectively. [Secura 2014]

# CHAPTER 7

## Male Reproductive Health

www.nim.nih.gov/medlineplus/teenhealth.html

Reproductive health is a term generally associated with women. Efforts are being made to include males in health education and outreach programs, acknowledging that men have important reproductive and sexual health needs of their own. Including men in discussions of contraception and STIs benefits their female partners as well.

### MEN AND SEXUAL EXPERIENCE

- Most adult men and almost half of adolescent men (46%) have had sexual intercourse. *[Guttmacher Inst.- 2008]*
- For men in the United States: Average age of first intercourse – 17.5
- In 2002, only 25% of adolescent males who had ever had sex had ever been tested for HIV
- 5% of males aged 15-19 have had sexual contact with another male. These young men may or may not have female partners as well
- 37% of 9th grade boys report being sexually experienced *[Youth Risk Behavior Survey-2003]*

### WHERE MEN GET THEIR REPRODUCTIVE HEALTH INFORMATION

- 2/3 had physical exams in the past year, and less than 20% received reproductive health counseling *[NSFG-2002]*
- One survey showed men get most of their STD/AIDS prevention information from the media rather than from a healthcare provider. *(Bradner, 2000)*
- Although most men get some form of sexuality education while they are in high school, for 3 out of 10 men this instruction comes too late – after they have begun having sexual intercourse. *(Sonfield, 2002)*

***What can healthcare providers do?***

- Make sure to talk to men about reproductive health at school and work physicals. Start early – many adolescents have sexual intercourse before age 17.
- When appropriate, talk to men about reproductive health issues such as STIs and contraception at doctor's visits for unrelated complaints – this may be the only time they visit a physician this year
- HPV vaccine, Gardasil, approved for males ages 9-26

### MEN AND CONTRACEPTION

When you come into contact with a man who is playing an active role in safely, effectively and carefully using contraceptives, go out of your way to give him positive reinforcement.

- Among sexually experienced adolescent males, 14% have made a partner pregnant and 2-7% are fathers. *(Marcell, 2003)*
- As men get older, condom use declines. 7 out of 10 men age 15-17 use condoms, compared to 4 out of 10 men in their 20s, and 2 out of 10 men in their 30s. *(Sonfield, 2002)*
- Vasectomy is a very effective male option for permanent birth control. However, it is estimated that approximately 500,000 men receive a vasectomy in the U.S. each year, in contrast to 700,000 women who have a female sterilization procedure. *(Hawes, 1998)* In only 4 countries throughout the world, Great Britain, Netherlands, New Zealand and Bhutan, do vasectomies exceed tubal sterilization as a method of birth control. Vasectomy has not been found to cause any long-term adverse effects

***Men's support of women's birth control methods matter***

- Education of adolescent males about birth control (including female methods) leads to improvement in use of the method by their partner(s) *(Edwards, 1994)*

## MEN AND SEXUALLY TRANSMITTED INFECTIONS

***How many men acquire sexually transmitted infections?***

- 17% of men aged 15-49 have genital herpes
- Among men in their 20s, there are 500-600 per 100,000 men new cases of gonorrhea and chlamydia per year *(Sonfield, 2002)*
- 8 out of 10 Americans living with HIV are men *(Sonfield, 2002)*
- Rates of STIs are higher among young, poor, and minority men

***Decreasing STI rates in men helps their female partner(s)***

- Treating men decreases initial infection rate and reinfection rate in women, which could decrease female complications such as pelvic inflammatory disease, ectopic pregnancy, and infertility.

***Decreasing STI rates in men helps themselves***

- While the link between gonorrhea and chlamydia infection and infertility in men has not been proven, there is some clinical evidence that it does have some effect:
  **gonorrhea/chlamydia infection ➤ urethritis ➤ epidymo-orchitis ➤ infertility**
  - If urethritis is treated promptly, there is less likelihood it will proceed to epidymo-orchitis *(Ness, 1997)*
  - The most common cause of epidymo-orchitis in men younger than 35 years old is gonorrhea and chlamydia infections *(Weidner, 1999)*

## MEN AND REPRODUCTIVE CANCERS

***Testicular cancer***

- "Testicular cancer is the most common solid malignancy affecting males between the ages of 15 and 35, although it accounts for only 1% of all cancers in men." *(Michaelson, 2004)*
- The number of deaths from testicular has dropped due to advances in therapy.
- Some signs or symptoms of testicular cancer are testicular enlargement, a dull ache in the abdomen or groin, scrotal pain, and fluid in the scrotum.
- The patient information website sponsored by the American Urological Association says that monthly testicular self exams are the most important way to detect a tumor early.
- The treatment for testicular cancer can be removal of the affected testicle. Removal of one testicle does not make a man infertile.

***Prostate cancer***

- The most important risk factor for prostate cancer is age. The older a man is, the greater his risk.
- Prostate cancer is screened for by digital rectal exam and prostate-specific antigen level.
- Some of the treatments for prostate cancer can affect male fertility. For instance, surgery to remove the prostate causes the male ejaculate to become "dry" so the ability to have children is usually lost. Prostate surgery can also cause erectile dysfunction

# CHAPTER 8

## Perimenopause and Menopause

www.menopause.org or www.nams.org

**PERIMENOPAUSE:** Perimenopause is marked by changes in the menstrual cycle and is a time that lasts through menopause. Characterized by fluctuations in ovarian hormones resulting in intermittent vasomotor symptoms, menstrual changes and reduced fertility. A perimenopausal woman should use contraception until she is truly menopausal (amenorrheic for one year).

- Average age of onset: 45
- Average duration: 3-5 years
- Women over 40 have second highest abortion ratio due to unintended pregnancy (# abortions/1000 live births), second to women under 15
- All methods of birth control are available to most healthy, nonsmoking women until menopause
- In US, 50% women >40 have been sterilized and another 18% have a partner with vasectomy
- Combined hormonal contraceptives have specific benefits for perimenopausal women: May regulate cycles, prevent osteoporosis, treat hot flushes. Usually should not be used for women >35 who smoke, have migraines or have significant cardiac risk factors
- Smokers > 35 or women with hypertension may use any non-estrogen containing methods, POPs, DMPA, IUDs or barriers unless they have other risk factors

**MENOPAUSE:** cessation of spontaneous menses x12 months. Retrospective diagnosis.

- Avg age: 51.1-51.4, earlier in smokers

***Common Physiologic Changes after Menopause:***

- Hot flashes (~ 75% women – only 15% severe) /sleep disturbances, mood swings
- Thinning of genitourinary tissue (atrophic vaginitis, urinary incontinence)
- Osteopenia, osteoporosis, increased risk for fracture
- Increased risk for cardiovascular disease, unfavorable lipid profiles

One health recommendation to make to all patients, with increasing importance to the aging, is to add regular exercise for its health benefits

**BENEFITS OF EXERCISE:**

- To decrease risk, gradually add exercise to daily routine rather than immediately starting strenuous activity
- Decreased all-cause mortality
- Decreased Cardiovascular disease (CVD): ↓VLDL, ↑HDL, ↓BP, ↓risk stroke
- Glycemic control: better glycemic control, insulin sensitivity. May prevent development of type 2 DM in high risk populations
- Cancer prevention: may reduce risk of developing breast and prostate cancer
- Prevents obesity: greater reduction in body fat and enhanced preservation of lean body mass than a weight loss diet alone
- Smoking cessation: vigorous exercise aids smoking cessation, and prevents weight gain
- Gallstones: decreases risk
- Function and cognition: improved in elderly who exercise

**HORMONE THERAPY:**

- Most effective treatment for hot flashes
- Recommended for relief of vasomotor sx and GU atrophy to be used at lowest dose that is effective for short durations. Short duration is not defined (some say 2-5 yrs); re-evaluate every 6 months or year. Not recommended for prevention of CVD
- Combination HT using premarin (0.625mg) and provera (2.5mg) per day associated with a small inc relative risk of CVD (1.29), stroke (1.41), invasive breast cancer(1.26), VTE (2.13) and a small protection against fractures (0.66) and colorectal CA at an average of 5 years of use (WHI data)

- Estrogen therapy alone 0.625mg associated with small increased risk of stroke (1.39) and DVT and small decreased risk of fracture (.61). No increased risk of CVD, PE or breast cancer, which had a small nonsignificant decreased risk 0.77 (0.59-1.01) (WHI data)

## PRESCRIBING PRECAUTIONS FOR HT:

- Pregnancy, undiagnosed abnormal vaginal bleeding, active liver disease
- Recent or active thrombophlebitis or thromboembolic disorders
- Breast cancer or known or suspected estrogen-dependent neoplasm
- Recent MI or severe CVD

## STARTING HORMONES FOR MENOPAUSAL WOMEN:

- Patient counseling is key to success with HT. May takes weeks for relief of hot flashes. Explain risks and side effects especially vaginal spotting and bleeding
- Usual well woman care measures should be provided – mammogram, pap test, lipid profile – but are not essential (except mammogram, which is) prior to providing HT. Endometrial biopsy not needed except when evaluating abnormal vaginal bleeding
- Consider starting with low doses and transdermal preparations (transdermal may have less of a risk for VTE)
- Re-evaluate need for HT/ET annually. The current products are:

| Generic names - Estrogens | Brand names |
|---|---|
| Conjugated estrogen tablets, USP | Premarin® |
| Synthetic conjugated estrogens, tablets | Cenestin®, Enjuvia |
| Esterified estrogens tablets | Menest® |
| Estropipate tablets | Ogen®, Ortho-est® |
| Estradiol tablets | Estrace® (micronized), Femtrace |
| Matrix estradiol transdermal systems | Alora®, Climara®, Vivelle™, Menostar, Vivelle-dot, Minivelle |
| Reservoir estradiol transdermal systems | Estraderm® |
| Topical estradiol | Estrasorb®, Estrogel®, Divigel®, Elestrin® |
| Transdermal spray | Evamist® |
| Vaginal estradiol | Vagifem® (tablet), Estring® (ring), Femring® (ring) |
| Vaginal conjugated estrogen | Premarin®, Estrace |

| Generic names - Progestins | Brand names |
|---|---|
| Medroxyprogesterone acetate (MPA) tablets | Provera® |
| Megestrol acetate tablets | Megace® |
| Norethindrone tablets | Micronor®, Nor-QD®, Errin®, Camila®, Jolivette®, Nora-Be® |
| Norethindrone acetate tablets | Aygestin® |
| Micronized progesterone capsules | Prometrium® |
| Progesterone vaginal gel | Crinone® |
| Levonorgestrel IUS | Mirena, Skyla |

| Generic names - Combined Products | Brand names |
|---|---|
| Estradiol and norgestimate tablets | Prefest® |
| Conjugated estrogens and MPA tablets | Premphase®, Prempro® |
| Esterified estrogens and methyl testosterone tablets | Estratest®, Estratest® H.S. |
| Ethinyl estradiol and norethindrone acetate tablets | Femhrt® |
| Estradiol and norethindrone acetate tablets | Activella™ |
| Estradiol/ norethindrone acetate transdermal systems/patch | CombiPatch™ |
| Estradiol + levonorgestrel patch | Climara Pro® |
| Estradiol + drospirenone tablets | Angeliq |
| Oral conjugated estrogen + bazedoxifene tablets | Duavee |

## FOLLOW-UP

- Be available to answer questions when there are media reports about HT
- Have the woman keep a menstrual calendar of any breakthrough bleeding or spotting
- If hot flashes continue, consider thyroid dysfunction and other causes before increasing dose or using other therapeutic approaches to hot flash treatment

# CHAPTER 9

## Prepregnancy Planning and Preparation

www.plannedparenthood.org or www.aidsinfo.nih.gov

***Women in the reproductive years should take 0.4 mg (400 micrograms) of synthetic folic acid daily. This easy, safe step significantly reduces the risk of neural tube defects in a developing fetus. All prenatal vitamins contain this minimum dose***

- ***400 micrograms of folic acid daily***
- ***Women with a history of spina bifida, women on antiseizure medication and insulin dependent diabetics need 4 mg folic acid daily***
- ***0.45 mg per day is now in 7 Beyaz and 7 Safyral oral contraceptive pills per cycle***

***Prepregnancy visit assess:***

- Reproductive, family and personal medical and surgical history with attention to pelvic surgeries
- Smoking, drug use, alcohol use: advise to stop and refer for help if needed. There is no safe level of alcohol use for pregnant women.
- Nutrition habits: identify excesses and inadequacies
- Medications: make adjustments in those that may affect fertility and/or pregnancy outcome. Advise patient not to make any changes without clinician's knowledge

  ***Review Medical History:***
  - Glucose control in diabetics before conception and in early pregnancy decreases birth defects and pregnancy failure
  - Hypertensive women on ACE inhibitors need to switch meds
  - Some antiepileptics are more teratogenic than others
  - Women on coumadin need to be transitioned to heparin or lovenox (low molecular weight heparin)
- Risk for sexually transmitted infection/infertility in both partners
- Impacts of any medications (over-the-counter, prescription, herbal). For example, Accutane and tetracycline (which are teratogenic) for acne requires extremely effective contraception and strong consideration of the use of 2 contraceptives correctly. Advise that patient delay pregnancy for at least one year after last Accutane. See Page 36. Helpful online databases include micromedex.com/products/hcs/demos/Part3.html
- Risk factors for preterm birth

**RISK FACTORS FOR PRETERM BIRTH:**

- non-white race
- age < 17 or > 35
- low socioeconomic status
- low prepregnancy weight
- maternal history of preterm birth - especially in second trimester
- vaginal bleeding in more than one trimester
- excessively physically stressful job (controversial)
- smoking
- twins

*Reference: ACOG Practice Bulletin, 2001*

***Offer Screening and/or Counseling for:***

- Infections (TB, gonorrhea, chlamydia, HIV, syphilis, hepatitis B & C, HSV as per CDC guidelines). Vaginal wet mount if discharge present
- Neoplasms (breast, cervical dysplasia, warts, etc.)

- Immunity (rubella, tetanus, chicken pox, HBV) HPV if applicable
- Alcohol use, tobacco use, substance abuse, obesity
- Advanced maternal and paternal age

***Provide Genetic Counseling:***
- For all women, but may need additional specialized counseling if going to be ≥ 35 y.o. when she delivers or has a significant personal or family history of genetic disorders, poor pregnancy outcome or partner of advanced paternal age
- Family history of mental retardation or genetic disorders such as sickle cell anemia, thalassemia, cystic fibrosis, Tay-Sachs, Canavan disease, neural tube defect
- High risk ethnic backgrounds: African Americans, Ashkenazi Jews, French Canadian, Cajun, etc
- Seizure disorders, Diabetes
- Other heritable medical problems

***Assess Environmental Hazards:***
- Chemical, radioactive and infectious exposures at workplace, home, hobbies
- Physical conditions, especially workplace
- Assess male partner as well!

***Assess Psychosocial Factors:***
- Readiness of woman and partner for parenthood
- Mental health (depression, etc.) and domestic violence
- Financial issues and support systems

***Recommend:***
- ***Ideally, planning a pregnancy should involve both a woman and her partner***
- Balanced diet
- Do not eat shark, swordfish, mackerel, tilefish or fish caught in local waters
- Eat at least 8 oz and up to 12 oz (2 average meals) of fish lower in mercury, which can include up to 6 oz of albacore tuna per week. Non albacore tuna has less mercury.
- Vitamin with folic acid 0.4 mg for all women planning pregancy or at risk for unintended pregnancy (women with previous pregnancy with a neural tube defect, insulin dependent diabetic, alcoholic, malabsorption or on anticonvulsants need 4 mg folic acid daily)
- Minimize STI exposure risk
- Weight loss, if obese (gradual loss until conception)
- Special planning for women with prior gastric bypass or current obesity
- Moderate exercise
- Avoiding exposure to cat feces (toxoplasmosis) if no known immunity
- Early in process of discussing pregnancy encourage breastfeeding as the best way to feed her baby
- Early prenatal care when pregnancy occurs

***Avoid***
- Raw meat (including fish) and unpasteurized dairy products
- Abdominal/pelvic X-rays, if possible
- Excesses in diet, vitamins, exercise
- Non-foods (pica), unusual herbs
- **Sex with multiple partners or sex with a partner who may be HIV-positive, have other STI or have other sex partner(s).** If in doubt, use condom consistently.

# CHAPTER 10

## Pregnancy Testing

**www.plannedparenthood.org, www.ovulation.com & 1-800-230-PLAN**

***Early testing gives a woman time to pursue pregnancy options***

- Prenatal care can be initiated promptly
- Unhealthy behaviors/exposures can be stopped sooner
- Ectopic pregnancies may be detected earlier
- Medical and surgical methods of abortion are safest at earlier gestations

### PREGNANCY TESTS

***Urine tests:***

- *Enzyme-linked immunosorbent assay (ELISA) test:*
  - Immunometric test uses antibody specific to placentally-produced HCG and another antibody to produce a color change. Commonly used in home pregnancy test and in offices and clinics. Performed in 1-3 minutes using urine samples
  - Most tests positive at levels of 25 mIU/ml. This level can be detectable 7-10 days after conception. May require 5-7 days after implantation to detect all pregnancies
  - Test results are positive for 98% of women 7 days after implantation
  - Tests can be positive as early as the day of the first missed menses.
  - Urine pregnancy tests are used in most clinical settings and are available for women to purchase over-the-counter; teach patients that no lab test is 100% accurate and that false negative tests (tests read as negative when a woman actually is pregnant) usually occur when done too early in the pregnancy and are far more common than false positive tests (tests read as positive when a woman actually is NOT pregnant)

***Serum tests (blood drawn):***

- *Radioimmunoassay:*
  - Uses colorimetry, which detects HCG levels as low as 5 mIU/ml
  - Results available in 1-2 hours
  - Offers ability to quantify levels of HCG to monitor levels over time when clinically indicated as for ectopic pregnancy diagnosis and treatment

### HCG QUICK FACTS

- β-HCG can be detected as early as 7-10 days after conception thereby, "ruling in" pregnancy, but pregnancy cannot be "ruled out" until 7 days after expected menses
- If needed for evaluation of early pregnancy, serial HCG testing should be done every 2 days until levels reach discriminatory levels of 1800-2000 mIU/ml, when a gestational sac can be visualized reliably by vaginal ultrasound. In normal gestations the levels of HCG double about every 2 days *[Stenchever MA-2001]*
- Average time for HCG levels to become non-detectable after first trimester surgical abortion ranges from 31-38 days

### MANAGEMENT TIPS

- Home tests can be misused or misinterpreted.
- Any test can have false-negative results at low levels. If in doubt, repeat urine test in 1-2 days or obtain serum tests with a quantitative HCG
- Recommend folic acid, 0.4 mg/day: every woman, every day (pregnancy test positive or negative)

## PREGNANCY TEST NEGATIVE: WANTS TO AVOID PREGNANCY NOW

A negative pregnancy test for a woman not wanting to become pregnant clearly provides the counselor or clinician with a teachable moment and perhaps an ideal time to offer a woman one of the forgettable methods: an IUD or implant.

***"What a relief! The pregnancy test is negative."*** **This must have been scary to worry that you might be pregnant.**

1. **If you haven't been using contraception, this is your "wake-up call." What contraceptive method would work best for you now? You may be able to start your contraceptive without a pelvic exam.**
2. **Don't try to become pregnant in order to see if you can become pregnant.**
3. **Don't take a chance from this moment on: never, just never, have intercourse without knowing that you are protected against both infection and unintended or unwanted pregnancy, unless you want to get pregnant.**
4. **Remember, your negative urine pregnancy test does not rule out conception from acts of intercourse in the past 2 weeks.**

*For Clinicians:*

5. **Learn about emergency contraceptive pills and emergency IUD insertion.**
6. **Discuss keeping emergency contraceptive pills at home for future use; can buy OTC if ≥ 17 years. Otherwise, provide prescription**

## PREGNANCY TEST POSITIVE: WANTS TO CONTINUE THIS PREGNANCY

The pregnancy test is positive and she wants to continue the pregnancy. Whether or not this pregnancy was planned and prepared for,* your patient has decided to continue this pregnancy, providing you, the counselor or clinician, with a teachable moment.

***The pregnancy test is positive and she is continuing her pregnancy to term***

1. **Start vitamins containing folic acid (0.4 mg) today. Buy vitamins on the way home.**
2. **Stop drinking alcohol or using any recreational drugs today.**
3. **Stop smoking today.**
4. **Ask: "Are you on any medication? Are you taking OTC products?**
5. **Use condoms if at any risk for HIV or other STIs.**
6. **Eat healthy foods. Gain 25-30 pounds during your pregnancy (if your weight is now normal).**
7. **Review current medical problems.**
8. **Learn about EC for the future**
9. **Establish prenatal care. Provide referral if needed**

*** If she doesn't want to continue pregnancy, discuss other options including adoption or pregnancy termination or refer her to someone who feels comfortable doing this.**

Counseling following a pregnancy test is important. If not done well, an important opportunity is lost. The steps above are the beginning of structured counseling for two pregnancy test results and two decisions a woman could make following her pregnancy test.

# CHAPTER 11

## Postpartum Contraception

www.avsc.org or www.fhi.org

**Planning for postpartum (PP) contraception should begin during pregnancy** and use should be initiated as early as possible postpartum. A newborn places many demands on a woman's time, so her method should be as convenient for her to use as possible, such as a LARC. In some women who are not breastfeeding, ovulation may return postpartum before a woman realizes she is at risk, which may be before her first period. **The 6-week postpartum visit is too late. The visit should be at 2-4 weeks. By 6 weeks postpartum, 50% of women as early as 26-28 days postpartum have had vaginal intercourse.** Involve her partner as often as possible. Advance provision of EC is always appropriate

- Pregnancies spaced at least 18-23 months apart are less likely to have: preterm delivery, low birth weight, and small for gestational age infants *[Zhv-2005]*

### AT DELIVERY

- Tubal sterilization may be performed (at C-section or after vaginal delivery)
- Be aware of need to sign consent form 30 days earlier in many situations
- Copper or levonorgestrel IUD may be inserted within 20 minutes of delivery of placenta (requires learning new technique) but rates of expulsion are higher than with insertion after uterine involution

### PRIOR TO LEAVING HOSPITAL

- Encourage breastfeeding. Reinforce education about lactational amenorrhea if patient is interested (see Chapter 14, Page 47)
- Pelvic rest (no douching, no sex, no tampons) is generally recommended for 4-6 weeks and/or until lochia stops. Many women choose NOT to follow this advice in spite of increased risk for infection, in which case condoms should be used. Some clinicians encourage women to become sexually active when they feel comfortable and ready
- At this time, sex may be the last thing the woman is thinking about. Nevertheless, encourage her to have a contraceptive plan for when she does intiate sexual activity. Options:
  - Tubal sterilization, vasectomy
  - Progestin-only methods: Depo-Provera (DMPA), progestin-only pills (POPs), Implanon or Nexplanon

    **NOTE:** There are three approaches to starting these progestin-only methods (all are off-label but are compatible with US MEC):

    1) When the patient leaves the hospital, start POPs, DMPA or receive Implanon or Nexplanon
    2) Since progestin-only methods may prolong bleeding wait 2-3 weeks to start them (no data). Women with history of or high risk for postpartum depression may also benefit from a delay in starting progestin-only methods. In breastfeeding women, progestin-only methods have no effect on milk production or composition or long-term growth of the infant *(Truit-2003)*
    3) Start at 4 weeks. Use condoms if intercourse prior to 4 weeks

    Label does not include use in first 6 weeks in nursing moms because many studies did not include such women, not because there is an established contraindication.
  - Male or female condoms to reduce risk of sexually transmitted infections

- Estrogen containing contraceptive may be prescribed for nonlactating women to start 3 weeks postpartum (increased risk of thrombosis associated with pregnancy reduced by that time). Recommend to start the Sunday after 21st day PP. Give a prescription when she leaves the hospital (to be started in 3 weeks)
- Provide EC in advance or advise to buy OTC

## AT POSTPARTUM VISIT (2-4 WEEKS) - see CDC MEC A-3

- Best time is likely at 2 weeks to coincide with infant's first exam. Waiting 6 weeks will miss important issues like resumption of sex, problems with breastfeeding, postpartum depression and adaptation at home to having a baby
- Ask if woman has resumed sexual intercourse
- Pregnancy is possible 3 months after delivery even if she is fully breastfeeding and 3 weeks if she is not
- Support continued breastfeeding if applicable
- Lactational amenorrhea follow-up. Provide condoms as transitional method and discuss other methods before transition to decreased breastfeeding
- Emergency contraception may be given if needed; IUD most effective EC
- Progestin-only methods may be provided (Depo-Provera, progestin-only pills, Mirena, Implanon). Provide back-up method as needed if initiated when not on menses
- COCs, patch or ring may be started after 3 weeks in non-breastfeeding women if no other risk factors for VTE. For breastfeeding women, start CHCs at 1 month PP, now a US MEC category 2. Provide backup method as needed
- IUD may be inserted if uterus well involuted (whether or not she is breast-feeding). Usually at 4 + weeks
- Condoms (male or female) may be given as primary or backup contraceptive to provide STI risk reduction; withdrawal can be used at any time
- Tubal sterilization via laparoscopy or transcervical (Essure) may be provided after uterine involution usually later than 4 weeks. Vasectomy may be provided anytime.
- Diaphragm, cervical cap may be fitted after pelvis/cervix return to normal configuration
- NFP and FAM should await resumption of normal cycles for at least 3 months
- Screen for postpartum depression

### A HARD LOOK AT MISTAKES MADE OVER AND OVER AGAIN

Often we see patients/clients who have made repeated mistakes; A postpartum woman who has already had several unplanned pregnancies, an individual with repeated infections who almost never uses a condom, a smoker, an abuser of alcohol or drugs, a person who eats far too much and exercises far too little. When this happens and the problem is inconsistent or incorrect use of a contraceptive we may want to share a message like this with our patient:

*"If you have made a mistake using a contraceptive method in the past, you may be able to learn to use it correctly in the future. BUT, you may also make the same mistake over and over again in the future. Such is human nature. We are creatures of habit. So, be very careful going back to a method that you have failed to use correctly in the past. This may be the time to think about using an IUD or implant, that is, one of the LARC or "Get It and Forget It" methods. If married and use of the pill is the problem, it may be the time to support a LARC method or taking combined pills continuously (or with only periodic two-day hormone free intervals). It may make sense as it eliminates the 7-day hormone free interval that may be prolonged when a woman fails to get her next cycle of pills on time. This may lead to ovulation."*

—Robert A. Hatcher

# CHAPTER 12

# Elective Abortion

www.prochoice.org/naf or www.earlyoptionpill.com

## OVERVIEW

Safe, legal, elective abortion procedures are important for fertility control since half of pregnancies in the U.S. are unintended and 22% of pregnancies end in induced abortion *[Jones-2002]*. In places where abortion is illegal, higher rates of morbidity and mortality from unsafe abortion exist. It is estimated that worldwide approximately 68,000 women die annually from unsafe abortions.

- In the U.S., serious complications and mortality are extremely rare
- Abortion related mortality is 0.6 per 100,000 compared to 8-10 per 100,000 for pregnancy related deaths (a rate 14 times higher) meaning having an abortion is much safer than continuing with pregnancy
- 60% of abortions are done at<9 weeks; 27% are <7 weeks
- Estimated mortality associated with medication abortion is 0.7 per 100,000 users
- Some states require women considering abortion to hear information that is biased to present abortion as more risky than pregnancy & childbirth
- Women deserve accurate information *[Raymond and Grimes, 2012]*

Despite having one of the highest abortion rates among developed countries, 87% of U.S. counties had no abortion providers or facilities, an increase from 78% in 2000. Many state laws impose mandatory restrictions, waiting periods, and consent requirements. For current information on your state's abortion laws (see page 14), contact Pro Choice America 202-973-3000 or www.naral.org/).

- 47% of all women in the US have had one or more elective abortions
- In 2002, about 2% of all women aged 15-44 had an abortion *[Fines, Hershaw-2005]*
- Half have had at least one previous abortion
- Each year about 10,000-15,000 abortions occur as a result of rape or incest

### Features of Medical Compared to Surgical Abortion

| Medical | Surgical |
|---|---|
| Generally avoids invasive procedure | Involves invasive procedure |
| Requires multiple visits | Usually requires one visit |
| Days to weeks until complete | Usually complete in a few minutes |
| Available during very early pregnancy | Available during early and later pregnancy |
| High success rate (94% - 97%) | Higher success rate (99%) |
| Requires follow-up to ensure completion of abortion | Does not require follow-up in most cases |
| May be more private in some circumstances; will vary for each individual patient | May be more private in some circumstances; will vary for each individual patient |
| Patient participation in multi-step process | Less patient participation in a single-step process |
| Analgesia available if desired | Allows use of sedation or anesthesia if desired |
| Does not require surgical training, but does require surgical back-up | Requires surgical training and sometimes licensed facility |

## ELECTIVE SURGICAL ABORTION

### DESCRIPTION

Voluntary termination of pregnancy using uterine aspiration in early intrauterine gestations. In later gestations (after 14 weeks) using instruments for tissue removal (standard dilation and evacuation [D & E] or intact dilation & extraction [D & X]).

### EFFECTIVENESS

- 98-99% effective; failures are mostly incomplete abortions with small amounts of retained tissue; rarely does the pregnancy continue

### PROCEDURE

- After informed consent obtained according to local law, type of procedure is determined by gestational age and patient preference
- Perform careful bimanual exam to assess size and position of uterus
- In second trimester, dilate the cervix with an osmotic dilator (laminaria, dilapan) OR with a prostaglandin analogue (misoprostol) with or without an osmotic dilator
- Two recent studies showed that same day cervical preparation with Dilapan or Misoprostol is associated with low complication rates and shorter operating time for gestations up to 21 weeks, 6 days. A same day dilation is more convenient for the patient. *[Lyons 2013], [Maurer 2013]*
- Peri-operative antibiotics reduce the risk of post-procedure infection. However, no studies demonstrate if a single regimen is better than others. The best study supports use of doxycycline. If chlamydia infection likely, a 7-day course of doxycycline, or a single dose of azithromycin 1 g may be given. If BV is present, treat with appropriate antibiotics
- Cleanse ectocervix and endocervix
- Administer cervical anesthesia; if desired, adjunctive sedation can also be used.
- Place tenaculum and mechanically dilate cervix if not previously dilated adequately
- Using sterile technique, insert a plastic cannula and apply suction to aspirate products of conception either with a machine, or manually with a manual vacuum aspiration (MVA) syringe
- May confirm adequacy of procedure by checking uterine cavity with a sharp curette (optional)
- Evaluate tissue to confirm presence of placental villi/gestational sac if early pregnancy. If more than 9 weeks should be able to visualize fetal tissue. If no villi, consider possibility of ectopic pregnancy
- Administer Rh immune globulin if woman is Rh negative

### ADVANTAGES

- Provides woman complete control over her fertility
- Ability to prevent an unwanted or defective birth or halt a pregnancy that poses risk to maternal health or other aspects of her life
- Safe and rapid; preoperative evaluation and procedure can usually be done in a single visit from a medical perspective (local legal restrictions may affect this)
- No increase in risk of breast cancer, infertility, cervical incompetence, preterm labor, or congenital anomalies in subsequent pregnancy after uncomplicated first-trimester abortion
- **Fewer risks to maternal health than continuing pregnancy**
- Can be provided as early as intrauterine pregnancy is diagnosed
- An IUD or implant may be inserted immediately after procedure

## DISADVANTAGES

- Cramping and pain with procedure; the noise of the vacuum machine (if electrical vacuum used) may cause anxiety.
- Possibility of later regret (regret is equally possible for undesired pregnancy that is continued)

## COMPLICATIONS

- Infection <1%, with an uncommon complication of infertility
- Incomplete abortion 0.5%-1.0%; Failed abortion 0.1%-0.5%
- Hemorrhage 0.03%-1.0%
- Post-abortal syndrome (hematometra) <1%
- Asherman's syndrome rare (more likely with septic abortion), with an uncommon complication of infertility
- Mortality: Elective surgical and medical abortion deaths <1 per 100,000

## CANDIDATES FOR USE

- Any woman requesting abortion. State laws often limit gestational age (typically available through 24 weeks). State laws may also affect access and consent procedures
  ***Adolescents:*** State laws vary regarding requirements and consent requirements (See Page 16)

## INITIATING METHOD

- Carefully discuss all pregnancy options, including prenatal care for continuing pregnancy or for adoption and programs available for assistance with each option
- If patient chooses abortion, discuss available techniques when applicable (surgical versus medical)
- Obtain informed consent after answering all questions
- Offer emotional support, education, pre- and post-procedural instructions, and contraception
- Usually perform procedure in outpatient setting unless woman has severe medical problems requiring more intense monitoring or deeper anesthesia
- Initiate contraception immediately after procedure including intrauterine contraception

## INSTRUCTIONS FOR PATIENT

- Fasting before abortions with low dose procedural sedation is not neccessary. No complications were identified in over 47,000 non-fasting patients with low dose procedural sedation. Avoiding fasting can decrease unnecessary stress. *[Wiebe et al. 2013]*
- Driving self home is not recommended
- Keep telephone number(s) nearby for any emergencies
- May resume usual activities same day if procedure done under local anesthesia
- One week pelvic rest (no tampons, douching or sexual intercourse)
- Use NSAIDs or acetaminophen for cramping, ergotamine (methergine) for heavy bleeding
- Showers are permitted immediately
- Seek medical care urgently if heavy bleeding, excessive cramping, pain, fevers, chills, or malodorous discharge

## FOLLOW-UP

- Have you had a temperature >100.4°F
- What has your bleeding been like since the procedure?
- Have you had any new abdominal or pelvic pain?
- Are you using a contraceptive?

## PROBLEM MANAGEMENT

***Infection***

- Always evaluate possibility of retained products and need for reaspiration
- Patients who develop endometritis can generally be treated using outpatient PID therapies described in the CDC Guidelines
- Cases that are more complicated may require hospitalization and IV antibiotics (uncommon)

***Persistent or excessive bleeding***

- *Possible causes* : uterine atony, retained products, uterine perforation, cervical laceration
- *Treat likely cause(s)*: Use uterine-contracting agents for atony (methergine, hemabate, misoprostol). Reaspirate if retained products. If uterine perforation, give antibiotics, and evaluate surgically if there is concern for bowel or vascular injury. Suture external cervical lacerations; tamponade endocervical lacerations
- *For significant hemorrhage (rare)*: transfuse if large blood loss. Provide blood factors to patients with coagulopathies. In extremely rare cases, uterine atery embolization, further surgery or hysterectomy may be necessary

## ELECTIVE MEDICAL ABORTION

## DESCRIPTION

- The first medication (mifepristone or methotrexate) is given to interrupt the further development of the pregnancy
- Misoprostol (MIS) is then given to induce expulsion of the products of conception (see protocol, Page 32)
- Misoprostol is a prostaglandin analogue which causes the cervix to soften and the uterus to contract. May be taken orally, vaginally or by sublingual or buccal routes, either at home or in the office. (Not as effective when given alone as when given with either mifepristone or methotrexate) *[Goldberg, Greenberg, and Darney-NEJM 2001]*
- Increasingly chosen as method of abortion; accounts for 23% of abortions ≤ 8 weeks gestation *[Pazol 2012]*

## INITIATING METHOD

- Discuss all pregnancy options, including prenatal care for continuing pregnancy or for adoption, and highlight programs available for assistance with each option
- If patient chooses elective abortion, discuss available techniques (surgical vs. medical)
- Review protocol, risks, benefits, and visit schedule
- Assess patient's access to provider if D&C is needed. Explain need for D&C if incomplete or if continuing pregnancy (some women think they can avoid surgery altogether)
- Obtain informed consent after all questions are answered
- Vaginal ultrasound to confirm dates if available

### Mifepristone (Ru-486) And Misoprostol (MIS)

**Most medical abortions in the U.S. and abroad now use mifepristone rather than methotrexate.** Mifepristone used as an abortifacient in France since 1988

***Mechanism*** - Mifepristone acts as an antiprogesterone to block continued support of the pregnancy. It blocks progesterone receptors. This causes decidual necrosis and detachment of products of conception. Mifepristone also causes cervical softening

***Dose of mifepristone*** - 600 mg is FDA approved dose - but 200 mg is just as effective in clinical trials and is commonly used

***Effectiveness*** - 92-98% effective depending on gestational age and MIS doses used: for gestational age up to 49 days if using oral MIS, up to 63 days if vaginal or buccal MIS. Process is generally more rapid than alternative regimens

***Contraindications*** - Not effective for ectopics. Not for use by chronic corticosteroid users, chronic adrenal failures, porphyrias, or with history of allergy to mifepristone or prostaglandins

***Protocol*** - (evidence-based regimens)

- ***Screening:*** Baseline labs including Rh, hemoglobin
- ***Mifepristone:*** administer 200 mg orally. Give Rh immune globulin if Rh negative at this time. Provide misoprostol for home use. Recent study supports home use of mifepristone *[Swica 2013]*
- ***Misoprostol:*** can be used vaginally, buccally or orally (800 mcg). Timing should be based on the woman's needs/schedule - a recent study of 400mcg buccal misoprostol found as effective as 800 mcg with 96% complete abortions in pregnancies up to 63 days with less side effects *[Chong 2012] [Swica 2013]*
- ***Follow-up:*** Can be performed 2-14 days after misoprostol use. If assessed at 14 days, can be just history and exam with ultrasound as indicated *[Chong 2012]*. If assessed at one week or less, ultrasound to establish absence of gestational sac. Alternative follow-up with serum hCG testing can be used. Perform D&C for heavy bleeding, signs of infection or continuing pregnancy. If gestational sac not expelled, can perform D&C or repeat misoprostol with return evaluation in 1-2 weeks.
  - At home over-the-counter pregnancy tests may be used for follow-up *[2012]*

**MIFEPRISTONE MEDICAL ABORTION AND INFECTION**

Serious infections and bleeding (rarely, fatal) occur following spontaneous, surgical, and medical abortions, including following mifepristone use. Ensure that the patient knows whom to call and what to do, including going to an Emergency Room if none of the provided contacts are reachable, if she experiences *sustained fever, severe abdominal pain, prolonged heavy bleeding, or syncope,* or if she experiences *abdominal pain or discomfort or general malaise* (including weakness, nausea, vomiting or diarrhea) more than 24 hours after taking misoprostol. A recent study supports option of taking mifepristrone at home. *[Swica et al. Acceptability of home use of mifepristone for mediacal abortion. Contraception 88 2013:122-127]*

***Atypical Presentation of Infection:*** Patients with serious bacterial infections (e.g. Clostridium sordellii) and sepsis can present without fever, bacteremia or significant findings on pelvic examination following an abortion. *Very rarely, deaths have been reported in patients who presented without fever, with or without abdominal pain but with leukocytosis with a marked left shift, tachycardia, hemoconcentration, and general malaise.* A high index of suspicion is needed to rule out serious infection and sepsis.

Revised Planned Parenthood protocol reduces risk of serious infections with medical abortion from 0.93/1,000 to 0.25/1,000 procedures. Their revised protocol is: 200 mg oral mifepristone followed 24-48 hours later by 800 mcg buccal misoprostal (400 mcg in each cheek for 30 minutes). All women receive prophylactic antibiotics: oral doxycycline 100 mg bid x7 days starting the day of mifepristone administration. *[Fjerstad M, Trussell J, Lichtenberg ES. Severity of infection following the introduction of new infection control measures for medical abortion. Contraception 83 (2011), 330-335]*

## ALTERNATIVE REGIMENS:

### Medical Abortion with Methotrexate (MTX) and Misoprostol (MIS)

Methotrexate prevents reduction of folic acid to tetrahydrofolate by binding to dihydrofolate reductase, which interferes with DNA synthesis. This action, in early pregnancy, prevents continued implantation (inhibits synctitialization of the cytotrophoblast). MTX 50 mg/m$^2$ IM or 50 mg PO is combined with MIS 800 mcg vaginally 3-7 days later in women up to 49 days gestation. Efficacy within 1 week is typically 70-80%. If the remaining non-continuing pregnancies are managed expectantly, the overall success rate is as high as 95%. Because of the significant delay in abortion for many women and the limit of efficacy to gestations only up to 49 days, the combination of MTX and MIS is generally not recommended for medical abortion.

## EARLY MEDICAL ABORTION WITH MISOPROSTOL ALONE

Misoprostol, when used without mifepristone or MTX, can cause abortion after 1-3 doses in women up to 56 days gestation. Treatment regimens typically include MIS 800 mcg vaginally at intervals ranging from every 8 hours to every 24 hours. Efficacy rates are generally around 70% with one dose of misoprostol, 80% after two doses and near 90% after three doses. Given the existence and availability of safe alternative regimens, MIS alone is generally not recommended for medical abortion. However, in situations where mifepristone is unavailable, MIS alone is an option

### CONTRACEPTION AFTER ABORTION

- All methods may be started on the day of an abortion procedure
- Advantages of starting immediately: know patient is not pregnant, immediate contraceptive protection
- If inserting IUD after second-trimester abortion procedure, may have slightly higher expulsion rate
- For medication abortions, start contraceptives on day of follow-up visit when termination of pregnancy confirmed.
- Vaginal rings were inserted within 1 week following surgical and medical abortions in 81 women and were found to be highly acceptable *[Fine-2007]*

# CHAPTER 13

## Choosing Among Contraceptive Methods

www.managingcontraception.com/choices , www.plannedparenthood.org/library

### THE BEST METHOD IS THE ONE THAT IS MEDICALLY APPROPRIATE AND IS USED EVERY TIME BY SOMEONE HAPPY WITH THE METHOD

- Women should consider the most effective methods, LARC, first
- Each contraceptive method has both advantages and disadvantages
- Be aware of your own biases
- Effectiveness and safety are important
- Convenience and ability to use method correctly influences effectiveness
- Protection against STIs/HIV needs to be considered for women and men at risk
- Effects of method on menses may be very important to a woman
- Ability to negotiate with partner may help determine method selected
- Religion, privacy, friend's advice and frequency of sex may influence decision
- Discuss all methods with patient, even those you may not use in your own practice
- Is partner supportive of contraception/condoms and will he help pay for them?
- Consider discussing with couple, particularly if there appears to be conflict

**EFFECTIVENESS:** measured by failure rates in 2 ways (see Table 12.2, Page 37)
***Correct and consistent use first year failure rate:*** The percentage of women who become pregnant during their first year of use when they use the method perfectly.
***Typical use first year failure rates:*** The percentage of women who become pregnant during their first year of use. This number reflects pregnancies in couples who use the method correctly and consistently and of those who do not. **This typical use failure rate is the relevant number to use when counseling new start users.**

- In spite of many very effective options, the U.S. has a high rate of unintended pregnancy. Just under 50% of all pregnancies in the U.S. are not planned. The U.S. also has the lowest rate of IUD use in the developed world. Our challenge is to help women and couples use available methods effectively

***Counseling about effectiveness:***

- Methods are divided into 3 groups:
  - A) *Highly effective:* female and male sterilization, Implants, IUDs
  - B) *Moderately effective:* pills (COCs and POPs), ring, patch, DMPA
  - C) *Less effective:* male latex condoms, diaphragm, cervical cap (no previous births or previous births), female condoms, spermicides (gel, foam, suppository, film), withdrawal, natural family planning (calendar, temperature, cervical mucus)

### KEY QUESTIONS

- ***What contraceptive did you come to this office today wanting to use?*** Data show that giving the method they ask for is more likely to result in continuation. *[Pariani S. et al. Stud Fam Plann, 1991]*
- ***Do you want one of the most effective methods?***

- ***When (if ever) do you want to have your next child?*** Helps teach need for preconceptional care and guides in selection of method. Consider IUDs for spacing. After first 1-2 years of use, most cost-effective method. If she definitely wants no further pregnancies, be sure to discuss sterilization in addition to the highly effective reversible methods
- ***Does your partner want to have children in the future? When?***
- ***Will your partner help you using condoms and/or paying for contraceptives? Using abstinence when you do not have another method?***
- ***What would you do if you had an accidental pregnancy? Is abortion an option or not?*** When abortion is not an option, highly effective methods should be stressed.
- ***What method(s) did you use in the past? What problems did you have with it/them?***
- ***What are you doing to protect yourself from STIs/AIDS?*** Inclusion of counseling about safer sex practices and condoms may be critical
- ***Do you know what emergency contraception is?*** Encourage her to purchase a package of ECPs to have on hand while encouraging use of a highly effective contraceptive thereby minimizing the potential need for EC
- ***Do you have any serious medical problems?***
- ***What side effects are you willing to accept?***

## COMPARING TYPICAL EFFECTIVENESS OF CONTRACEPTIVE METHODS

This chart available at www.who.int/reproductive-health/family-planning/tool.htm

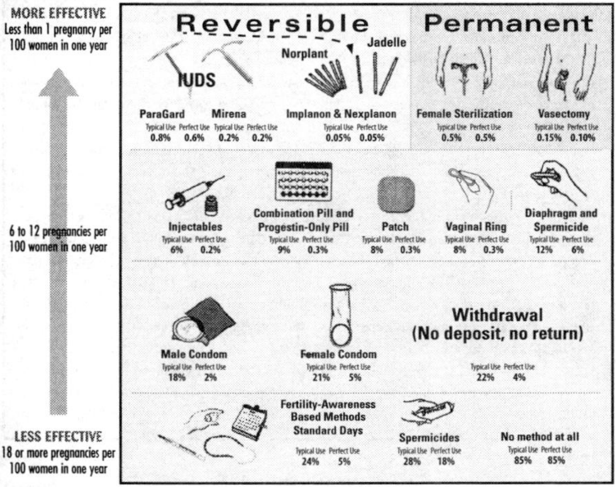


**Dual method use with condoms whenever there is risk of sexually transmitted infections.**

**TABLE 13.1 Comparative risk of unprotected intercourse on unintended pregnancies and STI infections***

| Unintended pregnancy/coital act | PID per woman infected with cervical gonorrhea |
|---|---|
| 17%-30% midcycle<br><1% during menses | 40% if not treated<br>0% if promptly and adequately treated |
| **Gonococcal transmission/coital act** | **Tubal infertility per PID episode** |
| 50% infected male, uninfected female<br>25% infected female, uninfected male | 8% after first episode<br>20% after second episode<br>40% after three or more episodes |

**Marrazzo JM and Cates W Jr. Reproductive tract infections. In: Hatcher RA, et al. Contraceptive Technology. 20th ed. New York: Ardent Media, 2011:573.*

### ACCUTANE SHOULD BE USED VERY CAUTIOUSLY IN REPRODUCTIVE AGE WOMEN

Accutane (isotretinoin) is a vitamin A isomer used in the treatment of extremely severe acne. If taken by a woman who is pregnant, it may cause a wide range of teratogenic effects including:

**CNS:** hydrocephalus, facial nerve palsy, cortical blindness and retinal defects

**Craniofacial:** low-set ears, microcephaly, triangular skull and cleft palate

**Cardiovascular:** transposition of the great vessels, atrial and ventricular septal defects

Important contraceptive messages for women considering Accutane use, in view of the fact that no method of birth control is 100% effective:

- **Use Two Methods:** In addition to compulsive, careful and consistent use of a very effective hormonal contraceptive, also use condoms consistently and correctly. Use of any combined (E/P) method is likely to have a beneficial effect on acne.
- **Repeated Pregnancy Tests:** Pregnancy tests are essential prior to initiating and on a monthly basis thereafter. This is particularly important since the critical time of exposure to Accutane is believed to be 2-5 weeks after conception *[Briggs-2002]*
- **Consider Abortion if Contraceptive Failure:** Should pregnancy occur, strongly consider an abortion. In the 22 months following its introduction, the manufacturer, FDA and CDC received reports on 154 Accutane-exposed pregnancies, of which 95 (61.7%) were electively aborted. Another 12 (7.8%) aborted spontaneously. 26 were born without major defects and 21 had major malformations *[Briggs-2002]* **Many clinicians will not provide this drug unless the woman agrees to have an abortion should a pregnancy occur**
- **Use Accutane Sparingly:** This drug is dangerous to a developing fetus and should not be used unless other approaches to managing acne have been used first AND unless the reproductive-age woman using it agrees to use contraception consistently and correctly.

**Table 13.2 Percentage of women experiencing an unintended pregnancy within the first year of typical use and the first year of perfect use and the percentage continuing use at the end of the first year: United States***

| | % of Women Experiencing an Unintended Pregnancy within the First Year of Use | | % of Women Continuing Use at One Year[1] |
|---|---|---|---|
| **Method** | **Typical Use[2]** | **Perfect Use[3]** | |
| Male Sterilization | 0.15 | 0.10 | 100 |
| Female Sterilization | 0.5 | 0.5 | 100 |
| Implanon | 0.05 | 0.05 | 84 |
| Intrauterine contraceptives | | | |
| ParaGard (copper T) | 0.8 | 0.6 | 78 |
| Mirena (LNg) | 0.2 | 0.2 | 80 |
| Depo-Provera | 6 | 0.2 | 56 |
| NuvaRing* | 9 | 0.3 | 67 |
| Evra patch* | 9 | 0.3 | 67 |
| Combined pill & Progestin-only pill | 9 | 0.3 | 67 |
| Diaphragm | 12 | 6 | 57 |
| Condom[8] | | | |
| Female (fc) | 21 | 5 | 41 |
| Male | 18 | 2 | 43 |
| Sponge | | | 36 |
| Parous women | 24 | 20 | |
| Nulliparous women | 12 | 9 | |
| Withdrawal | 22 | 4 | 46 |
| Fertility awareness-based methods | 24 | | 47 |
| Standard Days method[6] | | 5 | |
| TwoDay method[6] | | 4 | |
| Ovulation method[6] | | 3 | |
| Symptothermal method[6] | | 0.4 | |
| Spermicides[5] | 28 | 18 | 42 |
| No Method[4] | 85 | 85 | |

**Emergency Contraceptive Pills:** Treatment with COCs initiated within 120 hours after unprotected intercourse reduces the risk of pregnancy by at least 60-75%[9]. Pregnancy rates lower if initiated in first 12 hours. Progestin-only EC reduces pregnancy risk by 89%.

**Lactational Amenorrhea Method:** LAM is a highly effective, temporary method of contraception.[10]

Notes:

[1] Among typical couples who initiate use of a method (not necessarily for the first time), the percentage who experience an accidental pregnancy during the first year if they do not stop use for any other reason. Estimates of the probability of pregnancy during the first year of typical use for spermicides, withdrawal, fertility awareness-based methods, the diaphragm, the male condom, the oral contraceptive pill, and Depo-Provera are taken from the 1995 National Survey of Family Growth corrected for underreporting of abortion; see the text for the derivation of estimates for the other methods.

[2] Among couples who initiate use of a method (not necessarily for the first time) and who use it perfectly (both consistently and correctly), the percentage who experience an accidental pregnancy during the first year if they do not stop use for any other reason. See the text for the derivation of the estimate for each method.

[3] Among couples attempting to avoid pregnancy, the percentage who continue to use a method for 1 year.

[4] The percentages becoming pregnant in columns (2) and (3) are based on data from populations where contraception is not used and from women who cease using contraception in order to become pregnant. Among such populations, about 89% become pregnant within 1 year. This estimate was lowered slightly (to 85%) to represent the percentage who would become pregnant within 1 year among women now relying on reversible methods of contraception if they abandoned contraception altogether.

[5] Foams, creams, gels, vaginal suppositories, and vaginal film.

[6] The Ovulation and TwoDay methods are based on evaluation of cervical mucus. The Standard Days method avoids intercourse on cycle days 8 through 19. The Symptothermal method is a double-check method based on evaluation of cervical mucus to determine the first fertile day and evaluation of cervical mucus and temperature to determine the last fertile day.

[7] Without spermicides.

[8] With spermicidal cream or jelly.

[9] ella, Plan B One-Step and Next Choice are the only dedicated products specifically marketed for emergency contraception. The label for Plan B One-Step (one dose is 1 white pill) says to take the pill within 72 hours after unprotected intercourse. Research has shown that all of the brands listed here are effective when used within 120 hours after unprotected sex. The label for Next Choice (one dose is 1 peach pill) says to take 1 pill within 72 hours after unprotected intercourse and another pill 12 hours later. Research has shown that both pills can be taken at the same time with no decrease in efficacy or increase in side effects and that they are effective when used within 120 hours after unprotected sex. The Food and Drug Administration has in addition declared the following 19 brands of oral contraceptives to be safe and effective for emergency contraception: Ogestrel (1 dose is 2 white pills), Nordette (1 dose is 4 light-orange pills), Cryselle, Levora, Low-Ogestrel, Lo/Ovral, or Quasence (1 dose is 4 white pills), Jolessa, Portia, Seasonale or Trivora (1 dose is 4 pink pills), Seasonique (1 dose is 4 light-blue-green pills), Enpresse (one dose is 4 orange pills), Lessina (1 dose is 5 pink pills), Aviane or LoSeasonique (one dose is 5 orange pills), Lutera or Sronyx (one dose is 5 white pills), and Lybrel (one dose is 6 yellow pills).

[10] However, to maintain effective protection against pregnancy, another method of contraception must be used as soon as menstruation resumes, the frequency or duration of breastfeeds is reduced, bottle feeds are introduced, or the baby reaches 6 months of age.

*Adapted from Trussell J, Kowal D. The essentials of contraception. In: Hatcher RA, et al. *Contraceptive Technology*, 20th ed. New York: Ardent Media, 2011.
Updated from Trussel J. Contraception 83 (2011) 397-404
*Numbers for typical use failure of Ortho Evra and NuvaRing are not based on data. They are estimates based on pill data.

**Thank you, James Trussell, for this remarkable table!**

**Table 13.3 Major methods of contraception and some related safety concerns, side effects, and noncontraceptive benefits**

*Trussell J, Kowal D. The essentials of contraception. IN: Hatcher RA, et al. *Contraceptive Technology*. 20th ed. New York: Ardent Media, 2011:66. Slight adaptations from CT table.

| METHOD | NON-CONTRACEPTVE BENEFITS | SIDE EFFECTS | DANGERS |
|---|---|---|---|
| Combined hormonal contraception (pill, and presumably Evra patch, and NuvaRing.) | Decreases dysmenorrhea, menorrhagia, anemia and cyclic mood problems (PMS); protects against ectopic pregnancy, symptomatic PID, and ovarian, endometrial, and possibly colorectal cancer; reduces acne | Nausea, headaches, dizziness, spotting, weight gain, breast tenderness, chloasma | Cardiovascular complications (stroke, heart attack, blood clots, high blood pressure), depression, hepatic adenomas, increased risk of cervical and possibly liver cancers, earlier development of breast cancer in young women |
| Progestin-only pill | Lactation not disturbed | Less nausea than with combined pills | May avoid some dangers of combined hormonal contraceptives |
| IUD | Mirena decreases menstrual blood loss and menorrhagia and can provide progestin for hormone replacement therapy | Menstrual cramping, spotting, increased bleeding with non-progestin-releasing IUDs | Infection post insertion, uterine perforation, anemia |
| Male condom | Protects against STIs, including HIW; delays premature ejaculation | Decreased sensation, allergy to latex | Anaphylactic reaction to latex |
| Female condom | Protects against STIs | Aesthetically unappealing and awkward to use for some | None known |
| Implanon | Lactation not disturbed; decreases dysmenorrhea | Headache, acne, menstrual changes, weight gain, depression, emotional lability | Infection at implant site; may avoid some dangers of combined hormonal contraceptives |

| METHOD | NON-CONTRACEPTVE BENEFITS | SIDE EFFECTS | DANGERS |
|---|---|---|---|
| Depo-Provera | Lactation not disturbed; reduces risk of seizures; may protect against ovarian and endometrial cancers | Menstrual changes, weight gain, headache, adverse effects on lipids | Depression, allergic reactions, pathologic weight gain, bone loss |
| Sterilization | Tubal sterilization reduces risk of ovarian cancer and may protect against PID | Pain at surgical site, psychological reactions, subsequent regret that the procedure was performed | Infection; possible anesthetic or surgical complications; if pregnancy occurs after tubal sterilization, high risk that it will be ectopic |
| Abstinence | Prevents STIs, including HIV, if anal and oral intercourse are avoided as well | | None known |
| Diaphragm, Sponge | | Pelvic discomfort, vaginal irritation, vaginal discharge if left in too long, allergy | Vaginal and urinary tract infections, toxic shock syndrome; possible increase in susceptibility to HIV/AIDS acquisition if exposed to positive partner |
| Spermicides | | Vaginal irritation, allergy | Vaginal and urinary tract infections; possible increase in susceptibility to HIV/AIDS acquisition if exposed to positive partner |
| Lactational Amenorrhea Method (LAM) | Provides excellent nutrition for infants under 6 months old | | |

**Table 13.4 Routine Follow-Up After Contraceptive Initiation**

CDC Selected Practice Recommendations

| | Contraceptive method | | | | |
|---|---|---|---|---|---|
| **Action** | **Cu-IUD or LNG-IUD** | **Implant** | **Injectable** | **CHC** | **POP** |
| **General follow-up** | | | | | |
| Advise women to return at any time to discuss side effects or other problems or if they want to change the method. Advise women using IUDs, implants, or injectables when the IUD or implant needs to be removed or when a reinjection is needed. No routine follow-up visit is required. | X | X | X | X | X |
| **Other routine visits** | | | | | |
| Assess the woman's satisfaction with her current method and whether she has any concerns about method use. | X | X | X | X | X |
| Assess any changes in health status, including medications, that would change the method's appropriateness for safe and effective continued use based on U.S. MEC (i.e., category 3 and 4 conditions and characteristics) (Box 2). | X | X | X | X | X |
| Consider performing an examination to check for the presence of IUD strings. | X | — | — | — | — |
| Consider assessing weight changes and counseling women who are concerned about weight change perceived to be associated with their contraceptive method. | X | X | X | X | X |
| Measure blood pressure. | — | — | — | X | — |

Abbreviations: CHC = combined hormonal contraceptive; Cu-IUD = copper-containing intrauterine device; HIV = human immunodeficiency virus; IUD = intrauterine device; LNG-IUD = levonorgestrel-releasing intrauterine device; POP = progestin-only pill; U.S. MEC = *U.S. Medical Eligibility Criteria for Contraceptive Use, 2010.*

***CDC MMWR June 21, 2013, Vol. 62:No. 5***

## TIMING:

Couples considering contraceptives and their health care providers face myriad questions about the timing of contraceptive use. Sometimes our clients come to us with mistaken ideas. Sometimes we providers are actually the source of arbitrary misinformation about timing. In either case, timing errors, misconceptions, rigidity and oversimplifications can cause trouble; and trouble in family planning often can be spelled "unintended pregnancy". In most instances, more important than advice about the timing of contraceptives is rapid initiation and then correct, ***consistent*** use of contraceptives. Below are several suggestions to consider in helping patients with timing questions:

1. For many women, a practical way to start pills, the patch or the ring is on the first day of the next period. Even easier, sometimes, is the Quick Start method which is to start pills on the day you first see a patient if you ***can be reasonably certain that she is not pregnant*** [Westhoff-2002]. Recommend backup method for 7 days unless pills started during the five days after the start of menses or within 5 days of miscarriage. Women with unprotected intercourse in preceeding 5 days should also receive EC.
   The Quick Start approach to starting the use of pills, intrauterine devices, implants, injections has become one of the most important changes in how contraceptives are provided. EVERY method is less likely to be started if there is a delay in starting it.
2. Switching from one hormonal method to another can be done immediately as long as the first method is used consistently and correctly, or if it is ***reasonably certain that she is not pregnant***

***BOX 1. How to be Reasonably certain a woman is not pregnant - no symptoms and signs of pregnancy AND meets any of following criteria:***
- no intercourse since last menses
- has been using a reliable method consistently and correctly
- is ≤ 7 days after start of normal menses
- within 4 weeks postpartum
- is ≤ 7 days post abortion or miscarriage
- fully or near fully breastfeeding, amenorrheic and < 6 months postpartum
  Some experts recommend relying on lactational amenorrhea only through 3 months because 20% of fully nursing mothers ovulate at 3 months.
  *[CDC MMWR June 21, 2013 Vol. 62 No.5]*

3. Healthy women who tolerate pills well and do not smoke can continue pills until menopause unless a woman develops a complication or a contraindication to pill use. Periodic "breaks" from taking pills is still inappropriately recommended by some clinicians and is an unwise practice that can lead to unintended pregnancies and blood clots.
4. Extended use of combined pills with no pill free interval is an acceptable way for some women to take pills, with no increased risk of endometrial hyperplasia *[Anderson-2003]*.

5. The first Depo-Provera injection may be given at any time in the cycle if ***reasonably certain a woman is not pregnant (see Box 1)***. If the day of the first shot is NOT within 5 days of the start of a period, recommend that patient use a back-up contraceptive for 7 days; give EC and repeat pregnancy test in 2-3 weeks if recent unprotected intercourse
6. Avoid overly dogmatic advice regarding when postpartum women should start progestin-only pills and the progestin-only injection, Depo-Provera. US MEC category 1 for using progestin-only methods in the first month PP for non-breastfeeding women. US MEC category 2 for using progestin-only methods within the first month PP in breastfeeding women. There are clinicians and entire programs starting these two methods in each of the following 3 ways:
   - At discharge from hospital
   - 2-3 weeks postpartum
   - 6 weeks postpartum
7. Recommend that condoms be placed onto the erect penis OR onto the penis before it becomes erect. There are clear advantages and disadvantages to both approaches.
8. Offer Plan B (emergency contraceptive pills) to women in advance. Advance prescription of Plan B is one approach. Better yet, hand her the actual pills and instructions, or instruct her to purchase OTC and keep at home
9. Intrauterine contraceptives may be inserted at any time in a woman's menstrual cycle if reasonably certain she is not pregnant. If using an LNG-IUD, back-up is recommended for 7 days if not inserted in the first 10 days of the cycle. No back-up is needed for Copper IUD because of its high efficacy as an emergency contraceptive.
10. If in doubt about any timing question, use condoms until your timing questions have been resolved

## ➔ DECREASING UNINTENDED PREGNANCIES:

1. Use more forgettable methods or Long Acting Reversible Contraceptives. Today this means more intrauterine devices or implants.
2. ➔ Stop recommending or using emergency contraceptive pills as the "go to" approach to unprotected intercourse until we have emergency contraceptive pills that work. Now by far the best approach to emergency contraception is the Copper-T 380A interuterine device within 5 days of unprotected sex. Sometimes more than 5 days if date of ovulation is within 5 days.
3. To improve contraceptive effectiveness, to prevent sexually transmitted infections and to prevent infertility due to chlamydia infections and tubal sterilization, use condoms too.
4. Use the Quick Start approach to initiating almost all approaches to birth control.
5. Vasectomy and tubal sterilization are excellent options for some couples. Both should be ➔ considered 100 perent permanent. Close to half of sterilizations for women are done within 48 hours of postpartum.
6. ➔ To lower the 9% typical use failure rate of pills (one million women counting on pills become pregnant each year), switch to the continuous or the extended use of combined pills. If a pill free interval is desired for a withdrawal bleed, after at least 21 days active pills, 2-4 day break is sufficient.
7. ➔ Due to the less than 100% effectiveness of all contraceptives, carelessness, thoughtlessness, forced intercourse, and the cost of using some methods, unintended pregnancies will not be eliminated anytime in the foreseeable future and safe legal abortions must be available as a backup to our current contraceptives.

## Table 13.5 When to Start Using Specific Contraceptive Methods

CDC Selected Practice Recommendations

| Contraceptive method | When to start (if the provider is reasonably certain that the woman is not pregnant) | Additional contraception (i.e., back up) needed | Examinations or tests needed before initiation1 |
|---|---|---|---|
| Copper-containing IUD | Anytime | Not needed | Bimanual examination and cervical inspection[2] |
| Levonorgestrel-releasing IUD | Anytime | If >7 days after menses started, use back-up method or abstain for 7 days. | Bimanual examination and cervical inspection[2] |
| Implant | Anytime | If >5 days after menses started, use back-up method or abstain for 7 days. | None |
| Injectable | Anytime | If >7 days after menses started, use back-up method or abstain for 7 days. | None |
| Combined hormonal contraceptive | Anytime | If >5 days after menses started, use back-up method or abstain for 7 days. | Blood pressure measurement |
| Progestin-only pill | Anytime | If >5 days after menses started, use back-up method or abstain for 2 days. | None |

**Abbreviations:** BMI = body mass index; IUD = intrauterine device; STD = sexually transmitted disease

[1]Weight (BMI) measurement is not needed to determine medical eligibility for any methods of contraception because all methods can be used or generally can be used among obese women. However, measuring weight and calculating BMI at baseline might be helpful for monitoring any changes and counseling women who might be concerned about weight change perceived to be associated with their contraceptive method.

[2]Most women do not require additional STD screening at the time of IUD insertion if they have already been screened according to CDC's STD Treatment Guidelines (available at http://www.cdc.gov/std/treatment). If a woman has not been screened according to guidelines, screening can be performed at the time of IUD insertion and insertion should not be delayed. Women with purulent cervicitis, current chlamydial infection, or gonorrhea should not undergo IUD insertion. Women who have a very high individual likelihood of STD exposure (e.g., those with a currently infected partner) generally should not undergo IUD insertion. For these women, IUD insertion should be delayed until appropriate testing and treatment occurs.

*CDC MMWR June 21, 2013, Vol. 62:No. 5*

## CHAPTER 14

# Abstinence or Delaying Sexual Intercourse

www.managingcontraception.com or www.sexrespect.com

### DESCRIPTION

Abstinence means different things to different people. However, from a family planning perspective, the definition of abstinence is clear: it is delaying genital contact that could result in a pregnancy (i.e. penile penetration into the vagina). Some authors argue that abstinence is not a form of contraception, but is a lifestyle choice because a person not having intercourse needs no contraception. Regardless, abstinence is an important means of reducing unintended pregnancies and sexually transmitted infections. A woman or a man may return to abstinence at any time.

Close to 50% of young men and women would consider having intercourse on a first date and close to 50% have had vaginal intercourse on a first date reflecting a lack of commitment to abstinence.

### EFFECTIVENESS

***When abstinence is adhered to, there is no pregnancy***

### HOW ABSTINENCE WORKS

Sperm excluded from female reproductive tract, preventing fertilization

**COST:** None

**ADVANTAGES: Can be used as an interval method**
***Menstrual:*** none
***Sexual/psychological:*** May contribute to positive self image if consistent with personal values
***Cancers, tumors, and masses:*** Risk of cervical cancer far less if no vaginal intercourse has ever occurred
***Other:***

- Reduces risk of STIs (unless vaginal intercourse replaced with oral/anal)
- Many religions and cultures endorse
- May encourage people to build relationships in other ways

### DISADVANTAGES

***Menstrual:*** None
***Sexual/psychological:*** Frustration or possible rejection if abstinence not adhered to
***Cancers, tumors, and masses:*** None
***Other:***

- Requires commitment and self control; nonunderstanding partner may seek other partner(s)
- Patient and her partner may not be prepared to contracept if they stop abstaining

### COMPLICATIONS

- No medical complications
- Person may be in situation where she/he wants to abstain, but partner does not agree. Women have been raped/beaten for refusing to have intercourse

### CANDIDATES FOR USE

- Individuals or couples who feel they have the ability to refrain from sexual intercourse

***Adolescents:***

- Very appropriate method but need maturity to effectively use abstinence. Obtain information about contraceptive methods for future, understand the consequences of various sexual activities
- Counseling may include discussions on masturbation (solo or mutual) and also "outercourse" alternative ways of expressing affection/attraction/sexuality with partner

## MAINTAINING ABSTINENCE USUALLY REQUIRES OPEN COMMUNICATION

- Provide negotiating skills, how to say no or "not now", and how to resist peer (societal) pressures
- Recommend that patient ensure that partner explicitly agrees to abstain
- Stress that abstinence may just be a decision to delay intercourse. It may mean "not now", instead of "never". Remind her that she may use or return to abstinence at any time in life
- Prepare for time when (or if) decision to stop abstaining arises, contraceptive education
- Advise her to consider having condoms and emergency contraception in case of need

## PROBLEM MANAGEMENT

***Partner does not want to abstain:***

- Recommend continued communication and be available to discuss options with couples together
- Provide counseling in other forms of sexual pleasuring if patient interested (masturbation or outercourse)
- Seriously consider birth control method or another partner

## FERTILITY ISSUE

- Protects against upper reproductive tract infection preserving a woman's fertility

### Are Abstinence-Only Education Programs Effective?

In a review by Kirby (2001), only three evaluation studies of abstinence-only programs met the criteria established for inclusion in the review (e.g. random assignment, large sample size, long-term follow-up, measurement of behavior). **None of the studies demonstrated a significant programmatic effect on the initiation of sex, frequency of sexual activity, or the number of sexual partners.** A report released 4/07 of a long-term study commissioned by Congress, found that abstinence-only sex ed programs are not effective in preventing or delaying teenagers from having sexual intercourse, and have no impact on the likelihood that if they do have sex, they will use a condom.

In addition, these programs often provide misinformation and withold important information, e.g. about contraception, needed to make informed choices *[Santelli-2006]*.

Another recent study found the sexual behaviour of teenage virginity pledgers did not differ from matched non-pledgers, but pledgers were less likely to protect themselves from pregnancy and infection *[Rosenbaum-2009]*

- Recent survey of parents in NC found they overwhelmingly support (89%) comprehensive sexual education yet their state mandates abstinence education *[Ito-2006]*
- Society for adolescent medicine position paper (2006) states:
  Abstinence is a healthy choice for adolescents, but this choice should not be coerced. Instead, teens should be informed about sexual risk reduction including abstinence, correct and consistent condom use and contraception

*Source: Kirby, D. (2001). Emerging Answers: Research Findings on Programs to Reduce Teen Pregnancy. Washington, DC: The National Campaign to Prevent Teen Pregnancy.*

Please look at page 2 of *Choices*: Abstinence Tonight... Today... or Now!

## WAYS TO ENCOURAGE ABSTINENCE

*Ways to Think About Abstinence*

1. ***Primary Abstinence*** for a very long period of time

2. ***Return to Abstinence*** for a very long time

3. ***Abstinence "for a while" - for example, until***
   a) effective contraception has been achieved
   b) STD tests are negative and effective approach to prevention of STDs carefully discussed and agreed upon by both partners
   c) until 2, 4, or 6 week postpartum visit
   d) trust and communication (and monogamy) well established in relationship and consequences of sex including unplanned pregnancy can be negotiated

4. ***Abstinence right now - tonight or today.*** Every day there are some 10 million acts of intercourse in couples NOT wanting to become pregnant and 700,000 of those acts of intercourse are completely unprotected acts of sexual intercourse. Today 700,000 couples could decide NOT to have intercourse.

With each of those 4 time frames for abstinence (avoiding penis-in-vagina intercourse), couples may or may not choose any of a variety of sexual interactions sometimes called **outercourse** (holding hands, hugging, kissing, deep kissing, petting, mutual masturbation, oral-genital contact).

# CHAPTER 15

## Breastfeeding: Lactational Amenorrhea Method (LAM)

**www.lalecheleague.org or www.breastfeeding.com or www.ilca.org or www.gotmom.org**

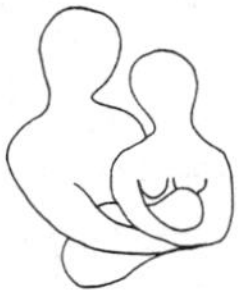

**DESCRIPTION:** The lactational amenorrhea method (LAM) is contingent upon nearly exclusive or exclusive, frequent breastfeeding. LAM is an effective method only under specific conditions:

- Woman breast-feeding exclusively; both day and night feedings (at least 90% of baby's nutrition derived from breast-feeding)
- The woman is amenorrheic (spotting which occurs in the first 56 days postpartum is not regarded as menses)
- The infant is less than 6 months old

In the U.S., the median duration of breast-feeding is about 3 months. It is important to provide a woman with another method to use when she no longer fulfills all the conditions. **The probability that ovulation will precede the first menstrual period in a lactating woman increases from 33-45% during the first 3 months to 64-71% during months 4 to 12 and 87% after 12 months. Among lactating women, 66% are sexually active in the first month postpartum and 88% are sexually active in the second month postpartum *[Ford - 1998]***

**EFFECTIVENESS: Controlled Studies**

***Life table pregnancy rate at 6 months:*** 0.45 and 2.45% in 2 published studies
***Uncontrolled studies:*** range from 0 - 7.5% *[Cochran Review-2008]*
At any time a woman is concerned, emergency contraception may be used by a nursing mother

**MECHANISM:** Suckling causes a surge in maternal prolactin, which inhibits ovulation. If ovulation occurs and fertilization occurs, the contraceptive effect of breastfeeding may be partly due to inhibiting implantation of a fertilized egg.

**COST:** None

**ADVANTAGES OF BREASTFEEDING**

***Menstrual:*** Involution of the uterus occurs more rapidly; suppresses menses
***Sexual/psychological:*** Breast-feeding pleasurable to many women

- Facilitates bonding between mother and child (if not stressful)

***Cancers, tumors, and masses:*** Reduces risk of breast, ovarian and endometrial cancer
***Other:***

- Provides the healthiest, most "natural" food for baby
- Protects baby against gastrointestinal and respiratory infecions, otitis media
- Facilitates postpartum weight loss
- No cost and less time preparing bottles and feedings

**DISADVANTAGES**

***Menstrual:*** Return to menses unpredictable
***Sexual/psychological:***

- Breastfeeding mother may be self-conscious in public or during intercourse
- Hypoestrogenism of breastfeeding may cause temporary atrophic vaginal changes
- Tender breasts may decrease sexual pleasure

***Cancers, tumors, and masses:*** None

***Other:***

- Working women need support to find time/place/resources to pump
- Effectiveness after 6 months is markedly reduced; return to fertility often precedes menses
- Frequent breastfeeding may be inconvenient or perceived as inconvenient
- No protection against STIs, HIV, AIDS
- If the mother is HIV+, there is a 14%-29% chance that HIV will be passed to infant via breast milk. Antiretroviral therapy decreases risk of transmission. Breastfeeding is not recommended for HIV+ women in the U.S.
- Sore nipples and breasts; risk of mastitis associated with breast-feeding

**COMPLICATIONS:** Risk of mastitis; return of fertility can precede menses

## CANDIDATES FOR USE

- Amenorrheic women less than 6 months postpartum who exclusively breast-feed their babies
- Women free of a blood borne infection which could be passed to the newborn
- Women not on drugs which can adversely affect their babies

## MEDICAL ELIGIBILITY CHECKLIST

Ask the patient the questions below. If she answers "NO" to ALL questions, she can use LAM. If she answers Yes to any questions, follow the instructions. Sometimes there is a way to incorporate LAM into her contraceptive plans; in other situations, LAM is contraindicated.

***1. Is your baby 6 months old or older?***

☐ No ☐ Yes Help her choose another method to supplement the contraceptive effect of LAM. Some experts recommend 3 months since 20% of breastfeeding women ovulate by that time

***2. Has your menstrual period returned? (Bleeding in the first 8 weeks after childbirth does not count)***

☐ No ☐ Yes After 8 weeks postpartum, if a woman has 2 straight days of menstrual bleeding, or her menstrual period has returned, she can no longer count on LAM as her contraceptive. Help her choose method appropriate for breastfeeding woman

***3. Have you begun to breastfeed less often? Do you regularly give the baby other food or liquid (other than water)?***

☐ No ☐ Yes If the baby's feeding pattern has just changed, explain that patient must be fully or nearly fully breastfeeding around the clock to protect against pregnancy. If not, she cannot use LAM effectively. Help her choose method appropriate for breastfeeding woman

***4. Has a health-care provider told you not to breastfeed your baby?***

☐ No ☐ Yes If a patient is not breastfeeding, she cannot use LAM. Help her choose another method. A woman should not breastfeed if she is taking mood altering recreational drugs, reserpine, ergotamine, antimetabolites, bromocriptine, tetracycline, radioactive drugs, lithium, or certain anticoagulants (heparin and coumadin are safe); if her baby has a specific infant metabolic disorder; or possibly if she carries viral hepatitis or is HIV positive. All others can and should consider breastfeeding for the health benefits to the infant. In 1997, the FDA advised the manufacturer of Prozac (fluoxetine) to revise its labeling; it now states that "nursing while on Prozac is not recommended." Multiple reviews conclude that women using SSRIs should be encouraged to continue breastfeeding *[Nulman Tetralogy, 1996][Briggs, 2002]* and that the overall benefits of SSRIs for depressed breastfeeding women outweigh the risks *[Edwards, 1999]*

**5. *Are you infected with HIV, the virus that causes AIDS?***

☐ No ☐ Yes Where other infectious diseases kill many babies, mothers should be encouraged to breastfeed. HIV, however, may be passed to the baby in breast milk. When infectious diseases are a low risk and there is safe, affordable food for the baby, advise her to feed her baby that other food. Help her choose a birth control method other than LAM. A meta-analysis of published prospective trials estimated the risk of transmission of HIV with breastfeeding is 14% if the mother was infected prenatally but is 29% if the woman has her primary infection in the postpartum period

**6. *Do you know how long you plan to breastfeed your baby before you start supplementing his/her diet?***

☐ No ☐ Yes In the U.S. the median duration of breastfeeding is approximately 3 months. Often breastfeeding women do not know when their menses will return, when they will start supplementing breastfeeding with other foods or exactly when they will stop breastfeeding their infant. It is wise to provide a woman with the contraceptive she will use when the answer to one of the above questions becomes positive and with a backup contraceptive and EC even during the period when breast-feeding is effective

## INITIATING METHOD

- Patient should start exclusively breastfeeding immediately or as soon as possible after delivery
- Ensure that woman is breastfeeding fully or almost fully (>90% of baby's feedings); feedings around the clock
- A woman working outside of the home requires a breastfeeding-friendly environment, and preferably on-site childcare so that woman can visit her child every few hours to breastfeed; otherwise, breast pumping is needed
- Encourage use of second method of contraception if any questions about LAM effectiveness

## INSTRUCTIONS FOR PATIENT

- Refer to lactation consultant/La Leche League for support/resources (www.lalecheleague.org)
- Breastfeed consistently, exclusively and correctly for maximum effectiveness
- Breast milk should constitute at least 90% of baby's feedings
- Think about methods that can be used once menses return or at 6 months

## PROBLEM MANAGEMENT

***Deficient milk supply:***

- The more a breast is emptied, the more it fills up, therefore, increase feedings or pumpings
- Commonly caused by insufficient nursing, use of artificial nipple (e.g. pacifier), fatigue or maternal stress
- Encourage woman to breastfeed often (8-10 times daily), eat well, get additional rest, drink lots of fluids and take prenatal vitamins and iron supplements
- Immediately postpartum women should breastfeed every 2-3 hours to stimulate milk production
- Seek assistance from a lactation specialist
- Avoid high-dose estrogen-containing contraceptives

*Sore nipples:*
- Commonly caused by incorrect application of the baby's mouth to the breast. Uncommonly caused by infection
- Check for correct ways of latching and suckling; be sure to break the suction before removing the baby from the breast
- Improve with practice; change the pressure points on the nipple by changing the baby's position for feeding
- Allow nipples to air dry with breast milk on the areola to reduce infection and nipple soreness. Apply lanolin to nipples after each feeding to decrease soreness after nipples have air dried
- Do not cleanse breasts other than with water at any time
- Cool gel packs are available to decrease soreness

*Sore breasts:*
- Wear a well-fitted, supportive nursing bra; avoid bras that are too tight or have underwire
- Apply heat on sore areas; some women apply teabag as compress on sore nipples
- Nurse frequently or use pump to get excess milk out of affected breast
- Use of an anti-inflammatory agent and a complex of bromelain/trypsin both significantly improved symptoms of engorgement. *[Cochrane Database of systematic reviews. Treatments for breast engorgement during lactation. 2008]*
- Encourage additional rest
- Seek medical evaluation if any erythema, fever or other signs or symptoms of infection develop

*Other:*
- Stress, fear, lack of confidence, lack of strong motivation to succeed at breastfeeding, lack of partner and/or societal support, and/or poor nutrition can cause problems

**FERTILITY AFTER USE:** Patient's baseline fertility (ability to become pregnant) is not altered once patient discontinues breastfeeding

## TEN STEPS TO SUCCESSFUL BREASTFEEDING

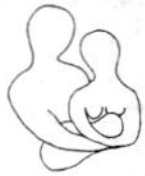

From: Protecting, Promoting and Supporting Breastfeeding: The special role of maternity services. (A joint WHO/UNICEF statement. Geneva, WHO, 1989)

***All healthcare facilities where childbirth is undertaken should:***

1. **Have a written breastfeeding policy that is routinely communicated to all health care staff.**
2. **Train all health care staff in skills necessary to implement this policy.**
3. **Inform all pregnant women about the benefits and management of breastfeeding.**
4. **Help mothers initiate breastfeeding within the first 30 minutes after birth.**
5. **Show mothers how to breastfeed and how to maintain lactation even if they are separated from their infants because of a medical reason.**
6. **Give newborn infants no milk feeds or water other than breast milk unless indicated for a medical reason.**
7. **Allow mothers and infants to remain together 24 hours a day from birth.**
8. **Encourage natural breastfeeding on demand.**
9. **Do not give or encourage the use of artificial nipples to breastfeed infants.**
10. **Promote the establishment of breastfeeding support groups and refer mothers to these on discharge from the hospital or clinic.**

**The importance of breastfeeding has been highlighted by the U.S. Department of Health and Human Services. Year 2010 goals: 75% of women will initiate breastfeeding and 50% will continue for 6 months**

# CHAPTER 16

# Breastfeeding and Contraceptive Decisions

www.lalecheleague.org OR www.breastfeeding.com

***All breastfeeding women should be provided contraception because:***

- Duration of breastfeeding in the U.S. is brief (median: under 3 months)
- Most couples resume intercourse a few weeks after delivery
- Postpartum visit should be no later than 3 weeks to ensure contraceptive coverage
- Ovulation may precede first menses
- LAM is an appropriate choice when fully breastfeeding

**Table 16.1** ***When to initiate contraception in breastfeeding women:***

| METHOD | WHEN TO START IN LACTATING WOMEN | EFFECT ON BREAST MILK |
|---|---|---|
| Condoms (Male & Female), Sponge | • Immediately | No effect |
| Cervical Cap, Diaphragm | • 4-6 weeks postpartum, after cervix and vagina normalized (need to be refitted for postpartum women) | No effect |
| Progestin-Only Methods<br>• Depo-Provera<br>• Progestin - Only Pills<br>• Implanon/Nexplanon | • New US Medical Eligibility Criteria 2010 (see appendix) allows for starting progestin-only methods in first month PP or before discharge from hospital.<br>They give this a category 2 which means method can be used because advantages outweigh theoretical or proven risks. | • No significant impact on milk quality or production<br>• Breast-feeding prolonged<br>• Breast fed children of DMPA users grow at normal rate |
| Combined Pills<br>Patch<br>Vaginal Ring | • American Academy of Pediatrics recommends use of low-dose combined hormonal contraceptives when infant' is not relying solely on breastmilk. No sooner than 3-6 weeks postpartum<br>• New CDC Medical Eligibility Criteria 2010 (see appendix) gives use of CHC in breastfeeding women a category 2 at 1 month PP meaning advantages outweigh disadvantages* | Quality and quantity of breast milk may be diminished if used prior to establishment of lactation. After lactation establishment, low-dose COCs have no significant impact |
| IUD:<br>• Copper<br>• Levonorgestrel | • May insert Copper or Levonorgestrel IUD within first 10 minutes after delivery of placenta with special technique<br>• Usually await uterine involution to insert (4-6 weeks) | No effect with Paragard. Mirena - same as other progestin-only methods |
| Tubal Sterilization | Usually done in first 24-48 hours postpartum, or await complete uterine involution for interval tubal sterilization (laparoscopy or Essure) (> 6 weeks postpartum) | No effect |

*Use of CHC at <1 month is a 3. <21 days in non-breastfeeding women is a 4.*

# CHAPTER 17

# Fertility Awareness Methods (FAM)

www.usc.edu/hsc/info/newman/resource/nfp.html
www.cyclebeads.com OR www.irh.org

**DESCRIPTION:** FAMs should only be used by women with regular menstrual cycles. They involve monitoring the cycle and having intercourse only during infertile phases or using another method, e.g. condoms, during fertile phases. A woman cannot identify the exact day of ovulation using FAM methods; rather she estimates when the fertile phase of her cycle begins and ends. A woman's fertile phase may begin 3-6 days before ovulation (because sperm can live in cervical mucus for 3-6 days) and ends 24 hours after ovulation

***For purposes of FAM, a woman's menstrual cycle has 3 phases:***

1. *Infertile phase:* before ovulation
2. *Fertile phase:* Approximately 5-7 days in the mid-portion of the cycle, including several days before and the day after ovulation;
3. *Infertile phase:* after the fertile phase

During the fertile phase, a couple should be abstinent or use a barrier method to avoid pregnancy. Of the FAM methods discussed, the Calendar Method, Standard Days Method, and the Cervical Mucus Method can be used to identify the beginning and the end of the fertile period; the BBT Method can only be used to identify the end of the fertile period. Thus, couples using the BBT Method could only safely have unprotected intercourse during the post-ovulatory period, as the method cannot be used to define the pre-ovulatory infertile phase. As couples using either the Calendar or the Cervical Mucus Methods can theoretically identify the beginning and the end of the fertile period, they may have unprotected intercourse during the pre-ovulatory infertile phase and the post-ovulatory infertile phase. However, in order to minimize the chance of an unintended pregnancy, some advocate that couples only have unprotected intercourse during the post-ovulatory infertile phase regardless of the method of FAM they are using.

Comparative efficacy of FAM methods is unknown due to poor subject retention in efficacy trials *[Grimes-2005]*

Techniques used to determine high-risk fertile days include:

***1. Calendar Method: To calculate the fertile days:***

- Record days of menses prospectively for 6-12 cycles
- Most estimates assume that sperm can survive 2-3 days and ovulation occurs 14 days before menses (motile sperm have been found as long as 7 days after intercourse and the extreme interval following a single act of coitus leading to an achieved pregnancy is 6 days *[Speroff-1999]*)
- Earliest day of fertile period = day # in a cycle corresponding to **shortest cycle length minus 18**
- Latest day of fertile period = day # in a cycle corresponding to **longest cycle length minus 11**

***2. Standard Days Method Utilizing Color-Coded Beads; cyclebeads™***

- For women with MOST cycles 26-32 days long, avoid UNPROTECTED intercourse on days 8-19 (white beads on CycleBead necklace). No need for 3-6 months of extensive cycle calculations
- 4.75% failure over 1 year with perfect use; 11.96% with typical use *[Arevalo-2002]*
- Resources available from the Institute for Reproductive Health, www.irh.org (CD, training manual, patient brochure, sample beads).

Beads can also be ordered from **www.cyclebeads.com**

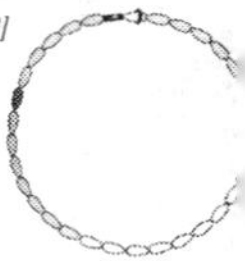

***3. Cervical Mucus Ovulation Detection Method***

- Women check quantity and character of mucus on the vulva or introitus with fingers or tissue paper each day for several months to learn cycle:
  - Post-menstrual mucus: scant or undetectable
  - Pre-ovulation mucus: cloudy, yellow or white, sticky
  - Ovulation mucus: clear, wet, stretches, sticky (but slippery)
  - Post-ovulation fertile mucus: thick, cloudy; sticky
  - Post-ovulation post-fertile mucus: scant or undetectable

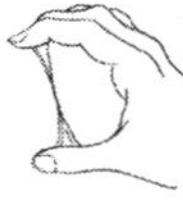

- When using method during preovulatory period, must abstain 24 hours after intercourse to make test interpretable as semen and vaginal fluids can obscure character of cervical mucus
  - Abstinence or barrier method through fertile period (ie abstinence for a given cycle begins as soon as the woman notices any cervical secretions)
  - Intercourse without restriction beginning 4th day after the last day of wet, clear, slippery mucus (post ovulation)

*4. TwoDay Method*
- Uses cervical secretions, but is much simpler
- Each day woman asks herself 1.) "Did I notice secretions today?" and 2.) Did I notice secretions yesterday?
- If no secretions two consecutive days, OK to have intercourse

*5. Basal Body Temperature Method (BBT)*

**Figure 17.1 Basal body temperature variations during a menstrual cycle**

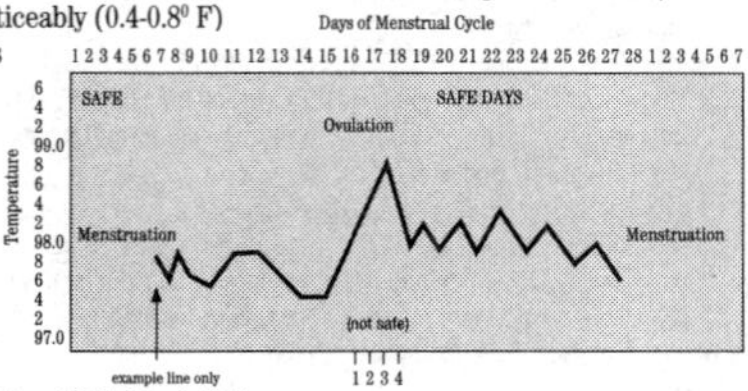


- Assumes early morning temperature measured before arising will increase noticeably (0.4-0.8° F) with ovulation; fertile period is defined as the day of first temperature drop or first elevation through 3 consecutive days of elevated temperature. Temperature drop does NOT always occur
- Abstinence begins first day of menstrual bleeding and lasts through 3 consecutive days of sustained temperature rise (at least 0.2° C or 0.4° F)

*6. Post-ovulation Method*
- Permits unprotected intercourse only after signs of ovulation (BBT, cervical mucus, etc) have subsided

*7. Symptothermal Method*
- Combines at least two methods — usually cervical mucus changes with BBT
- May also include mittelschmerz, change in libido, and changes in cervical texture, position and dilation to detect ovulation:
  - During preovulatory and ovulatory periods, cervix softens, opens and is moister
  - During postovulatory period, cervix drops, becomes firm and closes

*8. The Marquette Method (MM) of FAM*
- An online site that aids users who choose either electronic hormonal fertility monitor (EHFM), cervical mucus monitoring (CMM) or both.
- Recent RCT comparing the EHFM plus fertility algorithm vs. CMM plus algorithm found that over 12 months, EHFM (N=197) had 7 per 100 pregnant and CMM (N=164) had 18.5 per 100. *[Fehring 2013]*

**EFFECTIVENESS** (see Table 13.2, Page 37)

*NFP/FAM First-year failure rate (100 women-years of use)*

| *Method* | *Typical use** | *Perfect use* |
|---|---|---|
| Calendar | 25 | 9 |
| Standard Days Method | 12 | 5 |
| Ovulation Method | 25 | 3 |
| Symptothermal | 25 | 0.4 |
| Post-ovulation | 25 | 1 |
| TwoDay Method | 13.7 | 4 |

*FAM usually more effective than NFP *[Trussell IN Contraceptive Technology, 2011]*

**HOW FAM WORK:** Abstinence or barriers used during fertile period

**COST:** Training, supplies (special digital basal body thermometer, Cycle Beads, charts)

## ADVANTAGES

*Menstrual:* No change. Helps woman learn more about her menstrual physiology
*Sexual/psychological:* Men and women can work together in using this method. Men must be aware that abstinence or use of second method is essential during the fertile period
*Other:*

- May be only method acceptable to couples for cultural or religious reasons
- Helps couples achieve pregnancy when practiced in reverse

## DISADVANTAGES

*Menstrual:* No effect on menses
*Sexual/psychological:*

- Requires rigorous discipline, good communication and full commitment of both partners
- Requires abstinence, barrier method, or another contraceptive that does not change pattern of ovulation during 6-12 month learning/data-gathering period (unless CycleBead method is used)
- Complete abstinence in an anovulatory cycle, if using post-ovulation techniques. This method demands great self-control: either abstinence or use of another method must be used during long periods of time when woman is or may become fertile
- Requires abstinence at time of ovulation, which typically is the time of peak libido

*Cancers, tumors, and masses:* None
*Other:*

- Difficult to use in early adolescence, when approaching menopause, and in postpartum women when cycles are irregular (or absent)
- Even women with "regular" periods can vary as much as $\pm$ 7 days in any given cycle
- Cervical mucus techniques may be complicated by vaginal infections
- May not be helpful during time of stress
- Method very unforgiving of improper use
- Does not protect against STIs
- Relatively high failure rate with typical use
- Less reliable in settings of fever, vaginal infections, douching, and use of certain medications

**COMPLICATIONS:** None

## CANDIDATES FOR USE

- Women with regular menstrual cycles at minimal risk for STIs
- Women wanting to avoid hormones and devices
- Those with religious/cultural proscriptions against using other methods
- Highly motivated couples willing to commit to extensive abstinence or to use barriers during vulnerable periods

*Adolescents:* Not appropriate until regular menstrual cycles established

**MEDICAL ELIGIBILITY CHECKLIST:** Ask the woman the questions below. If she answers NO to ALL questions, she CAN use any fertility awareness-based method if she wants. If she answers YES to any question, follow the instructions. No conditions restrict use of these methods, but some conditions can make them harder to use effectively

***1. Do you have a medical condition that would make pregnancy especially dangerous?***

☐ No ☐ Yes She may want to choose a more effective method. If not, stress careful use of fertility awareness-based methods to avoid pregnancy and availability of EC

***2. Do you have irregular or prolonged menstrual cycles? Vaginal bleeding between periods? For younger women: Are your periods just starting? For older women: Have your periods become irregular?***

☐ No ☐ Yes Predicting her fertile time with only the calendar method may be hard or impossible. She can use basal body temperature (BBT) and/or cervical mucus, or she may prefer different method

***3. Did you recently give birth or have an abortion? Are you breastfeeding? Do you have any other condition that affects menstrual bleeding?***

☐ No ☐ Yes These conditions may affect fertility signs, making fertility awareness-based methods hard to use. For this reason, a woman or couple may prefer a different method. If not, they may need more counseling and follow-up to use the method effectively

***4. If you recently stopped using Depo-Provera or combined hormonal methods, are your periods still irregular?***

☐ No ☐ Yes If her cycles have not been re-established, she may need to use another method until cycles are regular

***5. Do you have any infections or diseases that may change cervical mucus, basal body temperatures, or menstrual bleeding—such as sexually transmitted disease (STD) or pelvic inflammatory disease (PID) in the last 3 months, or vaginal infection?***

☐ No ☐ Yes These conditions may affect fertility signs, making fertility awareness-based methods hard to use. Once an infection is treated and reinfection is avoided, however, a woman can use fertility awareness-based methods

## INITIATING METHOD

- Requires several months of data collection and analysis unless using CycleBeads
- Description of methods
- Formal training necessary. Couples may be trained together

**BUYER BEWARE** A woman considering use of the fertility awareness methods must be aware of several potential pitfalls, summarized in **the five "R's"**:

- **R**estrictions on sexual spontaneity (method requires periodic abstinence or the use of backup method)
- **R**igorous daily monitoring
- **R**equired training
- **R**isk of pregnancy during prolonged training period
- **R**isk of pregnancy high on unsafe days

## INSTRUCTIONS FOR PATIENT

- Requires discipline, communication, listening skills, full commitment of both partners. Mistakes using this method are particularly likely to lead to unintended pregnancies as intercourse is then occurring at the time in the cycle when a woman is *most* likely to become pregnant

- If using FAM, use contraception during fertile days
- If using NFP, abstain from sexual intercourse during fertile days
- Encourage other forms of sexual satisfaction

## FOLLOW-UP

- Have you had sexual intercourse during "unsafe" times during your cycle?
- Discuss use of emergency contraception if having sex during "unsafe" times during cycle
- Do you have emergency contraceptive pills at home?

## PROBLEM MANAGEMENT

***Inconsistent use and risk taking:*** Educate about emergency contraception when women start using method

**FERTILITY AFTER DISCONTINUATION OF METHOD:** No effect

# WORLD'S BEST BIRTH CONTROL
## AT YOUR HEALTH DEPARTMENT

### BIRTH CONTROL EFFECTIVENESS IN 10,000 WOMEN

MORE EFFECTIVE, LESS RISK

| Contraceptive Method | Pregnancies in first year |
|---|---|
| NEXPLANON | 5 |
| MALE STERILIZATION | 15 |
| MIRENA IUD | 20 |
| FEMALE STERILIZATION | 50 |
| PARAGARD IUD | 80 |
| DEPO SHOT | 600 |
| MINIPILL | 900 |
| COMBINATION PILLS* | 900 |
| CONDOM | 1,800 |
| WITHDRAWAL | 2,200 |
| NO METHOD | 8,500 |

* Estrogen increases risk for stroke, heart attack, and blood clots. When estrogen is combined with other risks like:

· Migraines with aura (visual or hearing changes) · Previous blood clots · Tobacco use
· Obesity · High blood pressure · Diabetes · Migraines without aura · Age over 40

*This ingenius method of explaining the differences in failure rates by placing the number of pregnancues in the first year of use by typical users over 10,000 women comes to you because of the creative genius of Dr. Claude Burnett in Athens, GA.*

*Burnetts pregnancy figures are derived form Contraceptive Technology, 20 ed. 2011, James Trussell, Typical Use Failure Rates in Hatcher, Trussell et al.*

# CHAPTER 18

## Condoms for Men

www.ppfa.org OR condomania.com OR askdurex.com OR www.ansell.com

**DESCRIPTION:** Condoms for men are sheaths made of latex, polyurethane or natural membranes (usually lamb cecum), which are placed over the penis prior to contact and worn until after ejaculation when the penis is removed from the orifice (vagina, mouth, anus). Latex condoms are available in only 2 sizes, in a wide variety of textures and thicknesses (0.03-0.09 mm), and come with or without spermicidal coating. Two brands of polyurethane condoms are currently available in the US. When used correctly and consistently, male latex condoms are highly effective in preventing sexual transmission of HIV and can reduce the risk for other STDs (ie gonorrhea, chlamydia and trichomonas). Natural membrane condoms (made from the intestinal cecum of lambs) may not provide the same level of STI protection. Condoms may be used as a primary contraceptive method, as a back up method, or with another method to provide STI risk reduction. **When used as a primary contraceptive method, it is important that condoms be coupled with advance provision/prescription/ advice to buy OTC emergency contraceptive pills (ECPs) since couples experience a condom break or slippage during approximately 3-5% of acts of intercourse.**

**EFFECTIVENESS** *[Trussell J IN Contraceptive Technology-2011]*

***Perfect use failure rate in the first year of use:*** 2% (See Table 12.2, Page 37)
***Typical use failure rate in the first year of use:*** 18%

- The most common reason for condom failure is not using a condom with every act of intercourse *[Werner-2004] [Steiner-1999]*
- Recent survey of condom users: the most common reason for nonuse of both condoms (44%) and EC (41%) was that the woman did not perceive she was at risk *[Nelson-2006]*.
- Dual use of a condom plus another contraceptive may dramatically reduce the risk of both pregnancy and STI. *[Warner-2004][Cates-2002]*.
- Although comparative testing has shown that latex and polyurethane condoms provide the same pregnancy protection, polyurethane condoms are more likely to slip or break (2.6 to 5 times more likely *[Gallo-2008]*) than latex condoms (1.6-1.7%)

**HOW CONDOMS WORK**

- Condoms act as a barrier; they prevent the passage of sperm into the vagina. Sheathing the penis also reduces transmission and acquisition of STIs, including HIV. **Spermicidal condoms are no longer recommended at all as they provide no additional protection against pregnancy or STIs!** Most condom manufacturers have stopped producing spermicidal condoms. A study of 145 couples using over 12,000 condoms found that applying spermicide AFTER the condom is placed on the penis reduces breaks and slips significantly. *[Gabbay-2008]*

**COST**

- Average retail cost for latex condoms is $0.50, but some designer condoms cost several dollars. Polyurethane condoms cost $.80-$2.00 each
- Some public health agencies and some college health services offer large numbers of free condoms.

**ADVANTAGES**

***Menstrual:*** No direct impact on menses, but a couple may feel more comfortable having sex while spotting or bleeding if using a condom

*Sexual/psychological:*

- Some men may maintain erection longer with condoms, making sex more enjoyable
- If the woman/partner puts the condom on, it may add to sexual pleasure
- Lubricated condoms are a good contraceptive option during breast feeding when some women are bothered by a dry vagina
- Male involvement is encouraged and is essential!
- Availability of wide selection of condom types and designs can add variety
- Makes sex less messy for the woman by catching the ejaculate
- Intercourse may be more pleasurable because fear of pregnancy and STIs is decreased

***Cancers/tumors & masses:*** Decrease in HIV and HPV transmission reduces risks of AIDS AND HPV-related malignancies

***Other:***

- Consistent condom use reduces risks of HIV transmission by approximately 10-fold *[Davis-1999] [Pinkerton-1997] [Warner-2004]* See Figure 17.2, Page 64
- Consistent condom use reduces risk of cervical and vulvovaginal HPV infection among newly sexually active women *[Winer-2006]*
- Readily available over the counter; no medical visit required
- Usually inexpensive for single use
- Easily transportable. Don't leave in wallet too long; probably ok for 1 month. It has been suggested that a condom be placed between photographs in a wallet to protect against damage
- Opportunity for couples to improve communication and negotiating skills
- Immediately active after placement
- May reduce risk of PID, infertility, ectopic pregnancy and chronic pelvic pain

**DISADVANTAGES: May break or fall off.** ***Options: see Fig. 18.3, Page 64***

***Menstrual:*** None

***Sexual/psychological:***

- Unless the woman puts the condom on as part of foreplay, condom use may interrupt love making
- Interruption of sex to put on a condom may cause man to lose erection
- Blunting of sensation or "unnatural" feeling with intercourse
- Plain condoms may decrease lubrication and provide less stimulation for woman (use water-based or silicone lubricant with latex condoms)
- Requires prompt withdrawal after ejaculation, which may decrease pleasure
- Makes sex messier for the man

***Cancers/tumors and masses:*** None

***Other:***

- Requires education/experience for successful use
- Either member of couple may have latex allergy or reaction to spermicide; polyurethane condom is appropriate alternative
- Users must avoid petroleum-based vaginal products when using latex condoms (Figure 17.1, p. 61). This is not a problem with polyurethane condoms
- Couples may be embarrassed to purchase or to apply condoms due to taboos about touching genitalia, stigma of concern about STDs/HIV

## COMPLICATIONS

- Allergic reactions to latex are rarely life threatening; 2-3% of Americans (men and women) have a latex allergy; up to 14% of individuals working with latex are latex sensitive. Polyurethane condoms do not cause allergic reactions
- Condom retained in vagina (uncommon) exposes woman to risk of infection as well as pregnancy. If this occurs: 1) try to remove by pinching with second and third fingers or 2) enlist partner's help or 3) go to clinician ASAP. Use EC ASAP

## PRECAUTIONS

- Men who are unable to maintain erection when they wear condoms; benzocaine condoms by Durex are now available to prevent premature ejaculation, but studies have not proven a benefit
- Woman whose partners will not use condoms
- Women who require high contraceptive efficacy should not be using condoms as their primary contraceptive method. They should, at a minimum, add another more effective method
- Couples in which either partner has latex allergy should avoid latex condoms; men can use Durex-Avanti or Trojan-Supra; women can use Reality female condom
- Couples in which either partner has spermicide allergy or is at high risk for HIV should avoid spermicide-coated condoms

## CANDIDATES FOR USE

- Anyone at risk for an STI; appropriate for most couples
- May be used alone or coupled with a second contraceptive method

***Special applications for infection control:***

- Non-monogamous couples (i.e. if either partner has multiple partners)
- During pregnancy as well as at all other times
- After delivery or pregnancy loss to reduce risk of endometritis (although abstinence is preferable)
- Couples with known viral infections (HIV, HPV, HSV-2) in areas completely covered by device

***Adolescents:*** Excellent option, especially when combined with another method

## INITIATING METHOD

Couples desiring to use condoms often benefit from concrete instructions. Can demonstrate on a banana or finger. Counsel new users about:

- Options among condom types
- Storage for safety and ready access
- How to negotiate condom use with partner and when to place condom *[Warner-2004]*
- How to open package and place correct side of condom over penis
- How to unroll and allow space for ejaculate (depending on condom design)

Provide ECPs to all couples relying on the condom for birth control to ensure immediate use in the event of condom mishap or problem. Breakage or slippage occurs in 3-5% of acts of intercourse.

- Specific instructions given to men on correct use decreases breakage and slippage *[Steines-2007]*

## INSTRUCTIONS FOR PATIENTS (See Figure 17.1, Page 63)

- ➔ If the woman puts the condom on the man, it can be fun for both partners
- Learn how to use a condom long before you need it. Both women and men need to know how. Practice with models: fingers or banana
- Buy condoms in advance, carry with you; Keep extra condoms out of sunlight and heat
- Try new condoms to find favorite size, scent, and texture and to add variety
- Check date on condom carefully. It may be an expiration date OR a date of production. If it is an expiration date, do not use beyond expiration date. If it is a date of production, condom may be used for several years from the date of production (2 years for spermicidal condoms, 5 years for nonspermicidal latex condoms)
- Open package carefully, squeeze condom out, avoid tearing with fingernails, teeth, scissors, etc.
- Use appropriate water-based or silicone-based lubricant with latex condoms (see Page 63). Never put lubricant inside the condom

**WHEN THE CONDOM BREAKS MORE THAN ONCE, FROM THEN ON, THAT COUPLE SHOULD ALWAYS USE TWO CONDOMS.**

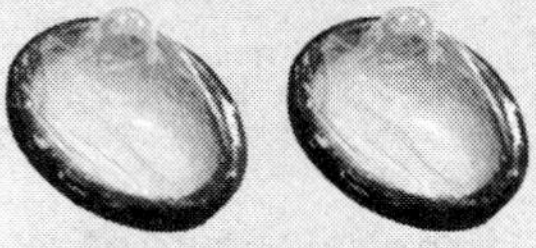

Albert AE, Warner DL, Hatcher RA, Trussell J, Bennett C. Condom use among female commercial sex workers in Nevada's legal brothels. Am J Publ Health 1995; 85:1514-1520.
When 2 condoms are used, place a water-based lubricant over the first condom before placing the second condom on.

- Place condom over penis before any genital contact. Either partner can put it on!
- Consider placing a second condom (larger size) over lubricated condom if history of previous breakage or if man has any evidence of STI
- If condom used for oral or rectal intercourse replace with a new condom prior to vaginal entry
- Vigorous sex can break the condom. Consider using 2 condoms at once
- Immediately after ejaculation (before loss of erection) hold rim of condom against shaft of penis and remove condom-covered penis from vagina (or anus). One study found only 71% of men held the rim of the condom during withdrawal and only 50% withdrew immediately after ejaculation *[Warner-1999]*
- Remove condom from the penis and inspect carefully for any breaks

If 14,000 acts of intercourse are protected by condoms, a mishap (breakage or slippage) will occur approximately 5% of the time or 700 times. If couples experiencing breakage or slippage identify this and use Plan B within one hour, only one of those 700 women will experience an unintended pregnancy. The failure rate of Plan B within one hour of unprotected sex is 0.14% or just about 1 in 700 *[Shelton-2002]*. Better yet get a CopperT IUD within 5 to 7 days after a condom mishap (see page).

- Dispose of used condom. Do not reuse.
- If a condom falls off, slips, tears or breaks, start using ECPs as soon as possible. Plan B is available OTC for women and men > 18 y/o. If you do not have ECPs, call 1-888-NOT-2-LATE or check www.not-2-late.com to find out how to get them. You can get EC from a pharmacist without a prescription. If any risk for STIs, seek medical care

## FOLLOW-UP

- Are you and your partner comfortable using condoms?
- Have you had any problems with using the condom? Breaking? Slipping off? Decreased sensation? Vaginal soreness with use? Skin irritation or redness during the day after using it?
- Have you had any post-coital "yeast infection" symptoms? (A woman may confuse an allergic reaction to the condom and/or spermicide with a candidal infection)
- Have you had intercourse—even once—without a condom?
- Did you have any questions about ECPs?
- Do you have Plan B ECPs at home?
- Do you plan to have children? OR Do you plan to have more children? When?

## PROBLEM MANAGEMENT

***Allergic reaction:*** *[See Warner-2004]*

- Beware that latex can induce anaphylaxis and that the severity of allergic reaction increases with continued exposure. More often a person who says he (or she) is ***"allergic"*** to condoms means condoms a) are difficult to put on or b) lead to loss of erection, c) the couple simply doesn't like condoms, d) is being irritated by a spermicide or lubricant or e) an ongoing infection may be causing irritation. Irritation can also be caused by thrusting during sex. Couple may try another brand of latex condoms

- If either a man or a woman is allergic to latex, switch to polyurethane condoms (Durex, 2 Avanti condoms or Trojan-Supra male condoms, Mayer Laboratories eZ-on, or female condom)
- Switch to another approach to reducing STI risk and contraception, such as the female condom for STI risk reduction and a hormonal method for contraceptive effectiveness

***Condom breakage:*** (Figure 17.3, Page 64) (1-2% for latex condoms)

- Ensure correct technique. Common problems: pre-placement manipulations (stretching, etc), use of inappropriate lubricant (placement inside condom), and prolonged or extremely vigorous sex
- May need to recommend larger condom. The largest are: Kimono, Kimono Microthin, Magnum, MAXX, and Trojan Very Sensitive
- If couple using polyurethane, consider switching to latex condom
- May need to switch method
- Confirm that woman is using ECPs and has supply available at home
- The risk of HIV transmission following a condom break is quite low, but treatment lowers it still further. Consult an HIV clinic immediately if this is a concern. See Page 184

***Condom slippage:*** (Figure 17.3, Page 64)

- Ensure correct technique. Common problems: condom not fully unrolled, lubricant placed incorrectly on inside of condom, and excessive delay in removing penis from vagina after ejaculation. Use of proper-sized condom is important (if condom is too large it may slip off). "Snugger fit" condoms are available
- Rule out erectile dysfunction. Condoms may not be appropriate if man loses erection with condom placement or use
- Confirm that woman is using ECPs and has supply available at home

***Decreased sensation:***

- Common causes: condom too small, too thick or too tightly applied; inadequate lubrication
- Suggest experimentation with different textured condoms or placing second (larger size) condom over inner lubricated condom. Thinner condoms now available
- Integrate condom placement into lovemaking (suggest partner place condom to help arouse/excite man)

## FERTILITY AFTER DISCONTINUATION OF METHOD

- Condoms do not affect fertility
- May protect fertility by reducing risk of STIs

*To purchase the 20th edition of **Contraceptive Technology**, with an excellent chapter on condoms by David Lee Warner (CDC) and Markus Steiner (FHI), call (770) 887-8383 or go to www.managingcontraception.com*

## Figure 18.1

# HOW TO USE A LATEX CONDOM

*(...Or rubber, sheath, prophylactic, safe, french letter, raincoat, glove, sock)*

Talk/Think about condom use with partner. Make the commitment, in advance, to use condoms without exception with each/every sexual act (vaginal, oral or anal). Have emergency contraceptive pills available in case you experience condom breakage or slippage.

↓

Keep a supply of condoms handy...Store condoms in a cool, dry place away from sunlight and check the expiration date **before** use

↓

Use NEW condom before each and every sexual contact

↓

**USE CONDOM CORRECTLY.**
Before putting on the condom, check to see which way the condom unrolls.
(If uncircumcised, pull back foreskin before unrolling condom.)
Unroll condom all the way down to the base of the penis (down to hair).
NOTE: A condom can be put onto a penis that is not fully erect.
Smooth out air bubbles. Make sure condom fits (condoms come in various sizes)

↓

Add WATER-based lubricant to outside of condom if desired

↓

Condom must be used throughout sex

↓

Change condom if penis exposed to different orifice

↓

**Immediately after ejaculation:**
Hold rim of condom and carefully withdraw penis before loss of erection

↓

**RELAX.** Check for breakage; Dispose of condom. (If condom breaks, slips, falls off or is not used, use EC. Go to pharmacy for OTC EC if $\geq$ 18, or call 1-888-NOT-2-LATE for EC.

### SAFE!

**WATER BASED OR SILICONE LUBRICANTS SAFE FOR USE WITH CONDOMS**

- Astroglide
- Water and saliva
- Glycerin
- All I-D Lubricants
- Aloe-9
- H-R Lubricating Jelly
- K-Y Jelly
- Prepair
- Probe
- AquaLube
- ForPlay
- Gynol II
- Wet
- Cornhuskers Lotion
- Silicone Lubricant
- deLube
- Spermicide*
- Slippery Stuff

**NOT RECOMMENDED!**

*Spermicidal condoms are no longer recommended although spermicides do not damage latex

### UNSAFE FOR USE WITH LATEX CONDOMS*

- Aldara cream
- Baby oil or Cold creams
- Edible oils (olive, peanut, corn, sunflower)
- Head and body lotions
- Massage oils
- Mineral oil
- Petroleum jelly
- Rubbing alcohol
- Shortening
- Suntan oil and lotions
- Whipped cream
- Vegetable oil and cooking oils
- Clindamycin 2% vaginal cream
- Vaginal yeast infection medications in cream or suppository form
  - Butoconazole cream
  - Clotrimazole cream
  - Clotrimazole vaginal tablet
  - Miconazole vaginal suppository
  - Terconazole ointment
  - Terconazole cream or vaginal suppository

*These lubricants/vaginal products can be used with polyurethane condoms*

**Figure 18.2 10 Studies demonstrating protective effect of latex condoms against HIV transmission in heterosexual couples**

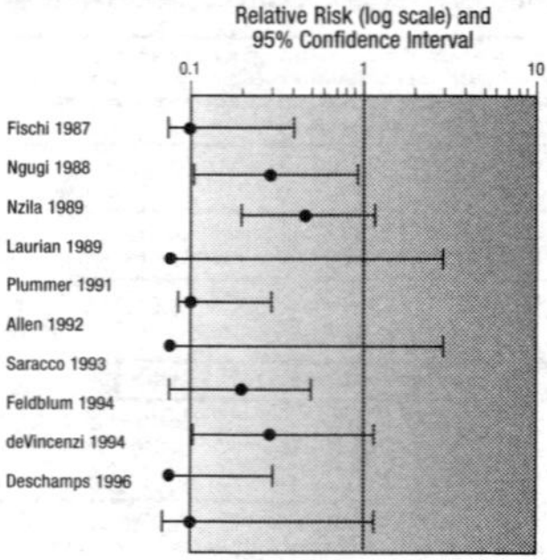


*[Feldblum et al., 1995]*

**Figure 17.3**

**CONDOM MISHAPS OR PROBLEMS**
**Provide ECPs to condom users in advance**

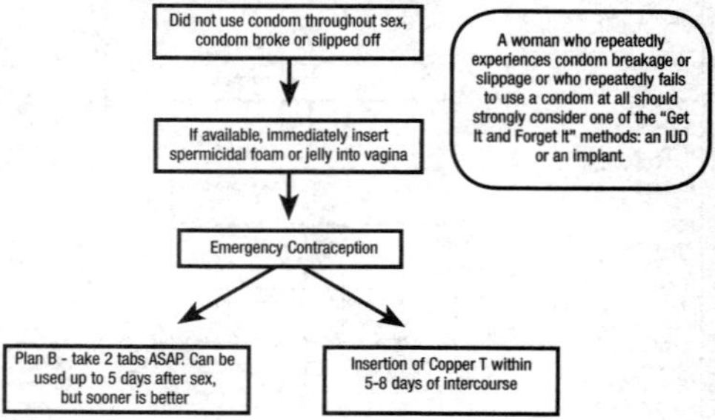

# CHAPTER 19

## Female-Controlled Barrier Methods

**www.femalehealth.com, www.cervcap.com, www.femcap.com, www.lea.com, www.plannedparenthood.org**

### DESCRIPTION

- Female-Controlled Barrier Methods include cervical caps, diaphragm, sponge and female condom
- Two cervical caps are FDA approved and currently available in the US: FemCap and Lea's Shield. Both caps are made of silicone rubber (latex-free), cover the cervix completely, and create suction between the cervix and the cap.
- The Ortho All-FlexTM diaphragm is now made of silicone; a dome-shaped device placed to cover the cervix, and held in place by the vagina. Currently, diaphragms must be fitted by a clinician. Both caps and the diaphragm are reusable, but should be replaced with any signs of wear and tear, or damage.
- The female condom: a disposable, single use, polyurethane (FC) or nitrile (the FC2) sheath placed in the vagina.
- When used as a primary method, these barrier methods should be coupled with counseling to have ECP on hand at home.

### EFFECTIVENESS

- The failure rate for the FemCap in the package insert is 29%
- A small study of women using Lea's Shield showed an 8.7% failure rate over 6 months with typical use *[Mauck-1996]*
- A recent Cochrane Review conducted by FHI found pregnancy rates during one year of use to be 11% to 13% for the diaphragm

| | | |
|---|---|---|
| **Diaphragm:** | ***Perfect use failure rate in first year:*** | 6% |
| | ***Typical use failure rate in first year:*** | 12% *[Trussell, 2011]* |
| **Female Condom:** | ***Perfect use failure rate in first year:*** | 5% |
| | ***Typical use failure rate in first year:*** | 21% *[Trussell, 2011]* |

**HOW THEY WORK:** Act both as a mechanical barrier to sperm migration into the cervical canal and as a chemical agent by applying spermicide directly to the cervix

### ADVANTAGES

***Menstrual:*** none

***Sexual/psychological:***

- Intercourse may be more pleasurable because fear of pregnancy is reduced
- Controlled by the woman
- Can be inserted several hours before sexual intercourse to permit spontaneity
- Can remain in place for multiple acts of intercourse up to 24 hours (diaphragm) to 48 hours (cervical cap) total from time of placement (except for female condom)

***Cancers, tumors and masses***

- Follow-up studies of earlier cervical caps show no associated increase in cervical dysplasia with use. Labeling of current cervical caps or diaphragms does not require additional pap smears

*Other:*
- May reduce risk of cervical infections, including gonorrhea, chlamydia, and PID, but offers no protection against HIV infection
- Immediately active after placement
- May be used during lactation

## DISADVANTAGES

*Menstrual:* none

*Sexual/psychological:*
- Requires placement prior to genital contact, which may reduce spontaneity of sex
- Some women do not like placing fingers or a foreign body into their vagina

*Other:*
- Lack of protection against HIV and some STD's. Must use condoms if at risk
- Higher failure rates than with hormonal contraception
- Odor may develop if left in place too long or if not appropriately cleaned (if reusable)
- Severe obesity or arthritis may make insertion/removal difficult

## COMPLICATIONS

- UTI's may increase
- Superficial cervical erosion may occur causing vaginal spotting and/or cervical discomfort and discontinuation
- No cases of toxic shock syndrome have been reported, but theoretically, the risk may be increased if these methods are left in too long or used during menses

**CANDIDATES:** Women NOT at high risk of HIV
- Women willing and able to insert device prior to coitus and remove it later
- Highly motivated women willing to use with every coital act
- Women with pelvic relaxation are better candidates for cap than for diaphragm
- Woman who is sensitive to use of hormones
- Women and partner(s) who have no sensitivity to spermicides

*Adolescents:* Appropriate, but requires discipline and preparedness to use consistently and correctly. If at risk for STI's use condoms in addition.

## INITIATING METHOD

- Given the high failure rates for these methods, it is important to provide ECP's in advance for use if needed or recommend purchase OTC for adults
- A speculum and bimanual exam is recommended before initiating use. Should not be used in the presence of vaginal infections, or vaginal or cervical abrasions
- Patient labeling for each device explains how to insert and remove. Demonstrate placement and removal during your exam, and allow the patient to demonstrate placement and removal before she leaves the office/clinic
- Additional spermicide is not necessary for additional acts of intercourse
- Encourage use of a back-up method for the first few uses until she is confident with correct use. Continual use of male condoms with these methods will reduce pregnancy and STI risk
- If device dislodges during use, EC should be used ASAP.
- For reusable devices, instruct the woman to wash with mild soap and water after each use, dry, and store in container until next use. The sponge and female condom should be disposed of after removal
- Recent gel use with a diaphragm, such as Replens, does not inhibit testing for HPV, urine GC/CT, or cervical cytology quality

## FOLLOW-UP

- Are you or your partner noticing any discomfort during sex?
- Do you notice an odor when you remove the device?
- Have you had any burning with urination, vaginal irritation or itching?
- Do you use the device every single time you have sexual intercourse?
- For the cap or diaphragm, do you always apply spermicide before insertion?
- Do you have ECP at home?

## PROBLEM MANAGEMENT

- Spotting/cervical or vaginal discomfort/erosion: Rule out infection; stop use to allow healing; consider different size or alternative method
- Urinary tract infections: Urinate postcoitally to reduce bladder contamination with vaginal bacteria. Check fit to be sure there is not excessive urethal pressure
- Odor upon removal: Rule out infection. Try Listerine soaks if reusable, shorten time left in place, or replace
- Dislodged during sex (ensure proper fit) or other failure to use correctly: Use EC. Provide ECPs to have on hand. Consider alternative method

## FERTILITY AFTER DISCONTINUATION

- Immediate return to baseline fertility

## THE FC - FEMALE CONDOM

- The "FC" is a polyurethane sheath. The FC2, available as of 2008, is a nitrile sheath that is cheaper to produce and buy
- Sold over-the-counter, without need for prescription ($3.30 - $6.00; $1.50 in public clinic)

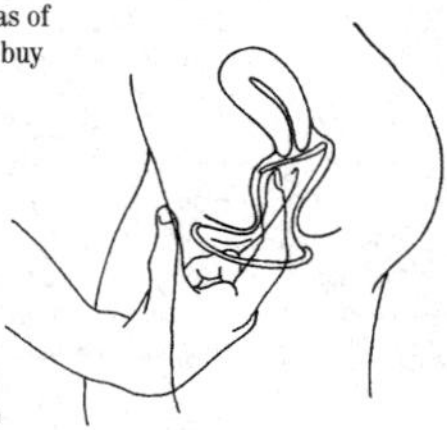

### *Instructions for Use:*

- Can be inserted up to 8 hours before sex to allow for spontaneity
- In squatting, leg-up, reclining or lithotomy position, compress inner ring and introduce into vagina guiding sheath high into vagina until outer ring rests against vulva. Rotate inner ring to stabilize device in vault
- Manually place penis in sheath
- Excessive friction between penis and device can cause breakage or device inversion
- Remove condom immediately after intercourse. Twist outer ring to seal off contents and then pull out of vagina. Test condom for patency, then discard
- If condom dislodges or breaks, or if any spillage of ejaculate occurs, use EC ASAP
- If a male latex condom is used with a FC, theoretically, there can be increased risk of breakage of either or both condoms

## CERVICAL CAPS

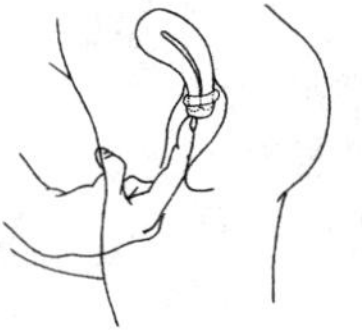

### *Lea's Shield:*

- Lea's Shield is held in place by the vaginal walls and muscles, so one size fits all
- Requires a prescription for use

### *Femcap:*

- Three sizes available. Approximately 85% of women can be assigned the correct size of FemCap based on their

obstetrical history: nulligravid women using the small (22mm) size, parous women who have not delivered vaginally using the medium (26 mm) size, and women who have delivered vaginally using the largest (30 mm) size
- Proper fit can be confirmed in the office or clinic by checking that: insertion instructions have been followed, the cervix is covered entirely, and the device is comfortable for the woman
- FemCap may be bought over the internet at www.femcap.com with recommendation for fit to be checked by clinician

### *Instructions for Use:*

***Instructions for use are similar for both types of cervical caps. Detailed instructions specific to each type can be found online at http://www.leasshield.com or www.femcap.com***
- Can be placed anytime before sex
- Coat the inside of the bowl and the rim with spermicide. Place a small amount of spermicide along the outer part of the cap.
- In the squatting, leg-up or reclining position, press the rims on each side of the bowl together and hold with the dome of the bowl pointing downward.
- Insert long/thick side first as far into the vagina as possible. Push the device over your cervix so that it covers the cervix completely. Then press upwards to create suction between the cap and your cervix. You might feel air venting out as the suction is created between the cap and the cervix.
- The device should be left in place for at least 6-8 hours after the last act of intercourse, up to 48 hours total.
- To remove, use fingers to grasp loop, twist or push on cap to break the suction (hearing a "pop"), and remove device from the vagina

## DIAPHRAGM

- As of 2008, the Ortho All-Flex™ diaphragm is now made of silicone (latex-free). Generic versions are no longer available in the U.S.
- Available only through manufacturer (coopersurgical.com). Current diaphragms need to be fitted by a clinician. The latest version has 4 sizes available.
- On bimanual exam, determine degree of version of uterus; not a good method for extremely anteverted or retroverted uterus. Introduce your third finger into the posterior fornix and and tilt your wrist upward to mark where your index finger/hand contacts the symphysis. Use that measurement as a guide and place a fitting diaphragm in the vagina
- Have woman walk around in your office to test its comfort
- Recheck the fit of the diaphragm each year during annual exam, and whenever there is a 20% weight change and/or pregnancy

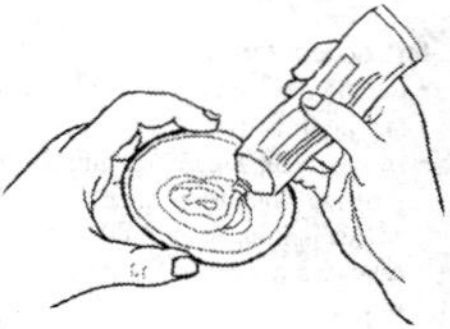

**Figure 18.1**
**Risk of pregnancy increases when a spermicide is not used. Put spermicide on outside and on inside**

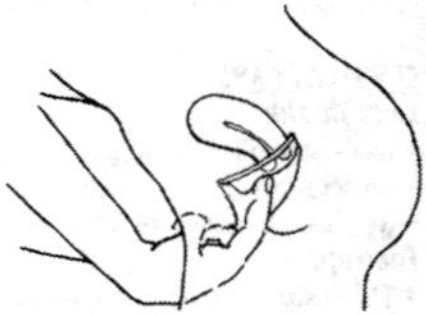

### *Instructions for Use:*

- Can be placed up to 6 hours before sex
- Fill inner surface of diaphragm 2/3 full with 2 teaspoons of spermicide

- In the squatting, leg-up or reclining position, press the rims on each side of the diaphragm together and hold with the dome of the bowl pointing downward.
- Insert with the dome side down as far into the vagina as possible. Push the diaphragm over your cervix so that it covers the cervix completely. Prior to each act of coitus, reconfirm correct placement. **For the second and each subsequent act, do not remove the diaphragm but use a condom for additional protection**
- Check to ensure diaphragm is lodged behind symphysis and completely covers the cervix. Bear down and digitally check to ensure that diaphragm does not move from behind pubic arch
- The diaphragm should be left in place for at least 6 hours after the last act of intercourse, up to 24 hours total from the time it was placed

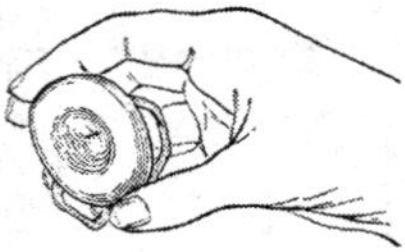

## TODAY™ CONTRACEPTIVE SPONGE

- The sponge is pre-filled with spermicide that is continuously released into the vagina during use

### *Instructions for Use:*

- Hold the sponge "dimple" side up and thoroughly wet sponge with tap water before insertion. Squeeze the sponge to produce suds
- In the squatting, leg-up or reclining position, press the rims on each side of the sponge together with the dimple still pointing upward
- Insert with the dimple first and loop last as far into the vagina as possible. Push the sponge over your cervix so that the dimple covers the cervix completely. To check positioning, squat or bear down to be sure it does not move
- The Today™ sponge should be left in place for at least **6** hours after the last act of intercourse, up to **24** hours total
- To remove, use fingers to grasp loop and remove device from the vagina. Dispose of sponge after use

# CHAPTER 20

## Spermicides

www.fhi.org OR www.avsc.org/contraception/cspe1.html OR www.microbicide.org

**DESCRIPTION: The search for an effective vaginal microbicide that would also kill sperm remains an important research priority, perhaps the most important research priority, in reproductive health.** In the USA, nonoxynol-9 (N-9) is available over the counter. In addition to N-9, patients around the world use menfegol, benzalkonium chloride, sodium docusate, and chlorhexidine (but these compounds are not available in the U.S.). Spermicides are available as vaginal creams, films, foams, gels, suppositories, sponges and tablets.

> Women at high risk of HIV should not use spermicides (US MEC:4). Nor should women who are HIV-infected (US MEC:4) Condoms without nonoxynol-9 lubrication are effective and widely available. Women at high risk of HIV infection should also avoid using diaphragms and cervical caps to which nonoxynol-9 is added (US MEC:3). The contraceptive effectiveness of diaphragms and cervical caps without nonoxynol-9 has been insufficiently studied and should be assumed to be less than that of diaphragms and cervical caps with nonoxynol-9. There is good evidence that N-9 does not protect against STI's and some evidence that it may be harmful by increasing genital irritation *[Cochrane Review-2008]*.

**EFFECTIVENESS** (See Trussell's failure rates, Table 12.2, Page 37)
***Perfect use failure rate in first year:*** 18%
***Typical use failure rate in first year:*** 28% *[Trussell J IN Contraceptive Technology, 2011]*
Failure rates are higher for spermicides than for any contraceptive currently available. While an application of a spermicide into the vagina is an appropriate backup contraceptive (including use with a condom), **spermicidal condoms are no longer recommended at all** as they provide no additional protection against pregnancy or STIs vs. condoms without spermicide. *[Warner-2004]*

- Cochrane review of spermicides for contraception found the probability of pregnancy varied widely in trials. A gel with 52.5 mg N-9 was significantly less effective than gels with higher N-9 doses (100 mg, 150 mg). Gel was liked more than film and suppositories in largest trial *[Grimes-2005]*

**MECHANISM:** As barriers, the vehicles prevent sperm from entering the cervical os. As detergents, the chemicals attack the sperm flagella and body, reducing motility

**ADVANTAGES**
***Menstrual:*** None
***Sexual/psychological:***
- Lubrication may heighten satisfaction for either partner
- Ease in application prior to sexual intercourse
- Either partner can purchase and apply; requires minimal negotiation

***Other:***
- Available over the counter; requires no medical visit
- Inexpensive and easy to use
- Foam and spermicidal jelly are immediately active with placement
- May be used during lactation

## DISADVANTAGES

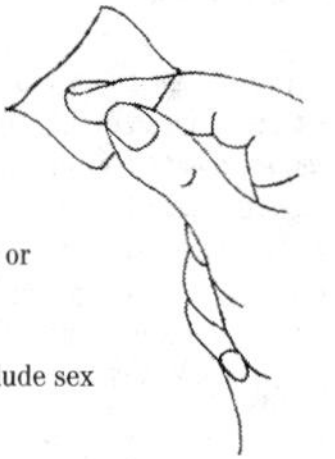

***Menstrual:*** None

***Sexual/psychological:***

- Films and suppository spermicides require 15 minutes for activation, which may interrupt or delay lovemaking
- Must feel comfortable inserting fingers into vagina
- Insertion is not easy for some couples due to embarrassment or reluctance to touch genitalia
- Some forms, e.g., foam, become "messy" during intercourse
- Possible vaginal, oral, and anal irritation can disrupt or preclude sex
- Taste may be unpleasant

***Cancers, tumors, and masses:*** None

***Other:***

- High failure rate means not effective enough to be used by women at risk for serious complications of pregnancy
- Relatively high failure rate among perfect and typical users and does not protect against transmission of HIV, GC or chlamydia (see p. 146 - statement from 2006 CDC STI Treatment Guidelines). Spermicides may, in women having frequent intercourse with multiple partners, enhance transmission of HIV by irritation of vaginal mucosa and by destroying vaginal flora, e.g., lactobacilli, in nonoxynol-9 concentrations as low as 0.1% *[Van Dame, Durban, 2000 found 1.7 RR of HIV transmission in users of spermicidal vaginal gel with 52.5 mg N-9] [Kreiss - 1992]*
- Allergic reactions and dermatitis in women and men that could decrease compliance

## COMPLICATIONS

- Women and men have confused fruit jelly, e.g., grape jelly, for spermicidal "jelly"
- Women and men have attempted to use cosmetics or hair products containing non-spermicidal octoxynols and nonoxynols (nonoxynol 4, 10, 12, and 14) in lieu of nonoxynol-9

## CANDIDATES FOR USE

- Willing to accept high failure rates
- Any woman and partner who presents with no prior allergy or reaction to spermicides

***Adolescents:***

- Readily available and not contraindicated for teens unless at high risk for HIV infection
- High failure rate should discourage long-term use as primary method

## INITIATING METHOD

- Except in cases where the patient, or partner, presents with pregnancy, allergy, or irritation, women can begin these methods at any time following product instructions
- Ensure ECPs are on hand at home

## INSTRUCTIONS FOR PATIENT

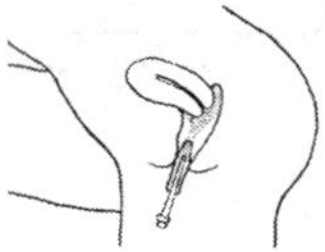

- Inserting person should wash and dry hands
- Spermicide has its greatest efficacy near the cervical os
- Water exposure, e.g. bathing or douching, within 6 hours after insertion or post-coitally can minimize effectiveness; reapply before next penetrative act

***Creams/foams/gels***

• Apply less than 1 hour prior to sexual intercourse. With foam, shake canister vigorously. Fill plastic applicator with spermicide. Insert applicator deeply into vagina and depress plunger. Immediately active. Finish sexual intercourse within 60 minutes of application

***Film, suppositories and tablets***

• Insert at least 15 minutes before sexual intercourse: with film, fold the sheet in quarters and then half again (this aids insertion). Using fingers or an applicator, the inserting partner places the spermicide applicator or film deep in the vagina, near cervix. Finish sexual intercourse within 60 minutes of application

## FOLLOW-UP

- Have you or your partner(s) experienced any rash or discomfort after using spermicides?
- Have you changed partners since beginning spermicides?
- Have you had sex—even once—without using spermicides?
- Would you like a more effective method?
- Did you have questions about ECPs?
- Do you have Plan B emergency contraceptive pills at home?
- Do you plan to have children? OR Do you plan to have more children? If yes, when?

## PROBLEM MANAGEMENT

***Dermatitis:*** Discontinue spermicides and offer another method. If spermicide was used as lubricant, recommend a water-based or silicone-based lubricant without nonoxynol-9

***Changed partners:*** Explain STI prevention, check for STIs, and recommend condoms

## FERTILITY AFTER DISCONTINUATION OF METHOD

- No effect on baseline fertility

# CHAPTER 21

# Coitus Interruptus (Withdrawal)

www.managingcontraception.com

**Thinking of completely unprotected sex tonight?** To avoid an unintended pregnancy, use outercourse, abstinence, a condom or withdrawal. Used perfectly one time, here's the math for withdrawal: a 4% failure rate for the perfect use of withdrawal for a year means: 4 pregnancies per 100 women each having sex about 80 times per year or 4/100 x 80 or 4 pregnancies per 8,000 acts of intercourse. That's 1 pregnancy per 2,000 acts of sex. **A 1 in 2,000 risk of pregnancy tonight if withdrawal is used once perfectly—that's not too bad!!!**

**Over the past two decades more, not less, woman have practiced withdrawal: 58% in 2006-2008: 41% in 1995, and 25% in 1992.** *[Mosher 2010]*

## EFFECTIVENESS

***Perfect use failure rate in first year:*** 4% (See Trussell's failure rates, Table 12.2, Page 37)
***Typical use failure rate in first year:*** 22% *[Trussell J IN Contraceptive Technology, 2011]*

Each night 700,000 to 1 million women who do not want to become pregnant have sex using no conraceptive at all. Condoms, withdrawal, outercourse and abstinence are far wiser options than proceding with unprotected sex.

**MECHANISM:** Withdrawal prior to ejaculation reduces or eliminates sperm introduced into vagina. Preejaculatory fluid is not generally a problem unless two acts of sexual intercourse are close together. It is very important that the penis is away from the introitus after withdrawal.

**Are there sperm in pre-ejaculate fluid? Possibly yes.**

In itself, the pre-ejaculate, a lubricating secretion produced by the Littre or Cowper's glands, presumably contains no sperm. Although two studies examining the pre-ejaculate for the presence of spermatozoa found none, two other studies found spermatozoa, though in small numbers. In one of these studies, 8 of 23 samples contained clumps of a few hundred sperm, which could theoretically have posed a risk of fertilization. In a recent study designed specifically to determine whether pre-ejaculate contained sperm potentially capable of fertilizing an egg, researchers examined the samples within 2 hours of production. The pre-ejaculate of 37% of men contained motile sperm, though the number of sperm in each sample was low. Because the number of sperm in each pre-ejaculate was low, the risk of pregnancy would be low, though not zero. Each man in the study was consistent in either leaking or not leaking sperm in with the pre-ejaculate fluid. *[Kowal D. Coitus interruptus (withdrawal) IN Hatcher, RA Contraceptive Technology 20th edition. p. 410]*

**COST:** None

## ADVANTAGES

***Menstrual:*** None
***Sexual/psychological:***

- No barriers
- Readily available method which encourages male involvement

***Cancers, tumors, and masses***: None
***Other:*** Surprisingly effective if used correctly

**DISADVANTAGES**

*Menstrual:* None

*Sexual/psychological*

- May not be applicable for couples with sexual dysfunction such as premature ejaculation
- Requires man's cooperation and control
- May reduce sexual pleasure of woman and intensity of orgasm of man
- Encourages "spectatoring" or thinking about what is happening during sexual intercourse

*Cancers, tumors, and masses:* None

*Other:* **Relatively high failure rate among typical users and poor protection against STIs.**

**COMPLICATIONS:** None

**MEDICAL ELIGIBILITY CHECKLIST**

- Man must be able to predict ejaculation in time to withdraw penis completely from vagina
- Premature ejaculation. A comon problem that makes method less effective
- Particularly appropriate for couples not at risk for STIs

**CANDIDATES FOR USE**

- Couples who are able to communicate during sexual intercourse
- Disciplined men who can ignore the powerful instinct, urging them to continue thrusting
- Couples without personal, religious or cultural prohibitions against withdrawal
- Women willing to accept higher risk of unintended pregnancy

*Adolescents:* Compliance may be a problem (as it is for couples of all ages); teens may have less control over ejaculation; advise use of condoms for better protection against pregnancy and STIs. While withdrawal is a relatively poor contraceptive option, especially if pregnancy prevention and infection control are very important, withdrawal is better than nothing

**INITIATING METHOD:** Can begin at any time; provide ECPs in advance

**INSTRUCTIONS FOR PATIENT**

- Practice withdrawal using backup method until both partners master withdrawal
- Wipe penis clean of the pre-ejaculation fluid prior to vaginal penetration
- Use coital positions that ensure that the man will be capable of withdrawing easily at the appropriate time
- Use emergency contraception (preferably an IUD) if withdrawal fails

**FOLLOW-UP**

- Does your partner ever ejaculate/begin to ejaculate before withdrawing?
- Do you want to use a more effective method?
- Did you have any Plan B at home?
- Do you plan to have children? OR Do you plan to have more children?
- Have you considered withdrawal early during intercourse, followed by putting on a condom, re-entering the vagina, then ejaculation.? In one study of college males, 43% reported using withdrawal during initial phases of intercourse and then applying a condom for intra-vaginal ejaculation. *[Crosby 2002]*

**PROBLEM MANAGEMENT**

*Failure to withdraw:* Use ECPs everytime. Withdrawal does not work! Consider another method or an IUD for EC.

**FERTILITY AFTER DISCONTINUATION OF METHOD:** No effect on fertility (except minimal protection against STIs)

# CHAPTER 22
## Emergency Contraception

www.not-2-late.com OR www.go2planb.com
1-800-330-1271

**Copper T IUD**
**NOT**
Emergency Contraceptive Pills

### EMERGENCY CONTRACEPTION WITH COPPER IUD: Ready for a paradigm shift

**Ten times fewer pregnancies than if emergency contraceptive pills are used**

### DESCRIPTION

- Insert Copper IUD, following the usual procedures, up to 5 days after ovulation
- Since day of ovulation is not always known, use is simplified to up to 5 days after unprotected intercourse
- If unprotected intercourse is 3 days before estimated ovulation, could be inserted as late as 8 days after intercourse
- More frequently used outside the U.S., where IUD costs are lower
- In the US, this method is generally restricted to use by women who intend to continue to use the IUD as an ongoing method
- Studies are underway to determine the effectiveness of the levonorgestrel IUD (Mirena).

### EFFECTIVENESS

- **The Copper-T IUD is the most effective postcoital contraceptive currently available**
- Failure rate just under 1 failure per 1000 Copper T insertions

**MECHANISM**: In the month it is inserted as an emergency contraceptive, it may act by interfering with implantation (see pages 81 and 88 for mechanisms of action of IUDs as routine, long-term contraceptive)

**COST**: In U.S. about $500. In Europe postcoital IUD insertion costs just $25 (Belgium) or is covered by health plan. Inexpensive in Europe or in the United States in comparison with costs (emotional and financial) of an unintended pregnancy

### ADVANTAGES

- The most effective post-coital method and may be used 2 days later than ECPs
- Provides long-term protection against pregnancy following insertion
- In one EC study, >80% continued use of IUD as their contraceptive *[Zhou-2001]*

**DISADVANTAGES:** Same disadvantages as when using Copper IUD as contraceptive (See Chapter 23)

- Expensive if only used for EC and removal expected soon thereafter, but much less expensive than an unintended pregnancy.

**COMPLICATIONS, CANDIDATES FOR USE, PRESCRIBING PRECAUTIONS, INITIATING METHOD, INSTRUCTIONS FOR PATIENT FOLLOW-UP, PROBLEM MANAGEMENT, FERTILITY AFTER USE:** Pretty much the same as when using Copper IUD as ongoing contraceptive (See Chapter 23)

## Table 22.1 Overview of Postcoital Methods Currently Available in U.S.

| Characteristic | Copper IUD | POPs | COCs* | Ulipristal acetate (UPA) |
|---|---|---|---|---|
| Timing of initiation after intercourse | Up to 8 days after ovulation. In practice, usually given up to 5 days after intercourse | ASAP but *can* be used up to 120 hours (5 days); Sooner is better | ASAP but *can* be used up to 120 hours (5 days); Sooner is better | ASAP but *can* be used up to 120 hours (5 days) |
| Dose | Place Copper IUD and leave in for ongoing contraception | Levonogestrel: 2 doses of 0.75 mg taken 12 hours apart or single dose of 1.5 mg | Two doses 12 hours apart of pills amounting to 100-120 mcg ethinyl estradiol and 0.5-0.75 levonogestrel (see chart, p. 80) | Single 30 mg tablet Ulipristal acetate |
| Pregnancies/100 women | 0.1% | Early start: 0.4% (<12 h)<br>Late start: 2.7% (1-3 days)<br>Average: 1.1% | Early start: 0.5% (<12 h)<br>Late start: 4.2% (1-3 days)<br>Average: 2 - 3.2% | • 0.9 - 1.4%<br>• Effectiveness maintained between 72 & 120 hours |
| Advantages | Effective long-term contraceptive for appropriate women | Fewer side effects than COCs; Product available for advance prescription<br>**Single dose** | Wide range of COCs available for use | More effective than LNG between 72 & 120 hours and in overweight women |
| Disadvantages | Expensive; must be appropriate candidate for IUD; Timing issues: counseling, testing, etc. Insertion procedure required | Less available than COCs that can be used to create an off-label EC regimen. Check for availability of Plan B at pharmacies near you at www.go2planb.com | Gastrointestinal side effects – can be reduced with antiemetic pretreatment<br>No dedicated product | Expensive; needs prescription; theoretically can interrupt early conception; no more than 1 dose per cycle; use barrier methods, not hormonal, for rest of cycle |
| Side effects | Pain, bleeding, expulsion | Spotting. Same hormonal side effects as COCs, but significantly less frequent and less severe | Nausea, vomiting, spotting headache, breast tenderness, moodiness, change in next menses | Nausea, vomiting, headache |
| Avoid use in pregnant women and women with other prescribing precautions | Prescribing precautions for IUD use (see p. 80) | Do not use in women with known pregnancy because the treatment will not be effective. Not a teratogen | Do not use in women with known pregnancy or current severe migraine. POPs a better option for all women with a history of DVT or PE | Do not use in pregnancy |

For more information about EC, phone numbers of EC providers, or **to become listed as an EC provider**, check out the web site www.not-2-late.com or call the EC Hotline at 1-888-NOT-2-LATE. Other good sources of information about EC are www.go2planB.com or call 800-330-1271.

* COCs using norgestrel are better studied. COCs with norethindrone may be used as ECPs, but failure rates are slightly higher as compared with COCs with norgestrel

## EMERGENCY CONTRACEPTION WITH ULIPRISTAL ACETATE (UPA)

### DESCRIPTION

A selective progestin receptor modulator that inhibits or delays ovulation. It is a compund derived from 19-norprogesterone and is similar to mifepristone, however it has less antiglucocorticoid activity.

### EFFECTIVENESS

- A meta-analysis of two trials of ulipristal found that it was as effective as levonogestrel at 24, 72 and 120 hours after unprotected intercourse *[Glasier AF, Cameron ST, Fine PM, Logan SJ, Casale W, Van Horn J, Sogor L, Blithe DL, Scherrer B, Mathe H, Jaspart A, Ulmann A, Gainer Lancet. 2010; 375 (9714): 555]*
- In the meta-analysis, at each time interval, the rate of pregnancy in patients receiving ulipristal was approximately 1 percent versus 2 percent after in patients receiving levonogestrel; these differences were statistically significant. Only 97 women were given ulipristal between 72 and 120 hours after unprotected intercourse, but it is encouraging that none of them became pregnant. By comparison, 106 women took levonogestrel in the same time frame and three became pregnant. There were relatively small numbers of women who received drug between 72 and 120 hours. There was no difference in the side effect profile of the two drugs.
- Further analysis from this meta-analysis revealed that the risk of pregnancy was more than threefold higher for obese women taking EC than non-obese, regardless of whether they took LNG or UPA, but the risk of pregnancy in obese women was greater if they took LNG EC. Highest risk was also related to having sex around ovulation or continued unprotected sex after taking EC. The authors recommend that women having unprotected sex around the time of ovulation, at greatest risk for pregnancy, who present for EC should be offered a copper IUD and women with body mass >25/kg/meter should be offered an IUD or UPA.
- Another study at Planned Parenthood sites examined 1,241 women presenting between 48 and 120 hours for EC who received 30 mg of UPA. 26 became pregnant for a rate of 2.1%. Effectiveness was steady throughout the windows of time ingested.
- Pooled data from phase III studies yielded a pregnancy rate of 1.9%, 41 pregnancies out of 2183 users. Pregnancy was more likely if women were obese or had future acts of intercourse in cycle. Lowest rate of pregnancy was 1.3% in nonobese women with no further acts of intercourse and highest was 8.3% in obese women with subsequent intercourse. *[Moreau, Trussell et al. Contraception 2012]*

**MECHANISM:** UPA delays or inhibits ovulation. In addition, UPA has some effects on the endometrium which may affect implantation.

### COST:

- Approximately $50.00

### ADVANTAGES

- All same as for other oral EC

### DISADVANTAGES

***Menstrual:*** Menses delayed by means of 2 days, which can create anxiety about pregnancy status

***Sexual/Psychological:*** Women who are uncomfortable with post-fertilization methods need reassurance that use is consistent with their beliefs if taken during the follicular phase. They need to know that if taken after ovulation, UPA may work as an interceptive.

***Cancer, tumors and masses:*** None

***Other:***

- Headache, nausea,abdominal pain possible.
- No protection against STIs, consider RX for STIs if exposed.
- Not recommended to start a hormonal contraceptive method immediately after UPA. Barrier methods for next 7 days or for remainder of cycle because of a theoretical concern that taking ulipristal could make either the ulipristal or the hormonal methos less effective by competitive binding to the progestin receptors.

**COMPLICATIONS:** None

**CANDIDATES FOR USE:** Same as for ECPS

**PRECAUTIONS:**

- pregnancy and ectopic pregnancy
- hypersensitivity to any compound of the product
- undiagnosed abnormal uterine bleeding (be suspicious of risk of ectopic pregnancy)
- not for repeated uses in single cycle
- barrier contraception is recommended immediately following UPA and throughout the same menstrual cycle; efficacy of hormonal contracetion may be decreased.
- drug interactions (see package label for more details): Conivaptan, CYP3A4 inducers, Deferasirox, herbs, Tocilizumab, St. John's Wort may decrease serum levels UPA

## EMERGENCY CONTRACEPTION PILLS

Emergency contraceptive pills can be provided from behind the counter (i.e. directly from the pharmacist without a prescription) for people ages 17 and older. An identification card is required. Even if providers do not have to write a prescription, they play a significant part in increasing patient education about emergency contraception and access to ECPs. Many pharmacies do not stock ECPs so having it in advance is important. *[French AC, Kauntiz AM]*

- Good news: Some data show increased availability after Plan B was awarded OTC status *[Geere-2008]*
- Tell **ALL** your patients about emergency contraception (EC)
- Provide EC pills or prescriptions in advance to your patients or advise to buy OTC
- Continue to write prescriptions for:
  - Women younger than 17
  - Women 17 and older with insurance coverage for EC
  - Women who may not have a government issued ID stating their age
  - Women who may be embarrassed to ask for EC without a prescription

## OVERVIEW

***Plan B and Next Choice now available OTC for people ≥ 17 years old. These should routinely be used as EC rather than combined pills***. The states with EC available direct from pharmacies for people of any age are Washington, California, Vermont, Alaska, Massachusetts, New Hampshire, New Mexico, Hawaii and Maine. In 34 countries, EC is available directly from pharmacies. Emergency contraception (EC) includes any method used after intercourse to prevent pregnancy. None of the current methods is an abortifacient and none disturbs an implanted pregnancy. There are currently 3 methods in widespread use worldwide:

- High-dose progestin-only contraceptive pills (POPs). PLAN B or Next Choice preferable to Ovrette or COCs
- Ulipristal acetate, Ella, now available (see Table 22.1)
- Yuzpe Method 13 brands of combined oral contraceptive pills (COCs)
- Copper IUD insertion (Paragard)

An estimated 51,000 pregnancies were averted by EC use in 2000 accounting for 43% of the decrease in abortions since 1994 *[Finer-2003]*. Only the two hormonal methods are utilized to any significant degree in the U.S. (all combined and progestin-only pills that may be used are on p. 80 of this book and in diagram on A-20). It is more effective to provide ECPs to patients in advance than to give them a prescription with refills in advance, but always do one or the other.

- Studies have found women getting EC in advance are not more likely to have unprotected sex
- Women in EC studies often underutilize EC. Inconvenience and fear of the side effects were reasons for non-use cited in one study *[Rocca-2007]*
- Increased access to EC enhances use but does not decrease pregnancy rates *[Raymond-2007]*

## EMERGENCY CONTRACEPTION WITH ORAL CONTRACEPTIVE PILLS

### DESCRIPTION

***POPs: more effective than COCs and less side effects***

- EITHER: Both Plan B or Next Choice tabs at once
  OR: Tab #1 followed by #2 in 12 hours
- EITHER: within 72 hours or 120 hours (5 days)
- BEST: 2 tabs at once as soon as possible or Plan B One-Step

- Plan B One-Step has both doses in a single pill
- Next Choice

***Yuzpe Method using any of the levonorgestrel-containing COCs:***

- Two large doses of COCs with at least 100 µg of ethinyl estradiol and either 100 mcg of norgestrel or .50 mg of levonorgestrel in each dose. Norethindrone pills have slightly less effectiveness as ECPs. Take first dose ASAP within 120 hours after inadequately protected sex; take second dose 12 hours later (second dose may be more than 120 hours after unprotected sex). Try to provide ECPs to women in advance (actual pills or prescription with refills if < 17 years old)

### EFFECTIVENESS

- In this large trial, starting treatment with a delay of 4-5 days did not significantly increase the failure rate compared to the efficacy of treatment begun within 3 days of unprotected intercourse. *[von Hertzen-2002]*. Failure rate was slightly higher when ECPs were taken on days 4 or 5. **Emergency contraceptive pills should be taken as soon as possible after unprotected sex**
- Taking more than number of pills specified is *not* beneficial and may increase risk of vomiting
- UPA significantly more effective than LNG at 72-120 hours
- LNG ECP significantly less effective in overweight and obese women
- UPA significantly less effective in obese women
- EC with POPs (eg Plan B) is virtually useless in women with a BMI of 26 or greater
- EC with Ella is useless (ineffective) in women with a BMI of 35 or greater *[Glaser, 2011]*

| | | | |
|---|---|---|---|
| ***EC with POPs*** ***PLAN B*** ***Next Choice*** | Only 1.1% of 967 women using POPs for EC became pregnant in a WHO multi-center study *[WHO task force on Postovulatory Methods of Fertility Regulation. Lancet Aug 8, 1998]* | 89% average reduction of pregnancy rate based on WHO perfect-use study population | 12 pregnancies per 1000 unprotected acts of sexual intercourse followed by POPs |
| ***EC with COCs*** | 2-3% failure rate | 74% average reduction of pregnancy rate (WHO perfect-use study) | 20-32 pregnancies per 1000 unprotected acts of sexual intercourse followed by Preven or COCs |
| ***EC with Ella*** | 1% pregnancy rate Most effective oral agent when taken between 72 and 120 hours after unprotected intercourse | 90% average reduction in pregnancy rate | Approximately 10 pregnancies per 1000 unprotected acts of intercourse followed by Ella |

**Plan B, Next Choice and other emergency contraceptive pills are NOT recommended for routine use as a contraceptive**

## HOW EMERGENCY CONTRACEPTIVE PILLS WORK:

- ECPs act by preventing pregnancy and never by disrupting an implanted pregnancy, i.e. never as an abortifacient
- If taken before ovulation, ECPs disrupt normal follicular development and maturation, blocks LH surge, and inhibit ovulation; they may also create deficient luteal phase and may have a contraceptive effect by thickening cervical mucus
- If taken after ovulation, ECPs have little effect on ovarian hormonal production and limited effect on endometrial maturation
- ECPs may affect tubal transport of sperm or ova

## COST

*POPs:*

- Plan B is available OTC in retail pharmacies for about $40- $50. Next Choice is less costly
- Non-profit and Title X agencies may purchase POPs at $4.50 - $8.00 per treatment
- Pharmacists in those states that may dispense without a prescription charge $50-$55 for counseling and medication

*Yuzpe method with COCs:*

- One cycle of COCs may vary from a few dollars to more than $50

*Other costs:*

- Cost prior to obtaining pills may vary from nothing (if already given) to cost of full exam and pregnancy test. This may increase total cost of EC to $45 to over $100

## ADVANTAGES

***Menstrual:*** None

***Sexual/Psychological:***

- Offers an opportunity to prevent pregnancy after rape, mistake, or barrier method failure (condom breaks or slips, diaphragm dislodges, etc.)
- Reduces anxiety about unintended pregnancy prior to next menses
- Process of getting EC may lead woman to initiate ongoing contraception

***Cancers, tumors and masses:*** None

***Other:***

- Estimated 40% of reduction in teen pregnancies ('95 to '99) due to EC

## DISADVANTAGES

*Menstrual:*

- Next menses may be early (especially if taken before ovulation), on time, or late
- Notable changes in flow of next menses seen in 10-15% of women
- **If no menses within 3 weeks (21 days) of taking ECPs, pregnancy test should be done**

*Sexual/psychological:*

- Women who are uncomfortable with post-fertilization methods need reassurance that use of EC with COCs or POPs is consistent with their beliefs if taken during the follicular phase. There are no data to show LNG may work after ovulation as an interceptive
- No STI protection

***Cancers, tumors and masses:*** None

***Other:***

- Breast tenderness, fatigue, headache, abdominal pain and dizziness
- No protection against STIs; consider treatment for possible STIs following exposure

***Nausea and vomiting:***

| | Nausea | Vomiting | Pretreatment with antiemetic |
|---|---|---|---|
| **POPs** | 23% | 6% | Many clinicians use only if Hx of past problems with nausea or vomiting |
| **COCs** | 50% | 19% | Can reduce symptoms by 30-50% |

## COMPLICATIONS

- Several cases of DVT reported in women using COCs as ECPs. No increased DVT risk with POPs

## CANDIDATES FOR USE

- All women who have had or who may be at risk for unprotected sex (sperm exposure) are candidates for ECPs for immediate or future use.
- As a backup method for barrier methods
- Forgotten pills, late for contraceptive reinjection, NFP miscalculation, failed withdrawal
- Failure to use methods: clouded judgment, sexual assault
- For the woman who has intercourse infrequently (1-2x/yr) Particularly effective if taken within one hour of otherwise unprotected sex
- NOTE: ECPs do not protect against pregnancy as well as ongoing methods

***Adolescents:*** appropriate back-up option. Having EC available does NOT make teens less likely to use regular contraception or more likely to have unprotected sex. *[Glasier-1998] [Raine-2000] [Ellertson-2001]*

## PRECAUTIONS

***Plan B/Next Choice:***

- Pregnancy (no benefit; no effect)
- Hypersensitivity to any component of product
- Undiagnosed abnormal vaginal bleeding

***Use of COCs for EC should be allowed for all women except those who:***

- Are pregnant; no benefit but also no dangers
- Are known to be hypersensitive to any component of the product
- Have acute migraine headaches at the time ECPs are to be taken (Use Plan B/Next Choice)
- Have history of DVT or PE (use Plan B/Next Choice)

## INITIATING METHOD: Pregnancy testing is optional, not required:

- Getting POPs OTC requires an ID. No evaluation is done by the pharmacist
- Offer ECPs routinely to all women who may be at risk for unprotected intercourse:

POPs (levonorgestrel) is better than combined pills
  - Advance provision and prescription increases use of EC but does not diminish use of primary method of contraception
  - Availability directly through pharmacists led to a thousand-fold increase in use of ECPs in selected pharmacies in the state of Washington
- Provide EC for all women who present after-the-fact, acutely in need. If you dispense off-label pills remove the inactive pills to reduce risk of mistake
- Patient history for prescribing EC after-the-fact:
  - LMP, previous menstrual period, dates of any prior unprotected intercourse this cycle, and date and time of last unprotected intercourse
  - Any problems with previous use of ECPs, COCs or POPs?
  - Breast-feeding or severe headaches now? History of DVT or PE? (Use POPs not COCs)
  - Any foreseeable problems if antiemetic causes drowsiness?
- No physical exam/labs needed on a routine basis:
  - No pelvic exam is necessary, now or in the past; No BP measurements needed
  - Pregnancy testing useful only if concerned that prior intercourse may have caused pregnancy. ***ACOG, IPPF and CDC do not include routine pregnancy testing in their protocols***
- Advise patient about possible side effects and consider other EC options (Copper IUD)
- If prescribing COCs, offer premedication with long-acting antiemetic one hour prior to first ECP dose. Take two 25 mg tablets of meclizine hydrochloride (over-the-counter Dramamine or Bonine). Other agents work, but do not have same duration of action. Avoid antiemetic if drowsiness will pose safety hazard. Antiemetics not needed prior to Plan B
- Tell her how to use appropriate number of tablets for particular ECP brand to reach adequate dose (see Figure 21.1 and p. A-20).
- **Both Plan B tabs may be taken at once.** If using COCs, encourage patient to take first dose ASAP and second dose approximately 12 hours after first dose. It is ok to take second dose in slightly less or more than 12 hours; realize that 72 hours after unprotected intercourse is NOT the absolute limit. ECP may be taken for up to 120 hours after unprotected sex
- Encourage patient to have available at home in case she has another need to use EC again OR provide prescription with refills if < 18 years old
- Inquire about desire to be checked for STI's (especially in cases of rape)

## STARTING REGULAR USE OF CONTRACEPTIVE AFTER USE OF ECPs

- Start using regular method immediately. ECPs offer no lingering reliable protection
- If missed OCs, restart day after ECPs taken (no need to catch up missed pills)
- If starting COCs, patch or ring, see COC precautions and then:
  - May wait for next menses or
  - Start OCs, patch or ring next day with 7-day backup method (this will affect timing of next menses). In office she may punch out a few pills at the beginning of a pill pack to correspond with the day of the week you are seeing her. This may reduce confusion
- If starting DMPA injections, can start immediately. If so, consider having patient return in 2-3 weeks for pregnancy test
- If starting barrier methods, start immediately.
- If starting NFP, use abstinence (or barrier/spermicide) until next menses

## SPECIAL ISSUES/FREQUENT QUESTIONS

- Give your patient a supply of EC at her annual visit. EC is more likely to be used if she already has it and need not visit a pharmacy *(Glasier 2001; Jackson 2003; Raine 2005)*
- When in cycle should EC be offered? Anytime
- How many times a year can a woman use ECPs? No limit, but be sure to ask her why her primary method is not working

- What if a patient has had unprotected intercourse earlier in the cycle? Do urine test to confirm no obvious pregnancy. Offer EC. If concerned that your test may miss an early pregnancy, give EC and have her return in 3 weeks (if no menses) for another pregnancy test. EC will not adversely affect a developing pregnancy
- What if she used EC earlier in the month? Offer it again; she may have just delayed ovulation. Review why her primary contraceptive is failing her and remedy the situation (perhaps with a new method). Consider performing pregnancy test in this setting even though it may be too early to have become positive; counsel her about this possibility
- What if the pharmacy is closed or does not carry EC? Plan ahead. Encourage her to have EC on hand at home. Check with local 24-hour pharmacies

## INSTRUCTIONS FOR PATIENT

- **EC works best if taken as soon as possible after sex. Women at risk of pregnancy need Plan B or Next Choice at home!** For advance prescription, have her fill her prescription (or obtain OTC) in advance and keep readily available.
- **It is now recommended that both doses of Plan B or Next Choice be taken at once**
- An antiemetic need <u>not</u> be taken prior to Plan B or Next Choice
- Start using contraception right away. ECPs do not reliably protect you beyond the day they are used
- Re-evaluate primary contraceptive method to make it more reliable
- Have her return for pregnancy testing if she has not had her menses 21 days after using ECPs

## FOLLOW-UP

- No routine follow-up needed
- Have patient return for pregnancy testing if no menses in 3 weeks
- If patient has persistent irregular bleeding or abdominal pain, she should return to rule out ectopic pregnancy

## PROBLEM MANAGEMENT

***Nausea/vomiting:***

- Antiemetic may be prescribed before or after taking combined COCs as ECPs (does not work as well when taken after EC)
- Vomiting that occurs due to ECPs probably indicates that enough hormones reached the bloodstream to have the desired contraceptive effect. Most experts (but NOT all) recommend a repeat dose of ECPs if vomiting occurs within 30 minutes of taking ECPs. ACOG recommends a repeat dose if vomiting occurs within two hours *[ACOG 2005]*
- POPs are preferable to COCs, but if repeating dose because of severe vomiting, switch from COCs to POPs or consider placing pills in vagina rather than mouth (off-label) or use of a copper IUD. Although uptake is slower with vaginal administration, this may also be possible for woman who has experienced extreme nausea while taking COCs in the past as her regular contraceptive. No data on effectiveness of vaginal COCs used as EC
- If severe vomiting occurs, consider IUD as emergency contraceptive

***Amenorrhea:*** If menses do not occur in 21 days (or more than 7 days beyond expected day for menses to begin), pregnancy test recommended

***Pregnancy in spite of using ECPs:*** If there is a pregnancy, the woman may be reassured that there is evidence that ECPs do not increase the risk of fetal anomalies, ectopic pregnancy or miscarriage

**FERTILITY AFTER DISCONTINUATION OF METHOD:** Must provide contraception for rest of cycle and beyond. If she starts using birth control pills or a vaginal ring, use a back-up (condoms) for the first 7 days. If she uses patches, use a back-up (condoms) for 9 days

**Figure 22.1**

## EMERGENCY CONTRACEPTION USING EMERGENCY CONTRACEPTIVE PILLS (ECPs)

**1-888-NOT-2 LATE; www.opr.princeton.edu/ec; www.go2planB.com**

**POPs (Plan-B/Next Choice): Behind the counter for men, women > 17 years old.** Educate/prescribe/provide emergency contraceptive pills (ECPs) **prior to the need** for them so that women and men have them available at home (or rapid access to them) in case they are needed. This is particularly important since some pharmacies will not dispense ECPs

↓

Start ECPs as soon as possible, after unprotected or inadequately protected sexual intercourse. **Can be used up to 5 days, but sooner is better; most effective if taken immediately or within 12 hours**

↓

No need to use anti-nausea medication if using POPs. If using a COC, first, take anti-nausea medication: 50 mg oral meclizine* has 24-hour duration of action

↓

| BRAND** | DOSE | |
|---|---|---|
| Plan B or Next Choice | 2 white tablets all at once*** | |
| *One hour after antiemetic, take first dose of ECPs. Choose one of the following:* | | |
| Ogestrel, Ovral | 2 white tablets per dose | |
| Levora, Low-Ogestrel, Lo/Ovral | 4 white tablets per dose | If vomiting occurs within 1 hour, repeat dose |
| Levlen, Nordette | 4 light-orange tablets per dose | |
| Tri-Levlen, Triphasil | 4 light-yellow tablets per dose | |
| Trivora | 4 pink tablets per dose | |
| Alesse, Levlite | 5 pink tablets per dose | |

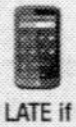

**CALL:** 1-888-NOT-2 LATE if you have any questions about emergency contraception OR if you need to hear about EC in Spanish or if you need phone numbers of 5 clinicians nearest you who will provide EC if you need a prescription (are < 17 years old).

↓

If using one of the other COC options, repeat the same dose of ECPs 12 hours later. In the case of Plan B or Next Choice, both tabs may be taken at once

↓

Patient should (re)start ongoing method immediately and restock ECPs at home

↓

Pregnancy test if no period in 3 weeks

NOTE: if anti-nausea medication is NOT taken prior to first dose of ECPs (which is recommended), it may be taken after the first dose, should nausea be severe or should woman vomit. Anti-nausea medication is usually not needed for women using POPs, as they do not contain estrogen.

* Meclizine hydrochloride is recommended because it has a 24-hour duration of action. It is available over the counter as Bonine and as Dramamine 2. Other medications to prevent nausea may be prescribed instead.

**Norethindrone pills recently shown to be effective but less than these levonorgestrel products.

One Plan B one-step pill or two Next Choice pills taken simultaneously deliver the same dose of hormone to prevent pregnancy. Should be used ASAP, as a single dose, after unprotected intercourse for maximum effectiveness.

## Emergency Contraceptive Pills 972 Million Times a Year? It will simply never happen. Not at $10 to $75 per ECP.

**MESSAGE:** People who need emergency contraception need it too often and use it too infrequently to significantly lower unintended pregnancies. In 15 out of 16 published articles, initiatives designed to increase use of emergency contraceptive pills led to no reduction at all in unintended pregnancies over the next year when compared to control groups of women. The magnitude of unprotected sex in the United States is explained in the following 3 paragraphs: We are talking about the potential need for emergency contraceptive pills some 972 million times a year.

1. Each night about 10 million women not wanting to become pregnant have sex. From 700,000 to 1 million of them use no contraception at all. Each night! That comes to upwards of **365 million each year.**

2. Women on pills miss about 4.5 pills per cycle or about 58 times a year. That means there are over 845 million missed pills each month. Each missed or even late pill may cause a woman to seek out emergency contraception. That comes to close to **585 million missed pills a year.**

3. Some 20 to 30% of women count partially or completely on condoms. Each night 19,000 condoms break and an even larger number of times, condoms fall off partially or completely. We can conservatively estimate that 60,000 times a night and **22 million times a year**, a couple using a condom experiences slippage or breakage.

4. 365 million plus 45 million plus 22 million equals **972 million times** when emergency contraceptive pills might be needed each year in the Unisted States.

**CASE:** Unprotected sex twice on day of ovulation -------> ECPs next day
Hi, I had unprotected sex twice on the very day ovulation was expected. I used an emergency contraceptive pill the next day. My period should have started 3 days ago. I am still period-free.

How long should I wait to do a pregnancy test? I'm really scared because I'm 17 (so is my partner), so there is not much I can do. I really can't go to my parents.

*She was encouraged to get a pregnancy test that day (now 19 days after unprotected sex).*

Final note, three days later: I'm pregnant; however my boyfriend and I worked with Planned Parenthood to schedule an abortion for the next week. We live in Washington, DC, and no parental involvement is necessary.

*Note: An emergency IUD probably would have prevented this pregnancy.*

**Figure 22.2**

## EMERGENCY CONTRACEPTION USING COPPER IUD*
## www.opr.princeton.edu/ec

Following unprotected or inadequately protected sexual intercourse, screen patient for candidacy for IUD use (generally not for women at risk for STIs)

↓

Insert Copper IUD within 5 days of the unprotected sexual intercourse**

↓

Menstrual period within 21 days?

↓ YES ↓

Ask if IUD is to be left in place OR remove IUD and initiate the contraceptive of her choice—a method she will use consistently and correctly

↓ NO ↓

Return for pregnancy test. If pregnancy test is positive, must remove IUD. If pregnancy test is negative, may continue to use IUD

*** There is no evidence that the levonorgestrel IUD, is effective for EC**

** The Copper IUD may be inserted up to the time of implantation—about 5 days after ovulation—to prevent pregnancy. Thus, if a woman had unprotected sexual intercourse 3 days before ovulation occurred in that cycle, the IUD could be inserted up to 8 days after intercourse to prevent pregnancy

Postcoital ParaGard insertion is the most effective emergency contraceptive. If a woman can use a Copper T 380 A IUD as her emergency contraceptive and leave it in as her ongoing long-term contraceptive, she may receive at least 10 or more years of excellent contraceptive protection.

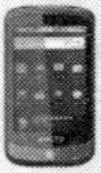

**CALL:** 1-888-NOT-2 LATE if you have any questions about emergency contraception OR if you need to hear about EC in Spanish or if you need phone numbers of 5 clinicians nearest you who will provide EC.

## ParaGard, the Copper T 380-A Device as an Emergency Contraceptive
## A failure rate of one in 1,000 sounds good!

**MESSAGE:** Today we have a superb emergency contraceptive. If the ParaGard IUD is tolerated well, it will provide ongoing contraception for 12 years (possibly longer).

1. In the literature, just over 12,000 copper T 380-A insertions for emergency contraception have been prescribed. Only 12 women became pregnant (1 pregnancy per 1,000 insertions).

2. After unprotected sex, a copper T IUD may be inserted for 5 to 8 days (see page 75, bullet 3).

3. There are no published studies of the use of the levonorgestrel IUD (Mirena). It is assumed that it has a contraceptive effect. If Mirena is used as an emergency contraceptive, an emergency contraceptive pill should also be used.

**CASE #1:** I had an abortion. My follow-up exam was scheduled for a month later. I had unprotected sex 3 days before that visit and took Plan B the next day. I also had unprotected sex the day before my post-abortion exam and was given Plan B again at my doctor's visit. Could I be pregnant?

*This woman would have been better served if an IUD had been placed immediately following her abortion or if a ParaGard had been inserted at her post-abortion exam (rather than being provided Plan B).*

**CASE #2:** *Perhaps no single practice could more quickly lead to increased use of Long Acting Reversible Contraceptives as the use of ParaGard IUD for emergency contraception. This is underscored by the following person writing in to the www.managingcontraception.com website.*

I take a morning-after pill every month. When we have sex my boyfriend usually pulls out. We had unprotected sex twice one morning and each time he pulled out. My ovulation test became positive 3 days later (when sperm could still have been alive and well in me). I figure my risk of pregnancy is fairly low. Is it safe to use morning-after pills as often as I am using them?

I read on your site that I could get an IUD inserted for emergency contraception. I told an OB/GYN who said they had never heard of this.

*So, this woman, were she to receive an emergency copper T insertion, it would be extremely effective both as an emergency contraceptive and as an ongoing contraceptive.*

# CHAPTER 23

## Intrauterine Contraceptives

www.popcouncil.org, www.engenderhealth.org, www.bayer.com, www.arhp.org, www.paragard.com

## IUD = IUC = IUCD

**OVERVIEW:** Three intrauterine contraceptives are available in the U.S.: the ParaGard® T 380A Intrauterine Coper IUD, the Mirena® levonorgestrel-releasing intrauterine system, and the slightly smaller levonorgestrel IUD called Skyla®.

- IUC among most effective methods, yet underutilized
- Clinician education/training important to increase utilization. *[Postlethwaite, 2007]* Program at California Planned Parenthood increased utilization by over 300%. *[Goodman, 2008]*
- Adolescents have minimal complications with IUD use and siliiar insertion success (96.4), expulsions (2.9% in first year), and high continuation rates. *[Bayer, 2012]*

**WOMEN MAY USE AN IUC IF THEY:**

- are nulligravid, nulliparous or multiparous
- are young or late in reproductive years
- immediately after abortion or miscarriage
- immediately after a vaginal or c-section delivery
- have had an STI in past
- have had an ectopic pregnancy in past
- are not in a monogamous relationship
- have fibroids that do not distort the uterine cavity
- need emergency contraception
- Copper IUD
- Hormonal IUD to help manage endometriosis, adenomyosis, fibroids and dysfunctional uterine bleeding (heavy or painful periods)

**Women must continue to:**

- protect themselves from STI's if not in mutually monogamous relationship

**CHOOSING BETWEEN THE TWO IUDS AVAILABLE:**

Your patient wants an IUD. Counsel her thoroughly about the advantages and disadvantages of each IUD available. Women need to know either IUD can be removed at any time.

**Copper IUD:**

- effective for at least 10 to 12 years
- no hormones, therefore, no hormonal side effects
- may cause heavier periods and/or more cramping
- can be used as an EC

**Hormonal IUD:**

- Mirena effective for at least 5 years
- Skyla effective for at least 3 years
- releases levonorgestrel, therefore, less pain and lighter to no periods. Irregular bleeding common in early months
- may cause hormonal side effects
- treats menorrhagia and dysmennorhea
- prevents and treats endometrial hyperplasia

### INTRAUTERINE COPPER CONTRACEPTIVE (ParaGard T 380A)

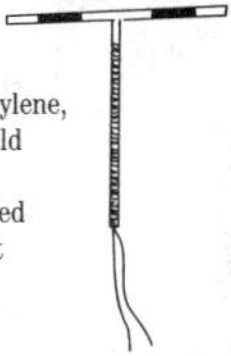

**DESCRIPTION:** T-shaped intrauterine contraceptive made of radiopaque polyethylene, with two flexible arms that bend down for insertion but open in the uterus to hold solid sleeves of copper against fundus. Fine copper wire wrapped around stem. Surface area of copper = 380 $mm^2$. Monofilament polyethylene tail string threaded through and knotted below blunt ball at base of stem creates double strings that protrude into vagina. This IUD has 2 straw colored strings.

**EFFECTIVENESS:** ***Think of IUDs/IUCs as "reversible sterilization"***
- Approved for 10 years use; effective for 12 years at least

***Perfect use failure rate in first year:*** 0.6% (see Table 12.2, Page 37)
***Typical use failure rate in first year:*** 0.8%
*[Trussell J IN Contraceptive Technology, 2004]*
***Cumulative 12-year failure rate:*** 2.1 - 2.8%

Use of IUDs decreases the risk of ectopic pregnancy by 70-80% vs. women not using contraception. But, if a woman gets pregnant with an IUD, you must rule out ectopic pregnancy. Of pregnancies with ParaGard in FDA trials, one out of 16 pregnancies was ectopic (WHO trial 1:9). For Mirena, 1 out of 2 was ectopic *[Furlong-2002]* although pregnancies rare

**HOW COPPER IUD WORKS:**
The intrauterine copper contraceptive works primarily as a spermicide. Copper ions inhibit sperm motility and acrosomal enzyme activation so that sperm rarely reach the fallopian tube and are unable to fertilize the ovum. The sterile inflammatory reaction created in the endometrium phagocytizes the sperm. Experimental evidence suggests that the copper IUDs do not routinely work after fertilization. They are not abortifacients. They primarily prevent pregnancy by killing sperm (spermicidal), and thereby preventing fertilization

**COST:** **$475.00**
- ParaGard units that are contaminated during insertion or are expelled or removed within first 3 months may be replaced free of cost. Contact Teva 877-727-2427. See Ordering and Stocking, Chapter 27, Page 164

**ADVANTAGES:** Effective long-term contraception from a single decision
***Menstrual:*** Period cycles remain regular
***Sexual/psychological***
- Convenient; permits spontaneous sexual activities. Requires no action at time of use
- Intercourse may be more pleasurable with risk of pregnancy reduced

***Cancers, tumors and masses***
- Probable protection against endometrial cancer (6 of 7 case control studies) *[Hubacher-Grimes-2002]*
- Possible 40% protection against cervical cancer *[Grimes-2004]*

***Other***
- Very effective
- Good option for women who cannot use hormonal methods
- Rapid return to fertility and private
- Convenient - single insertion provides up to 12 years protection (package labeling says 10 years)
- **Cost effective. Provides greatest net benefits of any contraceptive over a 5 year period.**
- Risk for ectopic pregnancy decreased
- **IUDs lead to highest level of user satisfaction of any contraceptive** *[Forrest-1996]*
- Can be used as an emergency contraceptive (see Page 75)

**DISADVANTAGES:**
***Menstrual***
- Average monthly blood loss increased by up to 50%; this may be diminished by NSAIDs
- May increase dysmenorrhea (removal rates for bleeding and pain first year = 11.9%)
- Spotting and cramping with insertion and intermittently in weeks following insertion

*Sexual/psychological*

- Some women (particularly young teens agers) uncomfortable with concept of having "something" (foreign body) placed inside them
- Some women are not at ease checking strings
- Strings palpable; if strings cut too short, may cause partner discomfort

***Cancers, tumors and masses:*** None

***Other***

- Requires office procedure for insertion and removal; both can be uncomfortable
- Some programs/protocols recommend a chlamydia/gonnorrhea check before insertion, others do not
- Some do a wet mount and test for GC/CT. Amplified PCR tests of cervix or urine can provide immediate results. If bacterial vaginosis or trichomonas, may still insert IUD and start treatment on the same visit (CDC 2010 MEC)
- Increased risk of infection in first 20 days after insertion (approximately 1/1000 women will get PID)
- Offers no protection from HIV/STIs; PID: see data in box below
- May be expelled obviously (with cramping and bleeding) or silently (unknowingly placing woman at risk for pregnancy). Rate of expulsion declines over time. At 5 years cumulative explusion rate (partial or complete) is 11.3%. Expulsion rate for the 5th year is 0.3%. Women who have expelled one IUD have about a one in three chance of expelling an IUD if another is inserted *[Grimes-2004]*

**COMPLICATIONS:** See PROBLEM MANAGEMENT section for details

| *Complication* | *Frequency* | *Risk factors* |
|---|---|---|
| PID within 20 days | 1/1000 | BV, cervicitis, contamination with insertion |
| Uterine perforation | 1/1000 | Immobile, markedly verted uterus<br>Breast-feeding woman<br>Inexperienced, unskilled inserter |
| Vasovagal reaction or Fainting with insertion | Rare | Stenotic os, pain<br>Prior vasovagal reaction |
| Expulsion | | Insertion on menses, immediately postpartum, not high enough in fundus or nulliparous |
| Pregnancy | | Poor placement, expulsion |

**CANDIDATES FOR USE:** ***Think of IUDs as reversible sterilization***

- See 2010 CDC Medical Eligibility Criteria, Page A1
- Currently recommended patient profile includes women who are not at high risk of STI's. The long acting reversible contraceptives (IUDs and implants) are best for women seeking longer-term (≥ 1 year) pregnancy protection due to their high initial cost
- Nulligravid women at low risk for STIs are candidates
- Women with history of PID are candidates if they currently are not at high risk
- Good option for women who cannot or do not want to use hormones

***Adolescents:*** Adolescents usually meet all the criteria for IUD use

- ➔ Counsel on menstrual cycle changes. Ask ***"Will a change in your menstrual bleeding pattern be acceptable to you?"*** Particularly important for women considering LNG-IUDs.

**PRESCRIBING PRECAUTIONS:** See US MEC, **Appendix**

- Pregnancy

- Uterus < 6 cm or > 9 cm (package insert, but may be able to use if >9 cm. Some clinicians use an upper limit of 10-12 cm) or greater especially if post abortion or delivery. Experienced clinicians occasionally do insert an IUD for a woman whose uterus only sounds 5.5 cm.
- Undiagnosed abnormal vaginal bleeding
- Severe anemia (relative contraindication) (levonorgestrel IUD would be a good choice)
- Active cervicitis or active pelvic infection or known symptomatic actinomycosis
- Women with current STI, STI within 3 months or women at risk (multiple sex partners)
- Recent endometritis (last 3 months)
- Allergy to copper; Wilson's disease
- Uterine anomaly or fibroid(s) distorting uterine cavity (US MEC 4) preventing fundal placement of IUD
- AIDS (US MEC: 3), HIV-infected (US MEC: 2), AIDS, clinically well on antiretoviral therapy (US MEC: 2), high risk of HIV (US MEC: 2) IUDs do not increase complications in women with HIV/AIDS *[Curtis - 2002]*
- Known or suspected uterine or cervical CA - Insertion (US MEC: 4), continuation (US MEC: 2)

## INITIATING METHOD

- Requires insertion by trained professional
- May be inserted at any time in cycle when pregnancy can be ruled out; lowest overall rates of expulsion are when insertion is at midcycle. No backup needed
- May be inserted immediately after induced, therapeutic spontaneous abortion if no infection (increased risk of expulsion if > second trimester)
- May be inserted immediately after delivery of the placenta or may await complete uterine involution postpartum, usually after 4 weeks
- May be inserted following second or third trimester loss (increased risk of expulsion)
- One IUD may be removed and a second inserted at the same visit
- Test for cervical infection, if indicated. Rule out BV; can start BV or trichomonas Rx and insert IUD the same day (US MEC 2)

## INSERTION TIPS: Each step should be performed slowly and gently

- All clinicians wanting to insert IUDs would benefit from training in IUD insertion
- Signed consent form
- May give NSAIDs one hour prior to insertion
- Be sure patient is not pregnant
- Routine antibiotic prophylaxis is not warranted; American Heart Association requires **no** antibiotic treatment for mitral valve prolapse, except for women at high risk for bacterial endocarditis
- Recheck position, size and mobility of uterus prior to insertion
- Cleanse upper vaginal, outer cervix, and cervical os and canal thoroughly with antiseptic
- Local anesthesia at tenaculum site: 3 approaches are 1) no anesthesia 2) apply benzocaine 20% gel first at tenaculum site then leave a gel-soaked cotton-tipped applicator in cervical canal for 1 minute before proceeding with IUD insertion 3) inject 1 ml of local anesthetic into the cervical lip into which the tenaculum will be placed
- Most women will NOT need a cervical anesthetic. However, can give 5 cc of local anesthetic at 3 and 9 o'clock
- Misoprostol (MIS) is sometimes recommended as a way to diminish pain and risk for a vasovagal reaction at the time of an IUD insertion and to make insertion easier. But the results are mixed. In one large study, there was no difference in pain and insertion was reported to be marginally easier *(Saav-2007)*. In another study, pain was actually greater in women receiving MPL and 50% of women receiving misoprostol experienced nausea *(Shafer-2010)* A recent RCT of Miso 400 mcg buccal 2-4h before procedure vs. placebo did not ease insertion in nulliparous women.
- Place tenaculum to stabilize cervix and straighten uterine axis.
- Sound uterus to fundus with uterine sound or pipelle; uterus should be between 6-9 cm.

**Figure 23.1 How to insert a Copper IUD**

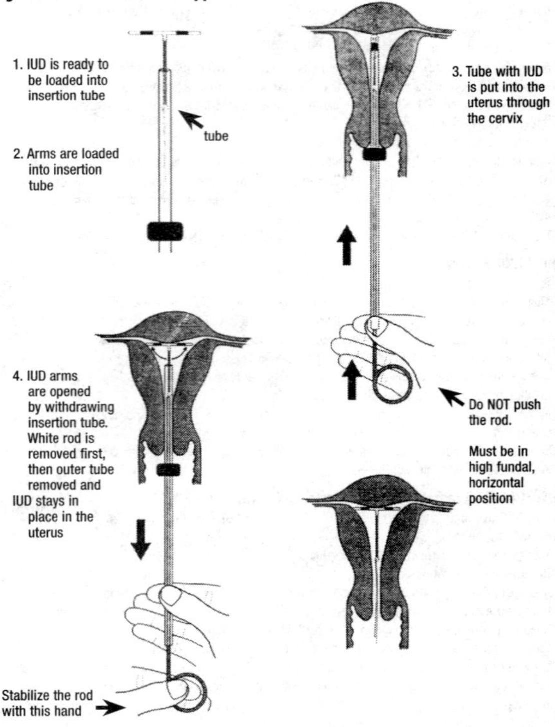


*[Speroff L, Darney P. A clinical guide for contraception. 4th ed. Baltimore: Lippincott, Williams & Wilkins, 2005:246.]*

- After insertion, trim strings to about 2" (3 1/2 cm). Mark length of strings on chart for later follow-up visits to confirm that length is the same. Also chart lot number
- If in doubt that IUD is at the fundus check with sonography

## POSTPLACENTAL & IMMEDIATE POSTPARTUM INSERTION

- Postplacental (preferably within 10 minutes after expulsion of the placenta) is a convenient, effective and safe time to insert Copper IUDs and can be done at ceserean section. Most studies are from developing countries
- Easiest to do in women with an epidural in place
- Expulsion rates for post-placental are higher (7- 15% at 6 months) and require that women receiving an IUD very soon after delivery be told how to detect expulsions and are instructed to return for reinsertion
- Unplanned pregnancy rates of post placental IUD insertion range from 2.0 - 2.8 per 100 users at 24 months *[O'Hanley-1992]*. After 1 year, one study found a failure rate of 0.8% following post-placental IUD insertion, comparable to interval insertions *[Thiery-1985]*
- The risk of infection is low following post-placental IUD insertion, with rates of 0.1% to 1.1% *[Lean-1967][Dharmeapanij-1970][Snidvongs-1970][Cole-1984]*. Rates of perforation are very low during post-placental IUD insertion, approximately 1 perforation in each study with patient populations ranging from 1150 to 3800 women *[Cole-1984][Edelman-1979][Phatak-1970]*
- Trim strings at level of cervix

**Figure 23.2 Two techniques of postplacental IUD insertion and proper location of IUD after insertion**

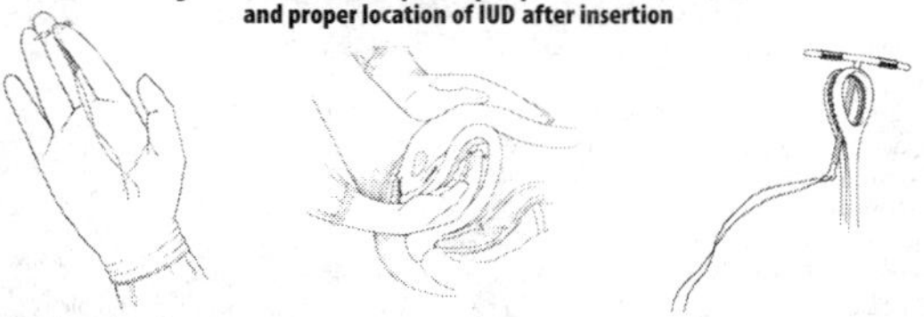

A) IUD strings placed in palm of hand | B) Manual insertion at top of fundus | C) Use of ring forceps to insert IUD

## INSTRUCTIONS FOR PATIENT

- Give patient trimmed IUD strings to learn what to check for after menses each month (strings may not be apparent until a few months after post-placental insertion)
- Advise patients to return if any symptoms of pregnancy, infection or IUD loss develop:

| *PAINS: "Early IUD Warning Signs"* | |
|---|---|
| **P** | Period late (pregnancy); abnormal spotting or bleeding |
| **A** | Abdominal pain, pain with intercourse |
| **I** | Infection exposure (STI); abnormal vaginal discharge |
| **N** | Not feeling well, fever, chills |
| **S** | String missing, shorter or longer |

**FOLLOW-UP:** Ask about risk for STIs. Offer condoms in large numbers to all women

- Have patient return for post-insertion check about 2 1/2 months after insertion to rule out partial expulsion or other problems requiring removal. Return earlier if any problems
- May be left in place during evaluation and treatment for cervical dysplasia
- Can you feel your IUD strings? Have they changed in length?
- Have you or your partner had any new partners since your last visit?

## PROBLEM MANAGEMENT

***Uterine perforation: All perforations occur or begin at insertion but may go unrecognized***

- Clinical signs: pain, loss of resistance to advancement of instrument and instrument introduced deeper than uterus thought to be on bimanual exam
- Perforation by uterine sound usually occurs in midline posterior uterine wall when there is marked flexion:
  - Remove uterine sound
  - Observe for several hours. Administer antibiotics. If no bleeding seen, stable BP and pulse, patient pain free and hematocrit stable for next several hours, she may be sent home. Provide alternate contraception
  - If any persistent pain or signs of other organ damage, take or refer immediately for laparoscopic evaluation (extremely rare)
- If IUD perforates acutely, attempt removal by gently pulling on strings
  - If resistance encountered, stop and do pelvic ultrasound and/or send to surgery for immediate laparoscopic IUD removal
- If IUD perforation noted and confirmed by ultrasound at later date, if asymptomatic, arrange for elective laparoscopic removal. Provide interval contraceptive. Can have IUD inserted later (i.e. not a contraindication to future IUDs)

***Spotting, frequent or heavy bleeding, hemorrhage, anemia:***

- All problems may be minimized with combined pills X 3 cycles or by NSAIDS.
- All may be managed by cycling with COCs for several cycles or by nonsteroidal anti-inflammatory agents (NSAIDS)
- Rule out pregnancy. If pregnant, rule out ectopic pregnancy
- Rule out infection, especially if post-coital bleeding
- Rule out expulsion or partial expulsion of IUD (see below)
- If anemic, provide iron supplement and deal with cause
- Consider replacement with the LNG-IUD

***Cramping and/or pain:***

- Rule out pregnancy, infection, IUD expulsion
- Offer NSAIDs with menses or just before menses to reduce cramping
- Consider copper IUD removal and use of LNG IUD or use another method if problem.

***Expulsion/partial expulsion:***

- If expulsion confirmed (IUD seen by patient or clinician), rule out pregnancy. May place a new IUD
- If expulsion suspected, use ultrasound to determine IUD absence or presence and location. Probe endocervical canal for IUD, remove if not properly placed. May replace immediately if patient not pregnant and does not have a purulent cervical discharge or PID
- If not seen on ultrasound, do abdominal x-ray to rule out extrauterine location
- If partial expulsion, remove IUD. If no infections and not pregnant, may replace with new IUD. If IUD not replaced, provide new contraceptive

***Finding missing strings in non-pregnant patients:***

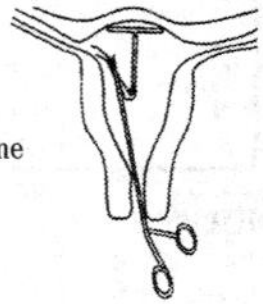

- Check vagina for strings. Assess string length. If normal, reassure and re-instruct patient how to feel for strings
- Twist cytobrush inside cervix to snag strings which may have become snarled in canal
- Ultrasound to determine IUD presence and exact location
- If IUD in endocervix, remove and offer to replace
- If IUD correctly in uterus, IUD may be left in place or removed.

- If decision is made to remove IUD after paracervical block, attempt to remove with IUD hook or alligator forceps (some clinicians obtain signed consent after reviewing risks of procedure) or refer for ultrasound to localize prior to attempted removal (provide interim birth control). A 5mm Novak currette (much more painful than alligator forceps) and/or concurrent sonography may be useful in removal of IUDs. In non-pregnant patients, removal may also be done under hysteroscopy
- After insertion following C-section, IUD stumps may come down through the cervix, remain in the uterus cavity or be retrieved
- 200 mcg vaginal misoprostol the night before attempted removal may cause strings to exit cervix and facilitate removal *[Cowman 2012]*

***Pregnancy with visible strings:***

- Visible strings in first trimester: advise removal of IUD to reduce risk of spontaneous abortion and premature labor
- Patient having miscarriage: Remove IUD. Consider antibiotics for 7 days

***Missing strings in pregnant patients:***

- Rule out ectopic pregnancy: 5-8% of all failures with the copper IUD are ectopic
- If intrauterine pregnancy, obtain ultrasound to verify IUD in situ
- If IUD is in uterus, advise patient she is at increased risk for preterm labor and spontaneous abortion but reassure her that fetus is not at increased risk for birth defects. May remove IUD at surgery if patient desires elective abortion. Otherwise, plan for removal at delivery

***Infection with IUD use:***

- *BV or candidiasis:* treat routinely
- *Trichomoniasis:* treat and stress importance of condoms to prevent STIs
- *Cervicitis or PID:* Give first dose of antibiotics to achieve adequate serum levels before removing IUD. IUD removal not necessary unless no improvement after antibiotic Rx. Patient may not be candidate for continued IUD use. (US MEC: 2 for continuation for both STI and PID)
- *Actinomycosis:* Cultures of asymptomatic women without an IUD AND of women with an IUD find that 3-4% of both are positive for Actinomyces *[Lippes, J. Am J Obstet Gyn-1999; 180-2 65-9]*. Often suggested by Pap smear report of "Actinomycosis-like organisms". True upper tract infection with this organism is very serious and requires prolonged IV antibiotic therapy with penicillin. However, less than half of women with such Pap smear reports have actinomyces and those that do usually have asymptomatic colonization only. Examine patient for any signs of PID (it can be unilateral). If signs of upper tract involvement, remove IUD and treat with antibiotics x 1 month. If patient has no clinical evidence of upper tract involvement, 3 options are available depending on patient's wishes and risk of infection:
  1. Conservative. Annual pap smears only. Advise patient to return as needed or if she develops PID symptoms or
  2. Treat with antibiotic penicillin G (500 mg qid p.o. x 2 weeks) or a tetracycline(tetracycline 500 mg qid p.o. for a month OR doxycyline 100 mg bid x 2 weeks) and repeat Pap smear or remove if no clearance of organism or
  3. Treat with antibiotic, remove IUD, and repeat Pap smear in 1 month. Reinsert if colonization cleared

**Figure 23.3**

## MANAGEMENT OF THE IUD WHEN A CU-IUD OR AN LNG-IUD USER HAS PID
### CDC Selected Practice Recommendations (SPR)

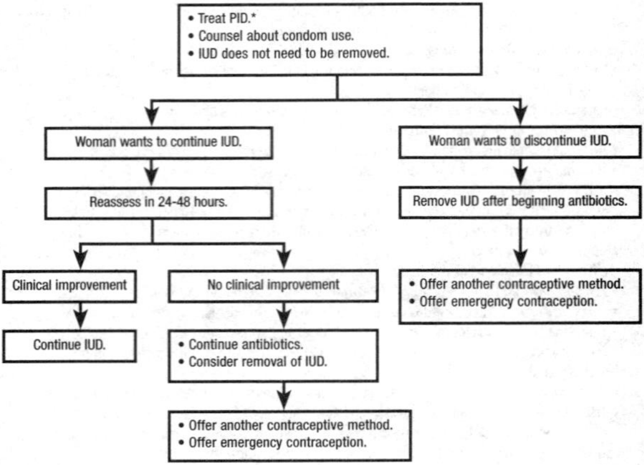


**Abbreviations:** Cu-IUD =copper-containing IUD; IUD= intrauterine device; LNG-IUD= levonorgestrel-releasing IUD; PID =pelvic infla matory disease.
* Treat according to CDC's STD Treatment Guidelines (available at http:/ lwww.cdc.govlstdl treatment).
*CDC MMWR June 21, 2013, Vol. 62:No. 5*

## REMOVAL
***Indications:*** Expelling IUD, infection, pregnant, expired IUD, complications with IUD, anemia, no longer candidate for IUD, patient request.
***Procedure:*** Grasp the strings close to external os and steadily retract until IUD removed
***Complications***
- Embedded IUD: Gentle rotation of strings may free IUD. If still stuck, may use alligator forceps removal with or without sonographic guidance (see Missing strings, Page 94). Hysteroscopic removal may be indicated in rare cases. A paracervical block reduces pain from removal of an embedded IUD
- Broken strings: Remove IUD with alligator forceps, IUD hook or Novak curette (more painful)

## FERTILITY AFTER DISCONTINUATION OF METHOD

Immediate return to baseline fertility

## LEVONORGESTREL INTRAUTERINE SYSTEMS (Mirena® and Skyla®)

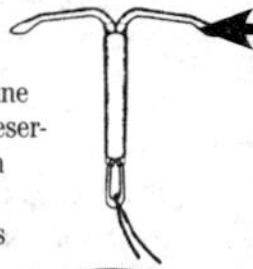

**DESCRIPTION:** Mirena is a T-shaped intrauterine contraceptive placed within uterine cavity that initially releases 20 micrograms/day of levonorgestrel from its vertical reservoir. Release falls to 14 mcg per day after 5 years. Concentrations of LNG are much higher in the endometrium than in the myometrium and the circulating blood *[Nilsson-1982]*. Product information/ordering: 1-866-647-3646. IUD has 2 gray strings

**EFFECTIVENESS: Mirena remains effective for at least 5 years, Skyla for 3 years**

*Perfect use failure rate in first year:* 0.1% (See Table 12.2, Page 37)

*Typical use failure rate of Mirena in first year:* 0.1% *[Trussell J. IN CT, 2004]*

*5-year cumulative failure rate of Mirena:* 0.7%

*7-year cumulative failure rate of Mirena:* 1.1% *[Sivin-1991]*

- 1-year continuation rate in Finland: 93%; 2 years: 87% *[Bachman-BJOG, 2000]*

**Now indicated and extensively used as contraceptive for women with heavy menstrual bleeding**

**HOW LEVONORGESTREL IUD WORKS:** Levonorgestrel works primarily by causing cervical mucus to become thicker, so sperm can not enter upper reproductive tract and do not reach ovum. Changes in uterotubal fluid also impair sperm and ovum migration. Alteration of the endometrium prevents implantation of fertilized ovum. This IUD has some anovulatory effect (5-15% of treatment cycles; higher in first years)

**COST:** $843.60. See Page 164 (Ordering and Stocking Device chapter). $0.00 if covered by Affordable Care Act.

- **The ARCH Foundation supplies Mirena intrauterine contraceptives to providers caring for economically disadvantaged women whose insurance does not cover Mirena. They also provide funds for removal to qualifying individuals. Go to www.archfoundation.com**
- **Mirena units that are contaminated or must be removed in first 3 months or are expelled *may* be replaced free of cost. Contact Bayer: 1-866-647-3646 or 1-888-842-2937**

## ADVANTAGES

*Menstrual:* **Dysmenorrhea generally improves**

- Menorrhagia improves (at 12 months, 90% less blood loss with LNG IUS; 50% with COCs; 30% with prostaglandin inhibitors). Among 44 menorrhagic women receiving Mirena, only 2 were still menorrhagic at 3 months. At 9 and 12 months 21 of 44 were amenorrheic *[Monteiro-2002]*
- After 3 to 6 months of menstrual irregularities (mostly spotting), Mirena decreases menstrual blood loss more than 70% (97% reduction in blood loss in one study) *[Monteiro-2002]*
- Amenorrhea develops in approximately 20% of users by 1 year and in 60% by 5 years
- Decreased surgery (hysterectomies, endometrial ablation, D & C) for menorrhagia, endometriosis, idiopathic causes of bleeding, leiomyomata or adenomyosis
- Indicated by product labeling for heavy menstrual bleeding

*Sexual/psychological:*

- Convenient: permits spontaneous sexual activity. Requires no action at time of intercourse
- Reduced fear of pregnancy can make sex more pleasurable

*Cancers, tumors and masses:*

- Protective effect against endometrial hyperplasia, endometrial cancer, fibroids
- Comparative cohort study of Mirena vs. oral progestogens for complex non-atypical or atypical endometrial hyperplasia found regression in 95% Mirena users vs. 84% oral progestogen users (OR 3.04 (95% CI 1.36-6.79, p=0.001) *[Gallos 2013]*

*Other: **Extremely effective; as effective or more effective than female sterilization***

- May be used as the progestin for endometrial protection with menopausal estrogen treatment
- ***Decreased*** risk for ectopic pregnancy by 80% *[Anderson-1994]*
  - Several studies show decreased PID, endometritis and cervicitis in LNG-IUS users
- Reduces symptoms e.g. pain of endometriosis *[Petta-2005]*
- May be used by women at increased risk for DVT or PE and by women with Factor V Leiden and other thrombogenic mitations (US MEC:2)

## DISADVANTAGES

*Menstrual:* **(Removal of LNG - IUD (Mirena) for any bleeding problem in first year: 7.6%)**

- Number of spotting and bleeding days is significantly higher than normal for first few months and lower than normal after 3 to 6 months of using levonorgestrel intrauterine system
- Amenorrhea (a negative if not explained, a positive for some women if explained well in advance) occurs in about 20% of women at one year of use
- May cause cramping following insertion
- Expulsion: 2.9% in women using Mirena exclusively for contraception; 8.9% to 13.6% in women using Mirena to control heavy bleeding *[Diaz-2000] [Monteiro-2002]*

***Sexual/psychological:***

- Same as Copper IUD except when spotting and bleeding may interfere with sexual activity
- Loss of menses means hard to keep track of menstrual cyclicity symptoms (e.g. PMS)

***Other:***

- Offers no protection against viral STIs like HPV or HIV
- Persistent unruptured follicles may cause ovarian cysts; most regress spontaneously
- Hormonal side effects: headaches, acne, mastalgia, moodiness including depression/anxiety
- Brief discomfort after insertion or removal

**COMPLICATIONS:** See 2010 US MEC - Appendix

- PID risk transiently increased after insertion (highest in first 3 weeks)
- Perforation of uterus at time of insertion (less than 1 in 1000)

**CANDIDATES FOR USE:** ***You can almost think of Mirena as a "forgettable" contraceptive***

- Women wanting effective, reversible long-term contraception including nulliparous women and women wanting to avoid tubal sterilization. While in place, as effective as laparoscopic or transcervical tubal sterilization
- Can be used in women with heavy menses, endometriosis, fibroids, cramps or anemia
- Menopausal women using estrogen, with intact uteri, who are unable to tolerate oral progestins are protected against endometrial carcinoma by using a levonorgestrel intrauterine contraceptive (off-label) *[Raudaskoski, 1995] [Luukkainen, Steroids - 2000]*
- Formal FDA approval is being sought for the use of the LNG IUS to treat menorrhagia
- 2010 CDC practice recommendations include post placental insertion of LNG-IUS up to 48 hours in women. Only a pilot study of 20 women is published on this topic *[Hayes-2007]*. Probably associated with a higher expulsion rate than interval insertion.

**PRESCRIBING PRECAUTIONS:** See CDC Precautions in Appendix

- May be used by woman with past history of ectopic pregnancy (CDC:1)

**INITIATING METHOD:** ***Each step should be performed slowly and gently***

- ***The one-hand insertion technique is different from current Copper IUDs. Training sessions may be set up by calling 1-888-84-BAYER.*** See Figure 25.3, pages 92-93
- If inserted within 7 days from LMP, no backup needed. She can have it inserted any other time of cycle if reasonably certain not pregnant, but add backup or abstinence x 7 days
- Insertion tube is 2 mm wider than for copper intrauterine contraceptives; may rarely need to dilate cervix
- Paracervical block may be required, especially for nulliparas

- Counsel in advance to expect menstrual cycle changes, including amenorrhea. Women using levonorgestrel contraceptive system who received information in advance about possible bleeding changes and amenorrhea were significantly more likely to be highly satisfied with the contraceptive. *[Backman-2002]*
- Advise NSAIDs for post-insertion discomfort. If pain persists, she must return

**INSTRUCTIONS FOR PATIENT:** Similar to copper intrauterine contraceptive, Page 93. Monthly string checks are particularly important for women using a levonorgestrol IUD for menorrhagia because of higher expulsion rates.

**FOLLOW-UP:** Same as Copper IUD

**PROBLEM MANAGEMENT:** Similar to Copper T 380-A; see Page 94

- ***Perforation:*** A case report from Israel actually looked at serum LNG levels from Mirena in the omentum following uterine perforation. They were higher than POP serum levels. So, theoretically, an abdominal Mirena IUD still provides adequate contraceptive effect until it is removed. Condoms and removal of IUD still recommended!

**FERTILITY AFTER DISCONTINUATION OF METHOD:** Immediate return to baseline fertility

### Figure 22.3 INSERTION TIPS: Each step should be performed slowly and gently

- All clinicians wanting to insert IUDs would benefit from training in IUD insertion
- Reconfirm signed consent
- May give NSAIDs one hour prior to insertion
- Be sure patient is not pregnant
- Routine antibiotic prophylaxis is not warranted; American Heart Association requires **no** antibiotic treatment for mitral valve prolapse, except for women at high risk for bacterial endocarditis
- Recheck position, size and mobility of uterus prior to insertion
- Cleanse upper vaginal, outer cervix, and cervical os and canal thoroughly with antiseptic
- Local anesthesia at tenaculum site: 3 approaches are 1) no anesthesia 2) apply benzocaine 20% gel first at tenaculum site then leave a gel-soaked cotton-tipped applicator in cervical canal for 1 minute before proceeding with IUD insertion (Speroff/Darney p. 245) 3) inject 1 ml of local anesthetic (1% chloroprocaine) into the cervical lip into which the tenaculum will be placed
- Most women will NOT need a paracervical block. However, can give 5 cc of local anesthetic at 3 and 9 o'clock
- Place tenaculum to stabilize cervix and straighten uterine axis.
- Sound uterus to fundus with uterine sound or pipelle; uterus should be at least 6 cm, but no strict limits.

**MIRENA® and Inserter**

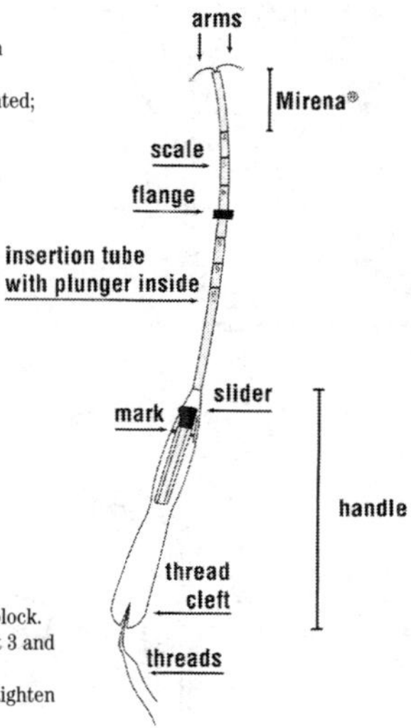

- Pick up Mirena and release the threads from slider so they hang freely
- Push slides in the furthest position away from you while pulling threads to load Mirena making sure arms stay horizontal
- Fix threads in cleft
- Set flange to depth measured by sound
- Keep thumb on slider as you insert Mirena into uterus
- Advance Mirena until the flange is 1.5 - 2 cm from external os
- Pull back slider until it reaches mark while holding inserter steady. Wait 30 seconds to allow arms to open within uterus
- Advance Mirena until flange touches cervix allowing Mirena to reach fundus
- Hold inserter in position while pulling slides down all the way. The threads should be released automatically from cleft. If not, manually remove the strings from the cleft
- Withdraw Mirena inserter from uterus
- Cut threads to 2 inches; requires care and sharp scissors to avoid dislodging Mirena
- Hand patient cut strings so she knows what to feel for during string check

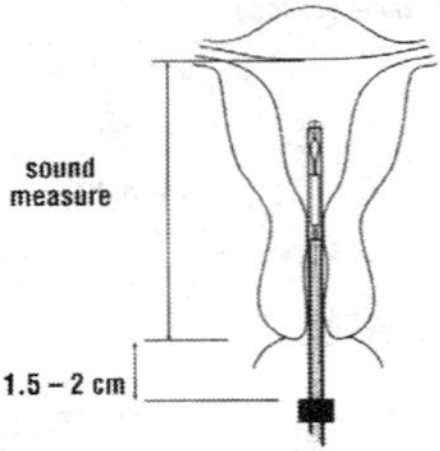


**Flange adjusted to sound depth**

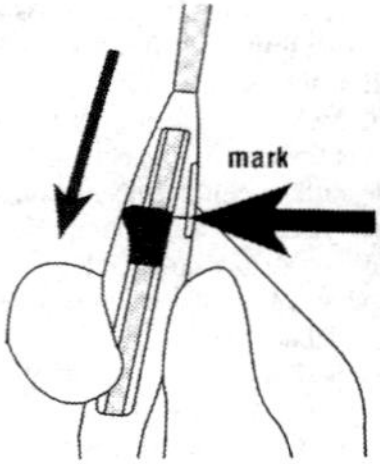


**Pulling the slider back to reach the mark**

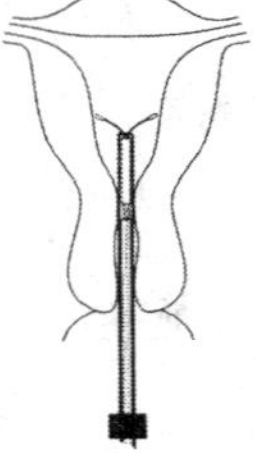

**The arms of the MIRENA® being released**

Teens in the contraceptive CHOICE project continue to use the LARC methods longer than the shorter-acting methods. 48% of the 9,256 women in this study chose to use the levonorgestrel IUD, Mirena.

## LEVONORGESTREL INTRAUTERINE SYSTEM (Skyla)

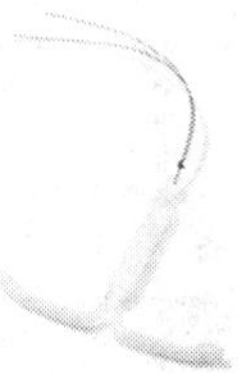

**DESCRIPTION:** T-shaped IUC, similar to Mirena, produced by the same manufacturer, but lower dose and smaller, and indicated for 3 years (vs. 5 to 7 years for Mirena). Skyla has a reservoir of 13.5mg of levonorgestrel, initially releasing 14mcg/day decreasing to 5mcg/day at 3 years of use. Product ordering same as Mirena.

**EFFECTIVENESS:** Effective for up to 3 years of use
***Perfect use failure rate in first year:*** 0.41%, 95% CI upper limit 0.96%
***Cumulative failure at 3 years:*** 0.9%, 95% CI upper limit, 1.7

### Differences from Mirena:

Skyla has much of the same profile as Mirena. Here are the differences:

| | Mirena | Skyla |
|---|---|---|
| Size | 32mm wide/32mm long | 28mm wide/30mm long |
| Hormone reservoir | 52mg LNG | 13.5mm LNG |
| Initial release rate | 20mcg/day | 14mcg/day |
| Inserter diameter | 4.75mm | 3.8mm |

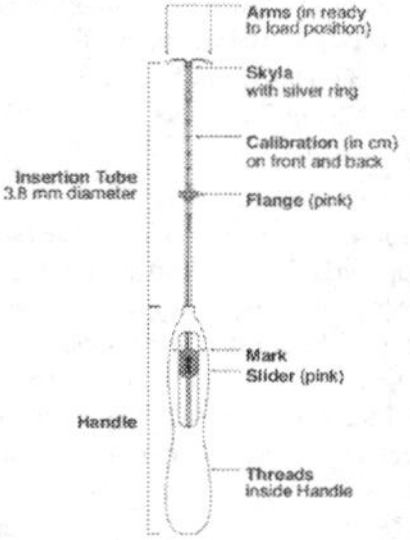


- Inserter of Skyla differs by having the strings preloaded inside inserter so no threads are hanging out of inserter. It is non-reloadable, arms are pre-aligned in inserter, and the diameter is narrower.
- Indication by product label: While Mirena label says recommended for women who have had at least one child, Skyla doesn't mention this and the clinical trial enrolled 39% nulliparous women. In practice, Mirena is used extensively by both nulligravid and nulliparous women.
- Bleeding profile: Bleeding profile similar to Mirena, but appears to have less reduction in menstrual blood flow

### Insertion Tips:

- A complete medical and social history should be obtained to determine conditions that might influence the selection of a levonorgestrel-releasing intrauterine system (LNG IUS) for contraception. If indicated, perform a physical examination, and appropriate tests for any forms of genital or other sexually transmitted infections.
- Follow the insertion instructions exactly as described in order to ensure proper placement and avoid premature release of Skyla from the inserter. <u>Once released, Skyla cannot be re-loaded.</u>
- Skyla should be inserted by a trained healthcare provider. Healthcare providers should become thoroughly familiar with the insertion instructions before attempting insertion of Skyla.
- Insertion may be associated with some pain and/or bleeding or vasovagal reactions (for example, syncope, bradycardia) or seizure in an epileptic patient, especially in patients with a predisposition to these conditions. Consider administering analgesics prior to insertion.

### Timing of insertion:

- Insert Skyla into the uterine cavity during the first seven days of the menstrual cycle or immediately after a first trimester abortion. Back up contraception is not needed when Skyla is inserted as directed.
- Postpone postpartum insertion and insertions following second trimester abortions a minimum of six weeks or until the uterus is fully involuted. If involution is delayed, wait until involution is complete before insertion.

**Tools for insertion:**

*Preparation*

- Gloves • Speculum • Sterile uterine sound • Sterile tenaculum
- Antiseptic solution, applicator

*Procedure*

- Sterile gloves • Skyla with inserter in sealed package
- Instruments and anesthesia for paracervical block, if anticipated
- Consider having an unopened backup Skyla available • Sterile, sharp curved scissors

**Preparation for insertion**

- Exclude pregnancy and confirm that there are no contraindications to the use of Skyla
- Ensure that the patient understands the contents of the Patient Information Booklet and obtain the signed patient informed consent located on the last page of the Patient Information Booklet.
- With the patient comfortably in lithotomy position, do a bimanual exam to establish the size, shape and postition of the uterus.
- Gently insert a speculum to visualize the cervix.
- Thoroughly cleanse the cervix and vagina with a suitable antiseptic solution.
- Prepare to sound the uterine cavity. Grasp the upper lip of the cervix with a tenaculum forceps and gently apply traction to stabilize and align the cervical canal with the uterine cavity. Perform a paracervical block if needed. If the uterus is retroverted, it may be more appropriate to grasp the lower lip of the cervix. The tenaculum should remain in position and gentle traction on the cervix should be maintained throughout the insertion procedure.
- Gently insert a uterine sound to check the patency of the cervix, measure the depth of the uterine cavity in centimeters, confirm cavity direction, and detect the presence of any uterine anomaly. If you encounter difficulty or cervical stenosis, use dilatation, and not force, to overcome resistance. If cervical dilatation is required, consider using a paracervical block.

**Insertion procedure**

**Proceed with insertion only after completing the above steps and ascertaining that the patient is appropriate for Skyla. The uterus should always be sounded —no exceptions.** Ensure use of aseptic technique throughout the entire procedure.

**Step 1: Opening of the package**

- Open the package. The contents of the package are sterile.
- Using sterile gloves, lift the handle of the sterile interior and remove from the sterile package.

**Step 2: Load Skyla into the insertion tube**

- Push the slider forward as far as possible in the direction of the arrow thereby moving the insertion tube over the Skyla T-body to load Skyla into the insertion tube. The tips of the arms will meet to form a rounded end that extends slightly beyond the insertion tube.
- Maintain forward pressure with your thumb or forefinger on the slider. DO NOT move the slider downward at this time as this may prematurely release the threads of Skyla. Once the slider is moved below the mark, Skyla cannot be re-loaded.

**Step 3: Setting the flange**

- Holding the slider in this forward position, set the upper edge of the flange to correspond to the uterine depth (in centimeters) measured during sounding.

**Step 4: Skyla is now ready to be inserted**

- Continue holding the slider in this forward position. Advance the inserter through the cervix until the flange is approximately 1.5-2 cm from the cervix and then pause. Do not force the inserter. If necessary, dilate the cervical canal.

**Step 5: Open the arms**

- While folding the inserter steady, move the slider down to the mark to release the arms of Skyla. Wait 10 seconds for the horizontal arms to open completely.

**Step 6: Advance to fundal position**
• Advance the inserter gently toward the fundus of the uterus until the flange touches the cervix. If you encounter fundal resistance do not continue to advance. Skyla is now in the fundal position. Fundal positioning of Skyla is important to prevent expulsion.
**Step 7: Release Skyla and withdraw the inserter**
• Holding the entire inserter firmly in place, release Skyla by moving the slider all the way down.
• Continue to hold the slider all the way down while you slowly and gently withdraw the inserter from the uterus.
• Using a sharp, curved scissor, cut the threads perpendicular, leaving about 3cm visible outside of the cervix (cutting threads at an angle may leave sharp ends). Do not apply tension or pull on the threads when cutting to prevent displacing Skyla.

Skyla insertion is now complete. Prescribe analgesics, if indicated. Keep a copy of the Consent Form with lot number for your records.

*Important information to consider during or after insertion:*
• If you suspect that Skyla is not in the correct position, check placement (for example, using transvaginal ultrasound). Remove Skyla if it is not positioned completely within the uterus. A removed Skyla must not be reinserted.
• If there is clinical concern, exceptional pain or bleeding during or after insertion, appropriate steps should be taken immediately to excludeperforation, such as physical examination and ultrasound.

## Today about half of all pregnancies are unintended and close to half of all unintended pregnancies lead to abortions. It was the same in 1966.

**If the world wants to avoid the consequences of unintended and unwanted pregnancies, we will need to approach sex and contraception *differently*. Just remember Albert Einstein's definition of *Insanity: doing the same thing over and over again and expecting different results.***

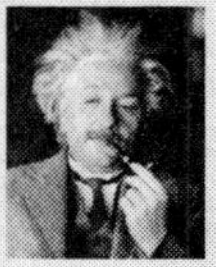

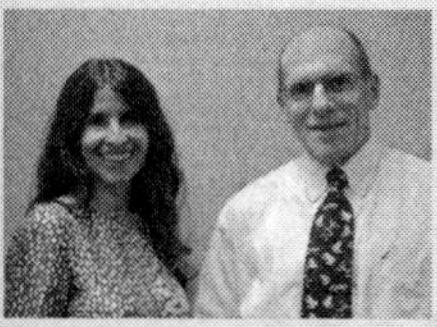

**Gina Secura and Jeffrey Peipert**

The remarkable **ST. LOUIS CONTRACEPTIVE CHOICE PROJECT** did provide contraceptives to **9,256** women very differently and **75%** of them chose to use one of the long-acting reversible contraceptives. How did they accomplish this on a completely voluntary basis? Gina Secura and Jeffrey Peipert suggest three answers:
1. The **effectiveness** of IUDs and implants is the first thing a woman is told about when she is considering entering this project. **"A woman is more than 20 times more likely to become pregnant if she uses pills, patches, or rings than if she uses an IUD or an implant."**
2. **Access.** At all the sites it was possible for women to receive an IUD or an implant. Trained personnel were there. The IUDs and implants were there. Delay was minimized.
3. **The price was right!** Contraceptives, screening for STIs and treatment for STIs if necessary, condoms for all contraceptors and pelvic exams when indicated were provided at **no cost at all.**
*(Winner, Peipert, NEJM 2012) (Renee Mestad, et al. Contraception, 2011) (Peipert Obstet Gynecol, 2012)*
Teen births fell to 6.3 per 1,000 in the Choice/St. Louis cohort vs. 34.3 per 1,000 in the U.S. *(Peipert, Madden Obstet Gynecol, 2012)*
The percent of abortions that were repeat abortions fell to less than half the average when compared to the national rate. *(Peipert, Madden Obstet Gynecol, 2012)*

**So what can we do to decrease unintended pregnancies? Seven possibilities:**

**1. Use more Long Acting Reversible Contraceptives: IUDs and implants.**

**2. ParaGard, the Copper T 380A IUD, is the emergency contraceptive of choice.** In one Asian study, IUD insertion within several days of unprotected sex led to **not one pregnancy in 1,963** women *(Godfrey 3 JOG 2010)* and provides them long term highly effective contraception. **Emergency contraceptive pills have almost no global effect at all.**

**3. Place IUDs or an implant right after delivery.** Within 10 minutes of the delivery of the placenta, whether delivery is by caesarian section or vaginally, a copper T IUD or a levonorgestrel IUD may be placed. This may be done for breastfeeding and non-breastfeeding women. This has been accomplished for 4,000 women delivering vaginally using a sponge forceps that is longer so that it reaches all the way to the top of the fundus. The expulsion rate was 1.6%, and the cost of the forceps is $7. Immediately following uterine aspiration for an induced abortion or a miscarriage, place an IUD or an implant. *(Bednarek NEJM June 9, 2011)*

**Planners of the St. Louis contraceptive CHOICE project estimated that 10% of the cohort of 10,000 women would choose an IUD and 3% an implant** *[Piepert, Madden 2012]*. **What transpired was completely different. Of 9,256 women enrolled, 46.0% chose a Levonorgestrel IUD, 11.9% a copper IUD, 16.9% chose an implant (78.4% chose a LARC or forgettable method).**

**4. Please accurately describe the duration of effectiveness of our contraceptive options:**

- ParaGard, the Copper T 380-A, is effective for at least 12 years
- Depo-Provera injections are effective for 15 weeks
- Mirena, the levonorgestrel IUD, is effective for at least 7 years
- NuvaRings, ethinyl estradiol and etonogestrel rings, prevent ovulation for 35 days
- Implanon, the etonogestrel implant, is effective for 4 years, possibly longer

**5. Quick start is the right way to start contraception.** Avoid delays: start each method NOW whenever possible.

**6. Tonight, use a condom, withdrawal, abstinence or outercourse.** Advice for anyone: if you are considering having unprotected sex when you do not want to become pregnant. **No mistakes. Not once. Not ever.**

---

What were the menstrual cycle distress factors analysed by Gupta *(Levonorgestrel intrauterine system versus medical therapy for menorrhagia, NEJM 2013, 368: 128-137)*

Heavy menstrual bleeding has several potential negative effects for women. This study analysed the effects of 6 treatments for heavy menstrual bleeding on the following areas of a woman's life:

- Practical life
- Family life
- Work and daily routine
- Psychological well-being
- Physical health

The LNG-IUS was compared to several "usual treatments" regimens which were:

- tranexamic acid
- mefenamic acid
- combined pills
- progestin-only pills
- Depo-Provera injections

**Scores were significantly more likely to improve in all 6 distress domains in women provided a Mirena IUD and the percent continuing to use Mirena at one year, 64%, was strikingly higher than the percent of women continuing to use the other treatments for heavy menstrual bleeding, 38%.**

---

# WORLD'S BEST BIRTH CONTROL
## AT YOUR HEALTH DEPARTMENT

### BIRTH CONTROL EFFECTIVENESS IN 10,000 WOMEN

MORE EFFECTIVE, LESS RISK

| Contraceptive Method | Pregnancies in first year |
|---|---|
| NEXPLANON | 5 |
| MALE STERILIZATION | 15 |
| MIRENA IUD | 20 |
| FEMALE STERILIZATION | 50 |
| PARAGARD IUD | 80 |
| DEPO SHOT | 600 |
| MINIPILL | 900 |
| COMBINATION PILLS* | 900 |
| CONDOM | 1,800 |
| WITHDRAWAL | 2,200 |
| NO METHOD | 8,500 |

**Note the absence of decimal points. This chart points out how much more effective Nexplanon is than pills.**

Nexplanon has a failure rate of 0.05%. Just what does 0.05% mean? This chart shows you!

* Estrogen increases risk for stroke, heart attack, and blood clots.

*This ingenius method of explaining the differences in failure rates by placing the number of pregnancues in the first year of use by typical users over 10,000 women comes to you because of the creative genius of* ***Dr. Claude Burnett*** *in Athens, GA. [Contraceptive Technology, 20 ed. 2011, James Trussell, Typical Use Failure Rates in Hatcher, Trussell et al.]*

# CHAPTER 24

# Combined (Estrogen & Progestin) Contraceptives

www.managingcontraception.com OR www.plannedparenthood.org OR www.noperiod.com

This chapter will describe the methods that provide both an estrogen and a progestin: combined birth control pills, the patch (Page 128) and the vaginal ring (Page 131)

## PILLS - DAILY "THE PILL" COMBINED PILLS

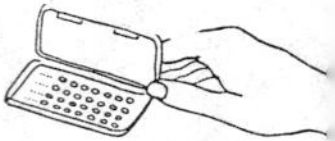

**DESCRIPTION:** Each hormonally active pill in combined pills contains an estrogen and a progestin. Ethinyl estradiol (EE) is the most commonly used estrogen; it is in most 50 µg pills and almost all of the sub-50 µg formulations. Mestranol, which must be metabolized to EE to become biologically active, is found in two 50 µg formulations (rarely prescribed). At least 7 progestins are used in the different pill formulations. Traditional packs have 21 active combined pills, with or without 7 additional pills (usually placebo pills or pills with iron). Many newer formulations have varying numbers of active pills and hormone free pills. For example, Seasonale has 84 consecutive hormonal pills followed by 7 placebo pills. Yaz and Loestrin-24 have 24 days of hormonal pills followed by 4 days of placebo pills. Lybrel, has no hormone free pills. Monophasic formulations contain active pills with the same amount of hormones in each tablet. Multiphasic formulations contain active pills with varying amounts of progestin and/or estrogen in the hormonal pills. All of the recently approved pills have less than 7 inactive pills per cycle

**EFFECTIVENESS** Women were 20 times more likely to become pregnant in one year in the St. Louis CHOICE project if they use contraceptive pills rather than an IUD or implant. *[Winner, Peipert, NEJM 2007]*

***Perfect use failure rate in first year:*** 0.3% (of every 1,000 women who take pills for 1 year, 3 will become pregnant in the first year use) (See Table 12.2, Page 37)

➔ ***Typical use failure rate in first year:*** 9% *[Trussell J IN Contraceptive Technology, 2004]*

**Annual pregnancy rates with typical use of oral contraceptives pills are estimated to be 9% for the general population, 13% for teenagers and 30% or higher for some high-risk subgroups.** *[Kost K, Sigah, Contraception 2008] [Fu H Family Planning Perspectives 1999]*

> **Given that approximately 1,000,000 women become pregnant each year while depending on pills, and 40% of those women choose to have an abortion, many of those women might be better served by taking their pills continuously (no hormone-free days or with 1 or 2 hormone free days per month).**

**HOW PILLS WORK:** Ovulation suppression (90% to 95% of time). Also causes thickening of cervical mucus, which blocks sperm penetration and entry into the upper reproductive tract. Thin, asynchronous endometrium inhibits implantation. Tubal motility slowed.

### COST

- Cost of one cycle: from a few dollars to more than $50. Most pharmacies charge $20-$42/cycle
- Costs differ from region to region, and pills with 50 mcg of estrogen often cost more.
- Generic brands are generally less expensive. They are not required to have clinical testing; they must only prove blood level equivalency (80–125% of parent compound's blood levels).
- Most major insurance companies cover at least some brands of pills
- The co-pay for Seasonale is as much as $60 per a package, but covers 3 months supply

## ADVANTAGES

***Menstrual:***

- Decreased blood loss and decreased anemia may decrease menstrual cramps/pain, and more predictable menses
- **Heavy menstrual bleeding (HMB)** affects 9-14% of women but closer to 30% of women consider their bleeding to be heavy [Nelson A. and Baldwin S. IN Hatcher Contraceptive Technology 20th ed., 2011]. Because of missed work, women with HMB earn an average of $1,692 less annually than women with normal menses [Cote I., et. al., Obstet Gynecol, 2002]. Diseases that may cause HMB: fibroids (leiomyomata), adenomyosis, endometrial and uterine polyps, endometrial hyperplasia and cancer, and diseases of disordered hemostasis. However, only about half of women with HMB have an anatomical pathology identified at hysterectomy [Clark A., et. al., Br J Obstet Gynecol, 1995]. The LNG IUD (Mirena) was found to be more effective than prostaglanin inhibitors combined pills, progestin only pills and Depo-Provero at decreasing HMB [Gupta, NEJM, 2013].
- Eliminates ovulation pain (Mittelschmerz)
- Can be used to manipulate timing and frequency of menses (see Choice of COC, Page 116 & Page 121)
- Reduces risk of internal hemorrhage from ovulation (especially important in women with bleeding diatheses or women using anticoagulants)
- Regulates menses and provides progestin for women with anovulation/PCOS (reducing risk of endometrial cancer)

***Sexual/psychological:***

- No interruption at time of intercourse; more spontaneous activity
- Intercourse may be more pleasurable because of reduced risk of pregnancy
- **Pelvic inflammatory disease** leads to subsequent infertility - 12% after one episode of PID, 23% after 2 episodes and 54% after 3 episodes [Westrom I., Am J Obstet Gynecol 1980]. Pills decrease the risk of hospitalization for PID by 50-60%, but at least 12 months of use of combined pills are necessary, and the protection is limited to current users [Eschenbach DA et al Am J. Obstet Gynecol 1977] [Panser LA et al Contraception 1991]. LNG IUDs, by thickening cervical mucus, having a strong protective effect against PID [Sivin I., et. al., Contraception 1991; Toivanen, Obstet Gynecol 1991]. Thickening cervical mucus in woman using Depo-Provera may prevent ascent of pathogens to the upper genital track [Lumbi Ganon, J. Obstet Gynecol, 1996]. Condoms are highy efective in protecting women against PID.

***Cancers/tumors/masses:***

- Low dose OCs offer the same 50% reduction in ovarian cancer risk as higher-dose formulations *[Ness-2000]*. COC users for 5 years have 50% reduction in risk; users for 10 years have 80% reduction. Protection extends for 30 years beyond last pill use; Significant reduction in risk also seen in some high risk women carrying BRCA mutations
- Decreased risk for **endometrial cancer** *[Grimes-2001]* (30 µg and higher dose pills)
  - COC users for 1 year have 20% reduction in risk; users for 4 years have 60% reduction
  - Protection extends for 30 years beyond last pill use *[Ness, AmJEpidemiol-2000]*
  - Particularly important for PCOS women, obese women, and perimenopausal women
- Decreased risk of developing or dieing from **colorectal cancer** *[Beral-1999]*
- Decreased risk of corpus luteum cysts and hemorrhagic corpus luteum cysts
- *Breast masses:* reduce risk of **benign breast disease** (including fibroadenomas)

## DO BIRTH CONTROL PILLS CAUSE BREAST CANCER?

- After more than 50 studies and 50 years, most experts believe ***that pills have little, if any, effect on the risk of developing breast cancer.***
- The Women's Care Study of 4575 women with breast cancer and 4682 controls found no increased risk for breast cancer (RR: 1.0) among women currently using pills and a decreased risk of breast cancer (RR: 0.9) for those women who had previously used pills. Use of pills by women with a family history of breast cancer was not associated with an increased risk of breast cancer, nor was the initiation of pill use at a young age *[Marchbanks - 2002]*
- However, several studies have shown that current users of pills are slightly more likely to be ***diagnosed*** with breast cancer (Relative Risk: 1.2). *[Collaborative Group; Lancet 1996]*
- Two factors may explain the increased risk of breast cancer being diagnosed in women currently taking pills: 1) a ***detection bias*** (more breast exams and more mammography) or 2) ***promotion*** of an already present nidus of cancer cells
- Ten years after discontinuing pills, women who have taken pills are at no increased risk for having breast cancer diagnosed. *[Collaborative Group; Lancet 1996]*
- Breast cancers diagnosed in women currently on pills or women who have taken pills in the past are more likely to be localized ***(less likely to be metastatic)***. *[Collaborative Group; Lancet 1996]*
- By the age of 55, the risk of having had breast cancer diagnosed is the same for women who have used pills and those who have not
- The conclusion of the largest collaborative study of the risk for breast cancer is that women with a strong family Hx of breast cancer do not further increase their risk for breast cancer by taking pills. *[Collaborative Group; Lancet 1996]* This was also the conclusion of the Nurses Health Study *[Lipnick-1986] [Colditz-1996]* and the Cancer and Steroid Hormone (CASH) study. *[Murray-1989] [The Centers for Disease Control Cancer and Steroid Hormone Study-1983]*
- ➔ While there are still unanswered questions about pills and breast cancer. The very positive overall conclusion is that pills do not cause breast cancer. ***"Many years after stopping oral contraceptive use, the main effect may be protection against metastatic disease."*** *[Speroff and Darney-2001] [Collaborative Group; Lancet 1996]*

## Advantages of combined pill over progestin-only pills:

Among the advantages of combined hormonal contraceptives over progestin only pills are the following:

- Regular withdrawal bleeding
- More dependable ovulation suprression
- Improvement in acne
- Documented reduced risk of both endometrial and ovarian cancer
- Combined pills are available at more pharmacies and in more clinics
- There is only ONE progestin only pill in the United States; Micronor.

***Other:***

- Reduces risk of ectopic pregnancy and risk of hospitalization with diagnosis of PID
- Treatment for acne, hirsutism and other androgen excess/sensitivity states
- Reduced vasomotor symptoms and effective contraception in perimenopausal women
- Possible increased bone mineral density. Pills with 35 micrograms of estrogen used by women in their 40s; have been associated with fewer postmenopausal hip fractures *[Michaelsson-1998; Lancet, 353:1481-1484]*. However, low dose pills do not affect fracture risk *[Vestergaard-2006]*
- Decreased pain and frequency of sickle cell disease crises

## DISADVANTAGES

NOTE: Many of the symptoms women complain of after starting pills (nausea, headaches, bloating) occur more frequently during the days a woman is on placebo pills. Therefore, ask women ***when*** they have these symptoms. **Symptoms occurring primarily during the placebo days may be an indication CONTINUOUS or EXTENDED use of pills** *[Sulak-2002]*

***"Nocebo" Phenomenon:***

- According to David Grimes and Ken Schulz, leading epidemiologists, counseling about side effects from OCPs and including them in the product label, is "unwarranted and probably unethical" since placebo-controlled randomized trials show no difference in side effects. They call this the "nocebo phenomenon:" if women are told to expect noxious side effects, they may occur due to power of suggestion. Or they may reflect prevalence of side effects in the population. *[Non-specific side effects of OCPs: nocebo or noise? Grimes DA, Schulz KF; Contraception 83 (2011) 5-9]*

***Menstrual:***

- Spotting, particularly during first few cycles and with inconsistent use
- Scant or missed menses possible, not clinically significant but can cause worry
- Post-pill amenorrhea (lasts up to 6 months). Uncommon and usually in women with history of irregular periods prior to taking pills

***Sexual/psychological:***

- Decreased libido and anorgasmia ARE possible.
- Mood changes, depression, anxiety, irritability, fatigue may develop while on COCs, but no more frequent than with placebos. Rule out other causes before implicating COCs
- In a longitudinal survey of over 9000 women in Australia, OCP use was not associated with depressive symptoms *[Duke-2007]*
- Daily pill taking may be stressful (especially if privacy is an issue)

***Cancers/tumors/masses:*** **Breast cancer - see comprehensive answer on Page 108**

- ***Cervical cancer:***
  - No consistent increased risk seen for squamous cell cervical carcinoma (85% of all cervical cancer) after controlling for confounding variables, such as number of sex partners, smoking and parity
  - Risk of adenocarcinoma, a relatively uncommon type of cervical cancer, is increased 60%, but no extra screening required other than recommended Pap screening
- ***Hepatocellular adenoma:*** risk increased among COC users (only in $\geq$ 50 µg formulations). Risk of hepatic carcinoma not increased, even in populations with high prevalence of hepatitis B

***Other:***

- No protection against STIs, including HIV.
- Shedding of HIV may be slightly increased with use of some antiretrovirals
- Nausea or vomiting, especially in first few cycles
- Breast tenderness or pain
- Headaches: may increase
- Increased varicosities, chloasma, spider veins
- Daily dosing is difficult for some women
- Average weight gain no different among COC users than in placebo users (see NOTE below)
- See COMPLICATIONS section below

***Most women on antiretrovirals should use condoms since:***

1) the meds may decrease the pill effectiveness if the antiretroviral induces cytochrome p 450 metabolism
2) GI side-effects from drugs may decrease OC effectiveness
3) It is important to avoid other infections that may facilitate HIV transmission

NOTE: Medical problems and symptom complaints are frequently attributed by patients and providers to COC use. While some women may be particularly sensitive to sex steroids, a recent placebo-controlled study found that the incidence of all of the frequently mentioned hormone-related side effects was not significantly different in the COC group than it was in the placebo group *[Redmond, 1999]* For example, headaches occurred in 18.4% of women on Ortho Tricyclen and in 20.5% of women in the placebo group. Nausea occurred in 12.7% of women on Ortho Tricyclen and in 9.0 % of women on placebo pills. Weight gain occurred in 2.2% of women on Ortho Tricyclen and in 2.1 % of women on placebo pills. For some women, however, these complaints may actually be related to pill use

## COMPLICATIONS

- *Venous thromboembolism (VTE)*
  - The risk of VTE with COC use is less than with pregnancy:

| | |
|---|---|
| No COC use | 50/100,000 women per year |
| COC use | 100/100,000 women per year |
| Pregnancy/Postpartum | 200/100,000 women per year |

  - DVT risk is associated with the dose of estrogen; the risk of VTE in 50 µg pills is greater than in 20-35 µg pills. The type of progestin may ***slightly*** influence DVT risk. A meta-analysis by Hennessy et al (2001) included 12 observational studies and found a summary relative risk of 1.7 (1.3) - 2.1; heterogenerty p = 0.09) but could not rule out confounding given nature of observational studies. If read, the excess risk was 11 per 100,000 women per year. The current labeling for desogestrel pills states that "several epidemiologic studies indicate that third generation OCs, including those containing desogestrel, are associated with a higher risk of venous thromboembolism than certain second generations OCs. In general, these studies indicate an approximate 2-fold increased risk. However, data from additional studies have not shown this 2-fold increase in risk." Neither the FDA nor ACOG recommends switching current users of desogestrel containing pills to other products. Underlying blood dyscrasias such as Factor $V_{Leiden}$ mutation and Protein S or C abnormalities increase risk of VTE significantly. However, in the absence of strong family history (see boxed message on p. 99), screening is not necessary. A very large well-designed prospective study of the risk of VTE with drospirenone found no relative increase in risk with the use of DRSP compared with LNG pills *(Dinger)*. Three recent large studies (one case-control, and one retrospective cohort and one claims based) did find small increases in risk with the use of DRSP pills compared with LNG pills *(Lidegaard, A van Hylckand, Sidney)*. A debate about whether these studies adequately controlled for confounding factors is ongoing
- *Myocardial infarction (MI) and stroke*
  - There is no increased risk of MI or stroke for young women who are using low-dose COCs who do not smoke, do not have hypertension and do not have migraine headaches with neurological findings
  - Women at risk:
    - Smokers over 35 shouldn't use COCs; all smokers should be encouraged to stop smoking. Smokers over 35 have MI rate of 396 per million COC users per year vs. 88 per million non-COC users per year
    - Women with hypertension, diabetes, hyperlipidemia or obesity
    - Women with migraine with aura (only stroke risk increases)

### ELEVATED BLOOD PRESSURE: A TEACHABLE MOMENT

*Each time you find an elevated blood pressure, several messages should reach the ears of your patient*:*

1. **If you smoke, stop smoking. This is by far the most important step you can take**
2. **Moderate exercise for 20-30 minutes each day, every day reduces blood pressure!**
3. **If overweight, lose weight. Reduce fat in your diet**
4. **Use salt in moderation**
5. **If you are on antihypertensive medications, take them regularly!**
6. **Work on reducing stress in your life (may be difficult and may take time)**

* *In addition to deciding if pills can be used*

- *Hypertension:* 1% of users develop hypertension which (usually) is reversible within 1-3 months of discontinuing COCs. Most users have a very small increase if any in blood pressure
- *Neoplasia:* COC users using early high dose pills are at higher risk of developing adenocarcinoma (rare) of the cervix and hepatic adenomas (rare). See boxed message on Page 108 for an answer to the question: Do birth control pills cause breast cancer?
- *Cholelithiasis/cholecystitis:* higher dose formulations were associated with increased risk of symptomatic gallbladder disease
  - Sub-50 mcg formulations may be neutral or have a slightly increased risk
  - Use COCs with caution in women with known gallstones. Asymptomatic (US MEC:2), treated by cholecystectomy (US MEC:2), symptomatic and being treated medically (US MEC:3), current and symptomatic (US MEC:3)
- *Visual changes:* Rare cases of retinal thrombosis (must stop pills). Contact lens users may have dry eyes. May need to recommend eye drops or need to switch methods

**CANDIDATES FOR USE:** See 2010 US MEC Medical Eligibility Criteria, Appendix
- Most healthy reproductive aged women are candidates for COCs
- Use of COCs is often decided on the basis of a balance of benefits and side effects
- In addition to medical precautions, real world considerations such as the need for privacy, affordable access to COCs, and the requirement for daily administration need to be considered when evaluating a woman for COC use

***Adolescents***
- May be excellent candidates for contraceptive benefits if patient is able to take a pill each day.
- Many of the non-contraceptive effects of OCs are particularly important for adolescent women – e.g. decreased dysmenorrhea (the most common cause of lost days of school and work among women under 25), and decreased acne, hirsutism, or hypoestrogenism due to eating disorders, excessive exercise, stress, etc.
- Failure rates are higher in teens using COCs. Help teens integrate pill taking into daily rituals (tooth brushing, cell phone, watch alarm, application of makeup, putting on earrings). Ask teenager how she will create a way to be successful. Suggest having her write down a plan. Ask if parents are aware that she is using contraception and if they are supportive. Consider continuous COC use. See p. 100
- Encourage teens to use condoms consistently and correctly
- Be sure she has a package of Plan B at home

## SPECIAL CONSIDERATIONS FOR USE
- Women with medical conditions that improve with COCs may find COCs a particularly attractive contraceptive option. This includes women with dysmenorrhea, endometriosis, menstrual migraine without aura, iron deficiency anemia, acne, hirsutism, polycystic ovarian syndrome (PCOS), ovarian or endometrial cancer risk factors, eating disorders or activity patterns that increase risk of osteoporosis. Consider continuous or extended COC use with a monophasic pill. See Page 98
- Women whose reproductive health would be improved by ovulation suppression or decreased menstrual blood loss should also consider COCs. This includes women with chronic amenorrhea (unopposed estrogen), and women who suffer menorrhagia or dysmenorrhea and some anticoagulated women (COCs decrease risk of internal hemorrhage with ovulation and menorrhagia)
- Women whose quality of life would be improved by reducing frequency of or eliminating menses with extended cycles or continuous COC use: See Page 98
- Women who have difficulty swallowing pills may benefit from the chewable formulation of Ovcon-35. OCs may potentially also be placed in the vagina for systemic absorption. Large studies are lacking

**PRESCRIBING PRECAUTIONS**

See US MEC Eligibility Criteria Appendix

- Thrombophlebitis, thromboembolic disease or history of deep venous thrombosis or pulmonary embolism (unless anticoagulated)
- Family history of close family members with unexplained VTE at early age (eg Factor $V_{Leiden}$ mutation)
- Cerebral vascular disease or coronary artery disease

> *The questions to ask are as follows:*
> - Has a close family member (parents, siblings, grandparents, uncles, aunts) ever had unexplained blood clots in the legs or lungs?
> - Has a close family member ever been hospitalized for blood clots in the legs or lungs? If so, did this person take a blood thinner? (If not, it is likely that the family member had a nonsignificant condition such as superficial phlebitis or varicose veins)
> - What were the circumstances in which the blood clot took place (eg. pregnancy, cancer, airline travel, surgery, obesity, immobility, postpartum, etc.)? *[Grimes - 1999]*
>
> "If the family history screening is positive - one or more close family members with a definite strong VTE history (young first - or second - degree relatives with spontaneous VTE) clinician might consider further laboratory screening for genetic conditions. Another alternative is to suggest progestin-only OCs or another non-estrogen-containing birth control method." *[Grimes - 1999]*

- Current breast cancer (US MEC: 4)
- Past breast cancer and no evidence of current disease for 5 years (US MEC: 3)
- Endometrial carcinoma or other estrogen dependent neoplasia (excluding endometriosis and leiomyoma)
- Unexplained vaginal bleeding suspicious for serious condition (before evaluation) (US MEC: 2)
- Cholestatic jaundice of pregnancy or jaundice with prior pill use
- Hepatic adenoma or carcinoma or significant hepatic dysfunction
- Smoking after age 35. CDC defines heavy smoking as $\geq$ 15 cigarettes/day (see Appendix)
- Complicated or prolonged diabetes, systemic lupus erythematosus (if vascular changes)
- Severe migraine with aura or other neurologic symptoms
- Breastfeeding women (without supplementation) until breastfeeding well established COCs have no adverse effects on babies of OC-using, nursing mothers
- Hypersensitivity to any components of pills
- Daily use of certain broadspectrum antibiotics. Although CDC (see Appendix) states that women using antibiotics other than grisiofulvin or rifampicin may use COCs (US MEC:1), patients are exposed to conflicting information. Many clinicians explain the differing opinons and let patient decide for herself. There are not convincing data that broad spectrum antibiotics increase the failure of COCs. Doxycycline and fluconazole *[Hilbert-2001]* do not lower the effectiveness of COCs *[Murphy AA-1991] [Neely JL-1991]*
- Hypertension with vascular disease $\frac{140\text{-}159}{90\text{-}99}$ = 3 (US MEC) $\frac{\geq 160}{\geq 100}$ = 4 (US MEC)

## EXTENDED USE OF PILLS MAY MEAN:

A. Manipulation of a cycle to delay one period for a trip, honeymoon, or athletic event
B. Use of active hormonal pills for more than 21 consecutive days) followed by 2 to 7 hormone-free days.
C. Continuous daily COCs for at least 21 pills, but after that, may break for 2-7 days if spotting or breakthrough bleeding is bothersome
D. Use of a monophasic pill indefinitely. BTB can occur at any time with this regimen. Eventually she develops an atrophic endometrium and breakthrough bleeding decreases.

### Cyclic symptoms that may improve from the extended use of pills:

***Symptoms usually occurring at the time of menses: (predicted benefits)***

- Abdominal, back or leg pain, dysmenorrhea
- If cyclic pills do not control symptoms of endometriosis *[Havada-2007]* continuous pills may work *[Vercellini-2003]*
- Bleeding abnormalities including menorrhagia
- Irritability or depression. Decreased libido
- Headaches including both menstrual migraine and other cyclic headaches *[Sulak-2000] [Kwiecien-2003]*
- Nausea, dizziness, vomiting or diarrhea
- Cyclic yeast or other infections or cyclic nosebleeds
- Cyclic seizures, arthritis, or recurrences of asthma at the time of menses
- Changes in insulin requirements
- Cyclic symptoms associated with polycystic ovarian disease

***Symptoms usually occurring at midcycle:(predicted benefits)***

- Spotting due to sudden fall in estradiol
- Sharp or dull pain (that precedes ovulation and is caused by high midcycle PG levels)

***Symptoms usually occurring just prior to menses: (predicted benefits)***

- Slight to more dramatic weight gain, bloating, swollen eyes or ankles
- Breast fullness or tenderness
- Anxiety, irritability or depression, nausea or headaches due to dropping estrogen
- Acne, spotting, discharge, breast fullness or tenderness
- Pain or cramping or constipation

### Most important advantages & disadvantages of taking COCs continuously:

***Advantages:***

- May be more effective as a contraceptive when taken daily
- May be easier to remember (do the same thing every day)
- Women wanting to avoid bleeding for an athletic event, special trip or any other reason
- Less frequent menstruation *[Sulak-2000] [Glasier-2003]* and less blood loss
- Recent Harris survey: three quarters of women prefer less frequent periods, although only 8% tried continuous pills. *[Harris-2008] Accessed at www.healthywomen.org/Documents/MenstrualManagementReport.pdf*
- Decreased expenses from tampons, pads, pain meds, and days of work missed

***Disadvantages:***

- More expensive and the extra packs of pills required may not be covered by insurance
- Unscheduled spotting or bleeding and the absence of regular menses
- Clinician must explain the difference: amenorrhea, while taking a progestin every day, is not harmful *[Miller-2003]*. Ammenorhea for a woman on no hormonal contraceptive, may lead to endometrial hyperplasia or cancer.

**MEDICAL ELIGIBILITY CHECKLIST**: Ask a woman on pills the questions below. If she answers NO to ALL of the questions and has no other contraindications, then she can use low-dose COCs if she wants. If she answers YES to a question below, follow the instructions

***1. Do you think you are pregnant?***

☐ No ☐ Yes Assess if pregnant. If she might be pregnant, give her male or female condoms to use until reasonably certain that she is not pregnant. Then she can start COCs. If unprotected sex within past 5 days, consider emergency contraception if she is not pregnant

***2. Do you smoke cigarettes and are you age 35 or older?***

☐ No ☐ Yes Urge her to stop smoking. If she is 35 or older and she will not stop smoking, do not provide COCs. Help her choose a method without estrogen

***3. Do you have high blood pressure? (see Appendix)***

☐ No ☐ Yes If BP below 140/90, OK to give COCs if no other comorbidities exist even if taking antihypertensive drugs. If BP is elevated, see Appendix, p. A-3. Consider IUD or progestin-only methods

***4. Are you breast-feeding your baby?***

☐ No ☐ Yes If yes, non-estrogen containing contraceptives are preferable. However, according to new CDC Medical Eligibility Criteria 2010 (see appendix) use of COCs in breastfeeding women is given a catagory 2 at 1 month PP meaning advantages outweigh disadvantages. CDC considering change to category 2 or 3 for the 3-6 week post partum period depending on a woman's risk factors for VTE.

***5. Do you have serious medical problems such as a heart disease, severe chest pain, blood clots, high blood pressure or diabetes? Have you ever had such problems?***

☐ No ☐ Yes Do not provide COCs if she reports heart attack or heart disease due to blocked arteries, stroke, blood clots (except superficial clots), severe chest pain with unusual shortness of breath, diabetes for more than 20 years, or damage to vision, kidneys, or nervous system caused by diabetes. Help her choose a method without estrogen. Consider POPs, LNg IUD, Copper T 380 A, Implanon, barriers, DMPA

***6. Do you have or have you ever had breast cancer? (see Appendix)***

☐ No ☐ Yes Do not provide COCs if current or less than 5 years ago. Help her choose a method without hormones. If disease free x 5 years, may consider COCs if there are no better option for her (CDC: 3)

***7. Do you often get bad headaches with blurred vision, nausea or dizziness?***

☐ No ☐ Yes If she gets migraine headaches with blurred vision, temporary loss of vision, sees flashing lights or zigzag lines, or trouble speaking or moving, or has other neurologic symptoms, do not provide COCs. Consider POPs, LNG IUD, Copper T 380 A, Implanon, barriers. Help her choose a method without estrogen. If she has only menstrual migraines without abnormal neurologic findings, consider COC use.

***8. Are you taking medicine for seizures or are you taking rifampin, griseofulvin or St. John's Wort?***

☐ No ☐ Yes If she is using St. John's Wort, rifampin, griseofulvin, topiramate (Topomax) phenytoin, carbamazepine, barbiturates, or primidone, guide her to a non-estrogen containing method or strongly encourage condom use as backup contraceptive. Use of valproic acid does NOT lower the effectiveness of COCs.

***9. Do you have vaginal bleeding that is unusual for you? (see Appendix)***

☐ No ☐ Yes If she is not likely to be pregnant but has unexplained vaginal bleeding that suggests an underlying medical condition, evaluate condition before initiating pills. Treat as appropriate or refer. Reassess COC use based on findings

***10. Do you have jaundice, cirrhosis of the liver, an acute liver infection or tumor? (Are her eyes or skin unusually yellow?) (see Appendix)***

☐ No ☐ Yes If she has serious active liver disease (jaundice, painful or enlarged liver, active viral hepatitis, liver tumor), do not provide COCs. Refer for care as appropriate. Help her choose a method without hormones

***11. Do you have gallbladder disease? Ever had jaundice while taking COCs or during pregnancy?***

☐ No ☐ Yes If she has acute gallbladder disease now or takes medicine for gallbladder disease, or if she has had jaundice while using COCs or during pregnancy, do not provide COCs. Consider a method without estrogen. Women with known asymptomatic cholelithiasis may use COCs with caution

***12. Are you planning surgery with a recovery period that will keep you from walking for a week or more? Have you had a baby in the past 21 days?***

☐ No ☐ Yes Help her choose a method without estrogen. If planning surgery or just had a baby, provide COCs for delayed initiation and another interim method

***13. Have you ever become pregnant on the pill?***

☐ No ☐ Yes Ask about pill-taking habits. Consider longer dosing hormonal methods or shortening or eliminating the pill-free interval while using COCs

**INITIATING METHOD** (see INSTRUCTIONS FOR PATIENT, Page 117)

- In asymtomatic women, **a pelvic examination is not necessary to start pills** *[Stewart-2001]*
- *Counseling is critical in helping women successfully use the pill*
  - Patients who are counseled well about how to use pills and what side effects may develop are usually better prepared and may be more likely to continue use
- *Timing of initiation* (see Table 23.1, Page 120)
  - First day of next menstrual period start
  - **"Quick Start"** (starting the day of the counseling clinic visit) is quite feasible to help women adapt to COCs *[Westoff-2002].* Provide 7 day backup. Bleeding is not increased in "quick starters". This is now the preferred method of starting pills
  - If using Sunday start, recommend back-up method x 7 days. Sunday start can result in no periods on weekends
- *Choice of pill*
  - The pill that will work best for the woman is the one that she will take regularly!
  - For special situations, some formulations offer advantages over others (see CHOOSING COCs FOR WOMEN IN SPECIAL SITUATIONS, Page 116)
    - In general, use the lowest dose of hormones that will provide pregnancy protection, deliver the non-contraceptive benefits that are important to the woman, and minimize her side effects

- Monophasic formulations are preferable if women are interested in controlling cycle lengths or timing by eliminating any or all pill-free intervals for medical indications or personal preference (see Choosing COCs, Figure 23.1, Page 121)
  - Triphasic formulations are preferred by some clinicians to reduce some side effects (such as premenstrual breakthrough bleeding) when it is not desirable to increase hormone levels throughout the entire cycle or when it is desirable to reduce total cycle progestin levels (e.g. acne treatment). There are no studies that support the superiority of triphasic pills for women with BTB
- *Choice of pattern of COC use*
  - 28-day cycling: Most common use pattern. Women have monthly withdrawal bleeding during placebo pills
  - *"First day start" each cycle:* Women can start each new pack of pills on first day of menses each cycle
  - *"Bicycling" or "tricycling":* Women skip placebo pills for either 1 or 2 packs and then use the placebo pills and have withdrawal bleeding after 6 weeks (end of 2nd pack) or after 9 weeks (end of 3rd pack). **Use monophasic pills**
  - You may prescribe 4 packs of low dose monophasic pills omitting the placebo pills or use Seasonale, Seasonique, LoSeasonique, Jolessa or Lybrel all pre-packaged for extended cycles
  - *"Continuous use":* Women take only active pills and have no withdrawal bleeding. Often women must transition through bicycling or tricycling to achieve amenorrhea. Must use monophasic pills. Need to counsel regarding BTB and spotting
  - Studies of extended cycles have found no increased risk of endometrial hyperplasia *[Johnson-2007]*

  *NOTE: the last three options may be particularly good for:*
    - Women with menstrually-related problems (menorrhagia, anemia, dysmenorrhea, menstrual mood changes, menstrual irregularity, endometriosis, menstrual migraine, PMS, PMDD)
    - Women on medications that reduce COC effectiveness (e.g. anticonvulsants, St. John's Wort). See further description on Page 117
    - Women who have conceived while on COCs or who forget to take them regularly
    - Women who are ambulatory but disabled and for whom menstrual bleeding may be particularly problematic
    - Women who want to control their cycles for their own convenience
- Provide or recommend EC for when/if needed

## CHOOSING COCs FOR WOMEN IN SPECIAL SITUATIONS

- *Endometriosis:* Pills taken continuously are most effective in reducing symptoms. Continuous use (no break) of ring may also be effective. See Page 98
- *Functional ovarian cysts:* higher dose monophasic COCs may be slightly more effective. Extended or continuous use of pills may also be more effective
- *Androgen excess states:* all COCs are helpful but pills with higher estrogen/progestin ratios are preferable to reduce free testosterone and inhibit 5 alpha-reductase activity.
- *Breastfeeding women:* progestin-only methods preferable to COCs in breastfeeding women. However, according to new US MEC Medical Eligibility Criteria, gives use of COC in breastfeeding women a catagory 2 at 1 month PP meaning advantages outweigh disadvantages.

- *Follow up:* offer condoms in large numbers to all women on pills, both to lower that 9% tpical user failer rate and to prevent infection.
- *Hypercholesterolemia:* Selection of pill depends on type of dyslipidemia:
  - Screening for lipids not necessary prior to prescribing COCs
  - Elevated LDL or low HDL: consider estrogenic pill (high estrogen/androgen rates)
  - Elevated triglycerides: Some clinicians recommend not prescribing COCs if triglycerides > 350 mg/dL because COCs increase triglycerides by approximately 30% and risk of pancreatitis increased (norgestimate may increase triglycerides less)
- *Hepatic enzyme-inducing agents (e.g. anticonvulsants except valproic acid, and St. John's Wort):* Options:
  - Prescribe high-dose COC (containing 50 µg EE)
  - Prescribe 30-35 µg pill with reduced pill-free interval (first-day start, bicycling with first day start, or continuous use)
- *Antibiotic use:* Concern that without intestinal flora to unconjugate the hormonal compounds produced by first hepatic processing, subsequent reabsorption of estrogen and progestin would not be possible. However, research on current dose pills suggests no significant difference in circulating serum levels of hormones when women used broad-spectrum antibiotics *[Murphy AA-1991][Neely-1991]*. Class OC labeling warns about potential antibiotic interactions. If patient has other risk factor (vomiting, diarrhea, forgetfulness) or is worried, do suggest back-up method for duration of antibiotic use. Rifampin **does** and griseofulvin **may** decrease pill effectiveness and a backup or alternative contraceptive is recommended. Check PDR for effects of antiretrovirals on steroid levels. Antiretrovirals receive a 2 (generally use the method) in the US MEC Medical Eligibility Criteria
- *Obese patients:* Current data do not suggest different prescribing for markedly overweight women but some studies show a higher failure rate and increased risk of DVT

**INSTRUCTIONS FOR PATIENT: Periodic "breaks" from pills are NOT recommended!**

- Key to successful pill use is a well-informed patient. Provide new-start patients with:
  - Clear instructions on pill initiation, preferably written and in her primary language. If reasonably certain that she is not pregnant, use Quick Start technique *[Westhoff - 2002]* *(See p. 102)*. Have her take the first hormonally active pill immediately and use all pills. This *may* delay onset of next period. This will not increase the number of days of menstrual bleeding nor the number of days of spotting.
  - Help her plan where to store pills, how to remember to take them and where to obtain refills
  - Explanation about possible transitional side effects (spotting, breast tenderness, headaches, etc.) and encouragement to call or return should any become troublesome (see PROBLEM MANAGEMENT). Also highlight noncontraceptive benefits
  - Warning about serious complications
  - There is no clinical data that suggests that generic OC's are less effective than branded OC's. Use the pill that is easiest to obtain (which may be the cheapest) *[ACOG Comm Opinion, Aug 2007]*
- Backup method: ensure patient has and knows how to use method if she needs to use one for interim protection, back-up, or as an alternate method if she ever discontinues COC use.
- Have patient return in 3 months for BP check and follow-up of any complaints (there is some debate about this recommendation especially if a woman can get the blood pressure determination elsewhere). Subsequently, only annual routine gynecologic exams are offered to low-risk patients
- Each woman on birth control pills needs a package of Plan B at home

## CHECKLIST FOR EACH RETURN VISIT FOR WOMEN USING PILLS

***Before you are seen by a counselor or clinician, please tell us your response to the following questions. Please check yes or no. Tell us if you have:***

| | | |
|---|---|---|
| Any problem you think could be caused by pills | Yes____ | No____ |
| Nausea or vomiting | Yes____ | No____ |
| Spotting or irregular vaginal bleeding | Yes____ | No____ |
| Occasional missed periods (no bleeding) | Yes____ | No____ |
| Breast tenderness or a breast lump | Yes____ | No____ |
| Any symptoms of pregnancy | Yes____ | No____ |
| Depression, severe anxiety or mood changes | Yes____ | No____ |
| Decreased interest in sex | Yes____ | No____ |
| Decreased ability to have orgasms | Yes____ | No____ |
| Gained 5 pounds or more | Yes____ | No____ |
| High blood pressure | Yes____ | No____ |
| Been smoking at all | Yes____ | No____ |
| Been taking medicines for seizures | Yes____ | No____ |
| Been taking over-the-counter herbs | Yes____ | No____ |
| Ever forgotten to take your pills | Yes____ | No____ |
| Forgotten to take pills quite often | Yes____ | No____ |
| Changed sexual partners | Yes____ | No____ |
| Experienced any of the following pill danger signals: | | |
| **A**bdominal pain? | Yes____ | No____ |
| Yellow skin or eyes? | Yes___ | No____ |
| **C**hest pain? | Yes____ | No____ |
| **H**eadaches which are severe? | Yes____ | No____ |
| **E**ye problems: blurred vision or loss of vision? | Yes____ | No____ |
| **S**evere leg pain? | Yes____ | No____ |

**"ACHES"** is a way for you to remember the pill danger signals.
***Please explain any question you have answered "yes" to:***

## PROBLEM MANAGEMENT

***Nausea/vomiting:*** **Rule out pregnancy, reassure that nausea usually improves**

- Prescribe lower estrogen formulation
- Suggest taking pills at night (evening meal or bedtime) to allow patient to sleep through high serum levels of hormones. Suggest taking pills with morning meal if experiencing bothersome nausea during the night
- If patient vomits within one hour of taking pill, suggest antiemetic prior to taking replacement pill. Use backup method for 7 days
- Consider change to a non-estrogen containing method
- Abdominal pain problems possibly related to COCs: thombosis of major intra-abdominal vessels, gallstones, pancreatitis, liver adenoma, Crohn's disease or porphyria

***Spotting and/or breakthrough bleeding:***

- See Fig. 23.2, Page 122 for women taking pills in the traditional 21/7 manner
- Do not double-up on pills!

***Women taking pills for an extended period of time:***

- Take first 21 pills every single day whether or not spotting occurs
- Thereafter, one approach to spotting is to stop active hormonal pills on first day of spotting (after having taken pills for at least 21 days). Take no pill for 2 or 3 days. Then restart pills daily until the next spotting day (again as long as pill has been taken for at least 21 days). With any pill taken continuously, the number of days with BTB will decrease over time

***Missed one pill:*** **Instruct patient to take missed pill ASAP and take next pill as usual**

***Missed two or more pills:***

- The most recent missed pill should be taken ASAP
- The remaining pills should be continued at usual time
- Backup for 7 days
- Consider emergency contraception (pills or a copper IUD)

***If patient uses ECPs:*** Instruct patient to resume taking pills in pack the next day after she finishes ECPs

***Missed withdrawal bleed on COCs (not on extended or continuous cycles):***

- Offer pregnancy test, especially if she missed any pills in last cycle or if she has any symptoms of pregnancy
- Offer emergency contraception if any intercourse in last 5 days
- Advise patient that there are no adverse clinical impacts of amenorrhea from COCs
- If patient prefers monthly withdrawal bleeding, consider switching to formulation with higher estrogen or lower progestin
- Otherwise, have her continue her COCs on usual schedule

***New onset or significant worsening of headaches on COCs:*** (see Figure 23.3, Page 124)

***Hot flashes on placebo-pill week:***

- Suggest starting on first day of withdrawal bleeding or continuous use of monophasic pills OR
- Offer low-dose of transdermal or oral estrogen during placebo-pill week (Mircette provides 5 days of estrogen during 4th week)
- Offer Seasonique, a formulation with 84 days of active pills, followed by 7 days of pills with 10 mcg EE or Lybrel, a formulation where all pills have hormones

If patient $\geq$ 50 years old, consider checking FSH level at least 2+ weeks off the pill (make sure she is using condoms) - see algorithm on p. 111

## MAKING THE TRANSITION FROM COCs TO HRT: (See Figure 23.4, Page 125)

## FERTILITY AFTER DISCONTINUATION OF METHOD

- Immediate return of fertility: Average delay in ovulation 1-2 weeks. Post-pill amenorrhea more common in women with a past history of very irregular menses; rarely persists for up to 6 months
- Women should initiate another method immediately after discontinuing COCs
- Women can be surprised to learn that their pattern of menses **prior** to starting pills (frequency, duration, flow, dysmenorrhea) **tends to return** once they stop COCs
- Taking pills for many years prior to trying to become pregnant may actually protect a woman from some of the causes of infertility such as endometriosis, endometrial cancer, uterine fibroids, polycystic ovarian disease and ovarian cancer

### Table 23.1 Starting Combined Oral Contraceptives*

| CONDITION BEFORE STARTING | WHEN TO START COCs? |
|---|---|
| Starting (restarting) COCs in menstruating women | • Immediately, if pregnancy excluded start with first pill in package; backup needed x 7 days<br>"QUICK START" *[Westhoff - 2002]* See Page 115<br>• First day of next menses<br>• If within 5 days after start of her menstrual bleeding, no backup required.**<br>• First Sunday after next menses begins.** Backup needed x 7 days |
| Starting (restarting) in amenorrheic women | Anytime if it is reasonably certain that she is not pregnant; abstain from sex or use backup method for the next 7 days |
| Postpartum and breastfeeding | According to US MEC Medical Eligibility Criteria 2010, use of COCs in breastfeeding women is a category 2 at 1 month postpartum meaning advantages outweigh disadvantages*** |
| Postpartum and not breastfeeding (after pregnancy of 24 or more weeks) | • Wait 3 weeks after delivery to allow hypercoagulable state of pregnancy to abate<br>• If has risk factor for VTE, CDC recommends waiting until 42 days |
| After 1st or 2nd trimester (≤ 24 weeks) pregnancy loss or termination | • Immediately - start the same day<br>No backup needed |
| Switching from another hormonal method | • Start COCs immediately if she has been using hormonal method correctly and consistently, or if it is reasonably certain she is not pregnant. No need to wait until next period. No additional contraceptive needed<br>• If previous method was an injectable, start COCs at the time repeat injection would have been given |
| Switching from a non-hormonal method (other than IUD) | • Can start immediately or at any other time if it is reasonably certain that she is not pregnant. Use backup method for the next 7 days unless it is the first day of menses |
| Switching from an IUD (including hormonal) | • Start pills within 5 days of start of mentrual bleeding, no additional contraceptive needed & IUD can be removed at that time<br>• Start pills at any other time if it is reasonably certain she is not pregnant. If sexually active in this menstrual cycle and more than 5 days since menstrual bleeding started, remove IUD at time of next menstrual period OR give EC, then start COCs immediately; backup x 7 days |
| After taking ECPs | • Day after ECP**<br>• First day of next menses } if using other interim<br>• Sunday of next menses** } method until menses |

* World Health Organization. Selected Practice Recommendations for Contraceptive Use. 2004

** Back-up method needed for 7 days after starting COCs if it has been more than 5 days since menstrual bleeding started

## Figure 24.1

### CHOOSING A PILL

**Woman wants to use "the Pill"**
**Does she have problem of:**

- Smoking & age 35 or older
- Hypertension (See appendix, A-3)
- Undiagnosed abnormal vaginal bleeding
- Diabetes with vascular complications or more than 20 years duration**
- DVT or PE (unless anticoagulated) or current or personal history of ischemic heart disease**
- Multiple risk factors for arterial cardiovascular disease**
- Headaches with focal neurological symptoms ** or personal history of stroke
- Current or past history of breast cancer**
- Active viral hepatitis or mild or severe cirrhosis**
- Breast-feeding exclusively at the present time**
- Major surgery with immobilization within 1 month
- Personal history cholestasis with COC use** or pregnancy

**YES:** history positive for one or more of above conditions.
→ May not be able to use COCs
→ Consider a LARC Method - IUD or implant. May also be eligible for a progestin only method, barrier or sterilization. If she has a serious medical condition, she should use a highly effective method because pregnancy may be more risky.

**NO:** history negative for all of above conditions
→ **May use any sub-50-microgram COC* continuously or cyclically**
→ Choose continuous or cyclic COC based on patient desires, availability, side effects, non-contraceptive benefits, cost, and prior experience of woman or clinician

- The World Health Organization and the Food and Drug Administration both recommend using the **lowest dose pill** that is effective. All combined pills with less than 50 μg of estrogen are considered "low-dose" and are effective and safe
- There are no studies demonstrating a decreased risk for deep vein thrombosis (DVT) in women on 20-μg pills. Data on higher dose pills have demonstrated that the less the estrogen dose, the lower the risk for DVT
- All COCs lower free testosterone. Class labeling in Canada for all combined pills states that use of pills may improve acne
- To minimize discontinuation due to spotting and breakthrough bleeding, warn women in advance, reassure that spotting and breakthrough bleeding become better over time. (See Figure 23.2, Page 122)

*The package insert for women on Yasmin and Yaz states *[Berlex-2001]*: "Yasmin is different from other birth control pills because it contains the progestin drospirenone. Drospirenone may increase potassium. Therefore, you should not take Yasmin if you have kidney, liver or adrenal disease, because this could cause serious heart and health problems. Other drugs may also increase potassium. If you are currently on daily, long-term treatment for a chronic condition with any of the medications below, you should consult your healthcare provider about whether Yasmin is right for you, and during the first month that you take Yasmin, you should have a blood test to check your potassium level: NSAIDs (ibuprofen [Motrin®, Advil®], naproxen [Naprosyn®, Aleve®, and others] when taken long-term and daily for treatment of arthritis or other problems]; potassium-sparing diuretics (spironolactone and others); potassium supplementation; ACE inhibitors (Capoten®, Vasotec®, Zestril® and others); Angiotensin-II receptor antagonists (Cozaar®, Diovan®, Avapro® and others); heparin"

**These are conditions that receive a US MEC:3 or a US MEC: 4 (See appendix)

## Figure 24.2

### SPOTTING/BREAKTHROUGH BLEEDING ON COCs 21/7

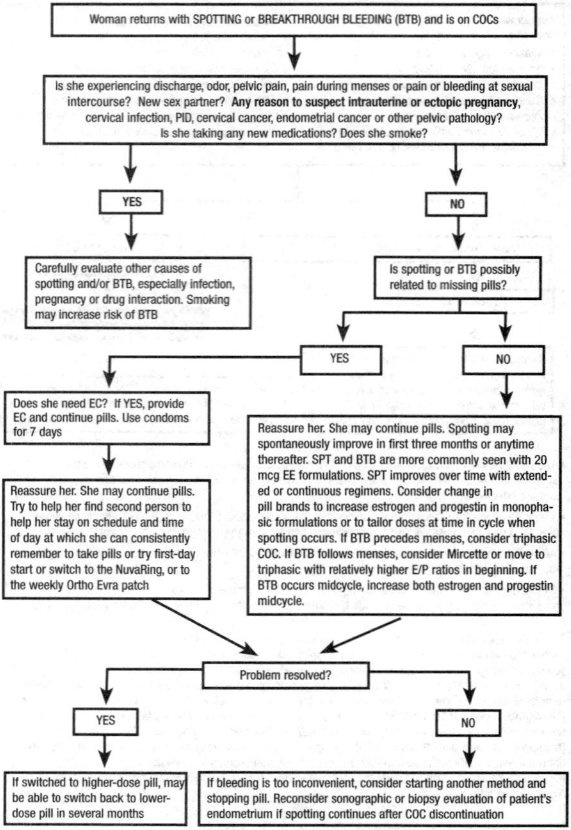

**Figure 24.3**

## MANAGEMENT OF WOMEN WITH BLEEDING IRREGULARITIES WHILE USING VARIOUS METHODS
### CDC Selected Practice Recommendations (SPR)

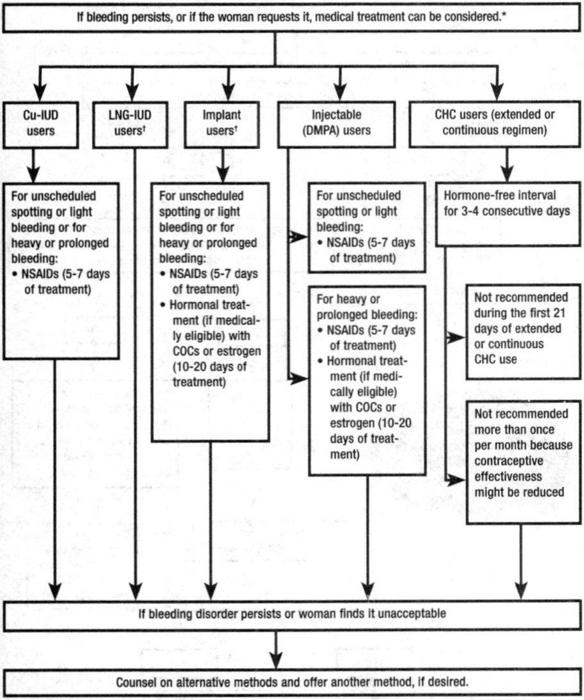


**Abbreviations:** CHC = combined hormonal contraceptive; COC = combined oral contracept ive; Cu-IUD = copper-containing intrauterine device; DMPA = depot medroxyprogesterone acetate; LNG-IUD= levonorgestrel-releasing intrauterine device; NSAIDs =nonsteroidal antiinflammatory drugs.

* If clinically warranted, evaluate for underlying condition. Treat the condition or refer for care.

† Heavy or prolonged bleeding, either unscheduled or menstrual, is uncommon.

*CDC MMWR June 21, 2013, Vol. 62:No. 5*

**Figure 24.4**

## NEW ONSET OR WORSENING HEADACHES IN COC USERS

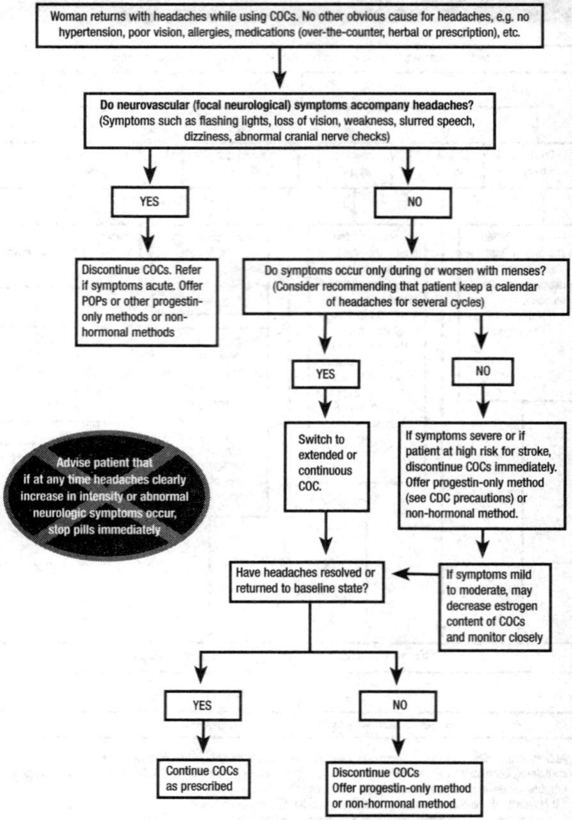

**Figure 24.5**

## MAKING THE TRANSITION FROM COCs TO MENOPAUSE, WITH OR WITHOUT HORMONE THERAPY (HT)

*The transition from COCs to menopause, with or without HT may be accomplished in a number of ways. Some reviewers of this algorithm switch to a 20 or 25-mcg pill if the patient is going to use COCs into their early 50s. A major concern is unintended pregnancy. Work together to determine a method for pregnancy prevention that is acceptable and effective*

*This algorithm does NOT include testing for a woman's menopausal status using FSH or LH tests**

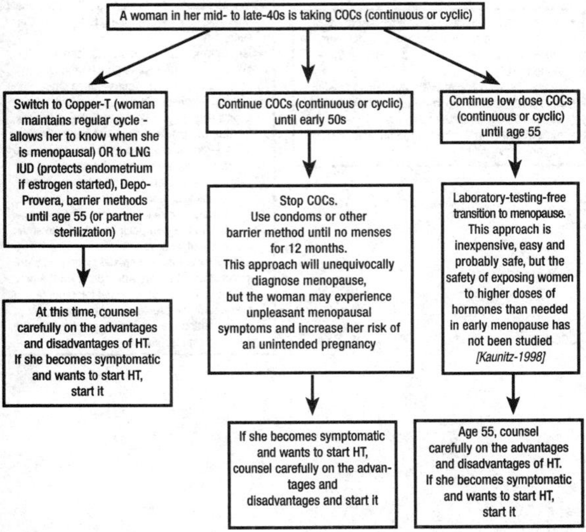


*FSH and LH testing are problematic because they show current status only. A perimenopausal woman can seem to be menopausal according to lab tests but ovulate unpredictably after that.

**Figure 24.6**

## RECOMMENDED ACTIONS AFTER LATE OR MISSED COMBINED ORAL CONTRACEPTIVE
## CDC Selected Practice Recommendations (SPR)

If one hormonal pill is late: (<24 hours since a pill should have been taken)

If one hormonal pill has been missed: (24 to <48 hours since a pill should have been taken)

- Take the late or missed pill as soon as possible.
- Continue taking the remaining pills at the usual time (even if it means taking two pills on the same day).
- No additional contraceptive protection is needed.
- Emergency contraception is not usually needed but can be considered if hormonal pills were missed earlier in the cycle or in the last week of the previous cycle.

If two or more consecutive hormonal pills have been missed: (≥48 hours since a pill should have been taken)

- Take the most recent missed pill as soon as possible. (Any other missed pills should be discarded.)
- Continue taking the remaining pills at the usual time (even if it means taking two pills on the same day).
- Use back-up contraception (e.g., condoms) or avoid sexual intercourse until hormonal pills have been taken for 7 consecutive days.
- If pills were missed in the last week of hormonal pills (e.g., days 15-21 for 28-day pill packs):
  - Omit the hormone-free interval by finishing the hormonal pills in the current pack and starting a new pack the next day.
  - If unable to start a new pack immediately, use back-up contraception (e.g., condoms) or avoid sexual intercourse until hormonal pills from a new pack have been taken for 7 consecutive days.
- Emergency contraception should be considered if hormonal pills were missed during the first week and unprotected sexual intercourse occurred in the previous 5 days. ·Emergency contraception may also be considered at other times as appropriate.

*CDC MMWR June 21, 2013, Vol. 62:No. 5*

## Figure 24.7

### RECOMMENDED STEPS AFTER VOMITING OR DIARRHEA WHILE USING COMBINED ORAL CONTRACEPTIVES
### CDC Selected Practice Recommendations (SPR)

**Vomiting or diarrhea (for any reason, for any duration) that occurs within 24 hours after taking a hormonal pill**

**Vomiting or diarrhea, for any reason, continuing for 24 to <48 hours after taking any hormonal pill**

↓

- Taking another hormonal pill (redose) is unnecessary.
- Continue taking pills daily at the usual time (if possible, despite discomfort).
- No additional contraceptive protection is needed.
- Emergency contraception is not usually needed but can be considered as appropriate.

**Vomiting or diarrhea, for any reason, continuing for ≥48 hours after taking any hormonal pill**

↓

- Continue taking pills daily at the usual time (if possible, despite discomfort).
- Use back-up contraception (e.g., condoms) or avoid sexual intercourse until hormonal pills have been taken for 7 consecutive days after vomiting or diarrhea has resolved.
- If vomiting or diarrhea occurred in the last week of hormonal pills (e.g., days 15-21 for 28-day pill packs):
  - Omit the hormone-free interval by finishing the hormonal pills in the current pack and starting a new pack the next day.
  - If unable to start a new pack immediately, use back-up contraception (e.g., condoms) or avoid sexual intercourse until hormonal pills from a new pack have been taken for 7 consecutive days.
- Emergency contraception should be considered if vomiting or diarrhea occurred within the first week of a new pill pack and unprotected sexual intercourse occurred in the previous 5 days.
- Emergency contraception may also be considered at other times as appropriate.

*CDC MMWR June 21, 2013, Vol. 62:No. 5*

## PATCHES - WEEKLY - ORTHO EVRA PATCH AND THE GENERIC PATCH XULAN (MYLAN)

**DESCRIPTION:** One Ortho Evra or Xulan patch is worn for one week for each of 3 consecutive weeks, on the lower abdomen, buttocks, upper outer arm or to the upper torso (except for the breasts). The fourth week is patch-free to permit withdrawal bleeding. This 4.5 cm square patch delivers 20 micrograms of ethinyl estradiol and 150 mcg of the progestin, norelgestromin (the active metabolite of norgestimate) daily. *[Grimes-2001]* It takes 3 days to achieve steady states or plateau levels of hormones after application of the patch and the patch contains sufficent hormone for 9 days though prescribing info states to remove after 7 days. The patch delivers about 60% more estrogen over a 21-day period than a 35 mcg EE COC and 3 times more than the ring. **The Ortho Evra patch was removed from the market in November 2014.**

**MECHANISM:** The patch prevents pregnancy in the same manner as combined pills

**COST:** 3 patches are slightly more expensive than one cycle of brand pills

**EFFECTIVENESS:** Among perfect users (users who apply transdermal contraceptive patches on schedule and each patch remains in place for the full week), only 3-6 in 1,000 women (0.3-0.6%) are expected to become pregnant during the first year (Table 12.2 on Page 37). Pooled data from three contraceptive efficacy studies (22,155 treatment cycles) using life table analysis found an overall failure rate of about 1% (0.8% or 8 pregnancies per 1000 women through 13 cycles). *[Zieman-2001]*

Of 15 pregnancies in the 3 clinical trials of the Ortho Evra Patch, 5 were in women who were markedly overweight (women more than 90 kilograms or 198 pounds). *[Zieman-2001]* (30% of failures in 3% of women) There are no reliable data available about typical failure rates, thus the typical failure rate is presumed similar to COCs *[Audet-2001]*

### ADVANTAGES

***Menstrual:*** Like combined pills

***Sexual/Psychological:***

- May enhance sexual enjoyment due to diminished fear of pregnancy
- Attractive for women who forget to take pills
- Does not interrupt intercourse

***Cancers/tumors and masses:*** No data yet; benefits probably comparable to combined pills

***Other:***

- Option throughout the reproductive years: Age is not a reason to avoid the Patch. Compliance among teens using patch is good. For some women compliance may be easier than taking a pill every day *[Audet-2001]*. Each patch contains enough hormone to suppress ovulation for up to 9 days.
- May bathe, swim and do normal activities

### DISADVANTAGES

***Menstrual:*** In the first cycle, about one-fifth of patch users experienced breakthrough bleeding or spotting. This improved with time

***Sexual/Psychological:*** Similar to pills, but use may be more obvious than pills. See p. 95

***Cancers/tumors and masses:*** Same as COCs

***Other:***

- Lack of protection against sexually transmitted infections (STIs)
- Among 812 women on the patch, 3 serious adverse events were considered possible or likely related to use of the patch, including 1 case of pain and paraesthesia in the left arm, 1 case of migraine and 1 case of cholecystitis *[Audet-2001]*
- Must remove and replace patch weekly. Application site problems include partial detachment (2.8%)

or complete detachment (1.8%) and skin irritation (1.1%) *[Audet-2001]*. **Pigment changes (hyper and hypo) have been noted under the site of patch application.** In a study of patch wear under conditions of physical exertion and variable temperatures and humidity, less than 2% of patches were replaced for complete or partial detachment. 2.6% of women discontinued using the patch because of application site reactions. Problems did not increase over time *[Audet-2001]*. Border of patch may become dirty, picking up lint, hairs or fabric. Able to remove with baby oil after patch is changed

- Nausea occurred in 20.4% of women on patch vs 18.3% of women using oral contraceptives; patch was discontinued by 1.8% of women because of nausea *[Audet-2001]*
- Breast discomfort was greater in women using the patch than in women on the pill. The difference was significant only in cycles 1 and 2 (15.4% vs 3.5% in cycle 1 and 6.6% vs 1.5% in cycle 2). For cycles 3-13, breast discomfort occurred in 0 to 3.2% of women using the patch and in 0 to 1.7% of women on pills (not statistically significant) *[Audet-2001]*
- Headaches were as likely in women on patch (21.9%) as in women on pills (22.1%)
- Irritation or an allergic skin reaction while using the patch (19%)

## COMPLICATIONS (See Page 186)

- Data demonstrate that patch users had average concentrations of EE at steady state that were ~60% higher than women using COCs with 35 mcg EE. They also had ~25% lower peak levels of EE. Based on data from oral contraceptives, higher levels of estrogen are associated with an increased risk of VTE and CV events. Epidemiologic data on the patch are limited so far. Several case control studies have reported odds ratios for VTE ranging from 0.9 to 2.4 meaning that there may be no increased risk or an approximate doubling of risk *[Jick-2006, 2007 Package Insert] [Cole-2007]*. Currently available data do not show an increased risk of MI or stroke. Women choosing the patch should be informed of **the possiblity** of an increase in risk of adverse events, particularly VTE.
- Other complications similar to COCs

## PRESCRIBING PRECAUTIONS

- Precautions for the patch are the same as those for combined pills (see Page 112 and A1-A8)
- **Women weighing more than 90 kg (198 lbs)** should be told that the patch is less effective as compared to its use in women < 198 lbs and that they should consider using a backup or another method. Should not be a "first-line" method for woman over 198 pounds

## CANDIDATES FOR USE

- Women wanting to avoid daily pill-taking or a sex-related method like condoms
- Women wanting regular menstrual periods. May be used by individuals allergic to latex

***Adolescents:* Excellent option, particularly for teenage women unable to remember to take pills daily** *[Archer-2002]*

## INITIATING METHOD

- With the 1st pack of patches, the patient is eligible for up to three free replacement patches. Write prescription for "replacement patch" with the first box of patches
- **A pelvic examination is not necessary prior to starting this method** *[Stewart-2001]*
- Ask patient, "What day of the week is the easiest for you to remember?" and start then if you are reasonably certain she is not pregnant. Unlike pills, the time of day doesn't matter!
- Women switching from pills can switch to the patch any time in cycle. They need not wait to complete pack of pills
- Women switching from DMPA should start when the next injection is due
- But as with pills, the patch can be started anytime with backup for 7 days, if you are reasonably sure the woman is not pregnant. If started on day one of cycle, backup not needed
- Quick Start initiation of the patch resulted in no increase in pregnancy or BTB *[Murthy-2005]*
- Provide or recommend EC for when/if needed

**INSTRUCTIONS FOR PATIENT**

- If the PATCH-FREE interval is more than 9 days (late restart), apply a new patch and use backup contraception for 7 days
- No band-aids, tatoos, or decals on top of patch as this might alter absorption of hormones
- Smooth the edges down when you first put it on
- Avoid placing patch on exactly the same site 2 consecutive weeks
- Location of patch should not be altered in mid-week
- Women should check the patch daily to make sure all edges remain closely adherent to skin
- Single replacement patches are available through pharmacists. The manufacturer will reimburse a woman for up to $12 for the replacement patch
- Disposal: fold over self. Place in solid waste, preferably in a sealed plastic bag to minimize hormone leakage into waste site. Do not flush down toilet

## ➔ Figure 24.8

**RECOMMENDED ACTIONS AFTER DELAYED APPLICATION OR DETACHMENT WITH COMBINED HORMONAL PATCH**
**CDC Selected Practice Recommendations (SPR)**

Delayed application or detachment* for $<48$ hours since a patch should have been applied or reattached

↓

- Apply a new patch as soon as possible. (If detachment occured $<24$ hours since the patch was applied, try to reapply the patch or replace with a new patch.)
- Keep the same patch change day.
- No additional contraceptive protection is needed.
- Emergency contraception is not usually needed but can be considered if delayed application or detachment occurred earlier in the cycle or in the last week of the previous cycle.

Delayed application or detachment* for $\geq 48$ hours since a patch should have been applied or reattached

↓

- Apply a new patch as soon as possible.
- Keep the same patch change day.
- Use back-up contraception (e.g., condoms) or avoid sexual intercourse until a patch has been worn for 7 consecutive days.
- If the delayed application or detachment occurred in the third patch week:
  - Omit the hormone-free week by finishing the third week of patch use (keeping the same patch change day) and starting a new patch immediately.
  - If unable to start a new patch immediately, use back-up contraception (e.g., condoms) or avoid sexual intercourse until a new patch has been worn for 7 consecutive days.
- Emergency contraception should be considered if the delayed application or detachment occurred within the first week of patch use and unprotected sexual intercourse occurred in the previous 5 days.
- Emergency contraception may also be considered at other times as appropriate.

* If detachment takes place but the woman is unsure when the detachment occurred, consider the patch to have been detached for : $\geq 48$ hours since a patch should have been applied or reattached.

*CDC MMWR June 21, 2013, Vol. 62:No. 5*

**FOLLOW UP**
- What is happening to your menstrual periods?
- Have you experienced skin irritation?
- Has your patch ever come off partially or completely?
- Have you had problems remembering to replace your patch on schedule
- Offer condoms in large numbers to all women

**PROBLEM MANAGEMENT** (See Page 119)

**FERTILITY AFTER DISCONTINUATION OF METHOD:** Likely the same rapid return of fertility as COCs

## VAGINAL CONTRACEPTIVE RING - MONTHLY - NuvaRing

**DESCRIPTION:** (also see www.nuvaring.com) The NuvaRing is a combined hormonal contraceptive consisting of a 5.4 cm (2 inches) diameter flexible (not hard) ring, 4 mm (1/8 inch) in thickness. The ring is made of ethylene vinylacetate polymer. It is left in place in the vagina for 3 weeks (or 1 month) and then removed for a week to allow withdrawal bleeding. It may be used continuously with no hormone-free days, but this is off-label. **It is generally recommended that it not be removed for intercourse. If it must be, however, it should be replaced within 3 hours.** Douching is discouraged but topical therapies (antifungal agents, spermicides, etc) are allowed. NuvaRing releases low doses of ethinyl estradiol (15 micrograms daily) and etonogestrel, the active form of desogestrel (120 micrograms daily). With oral hormones there is a daily spike in hormone levels after the woman swallows each dose, followed by a gradual drop throughout the rest of the day. A single vaginal ring maintains a steady, low release rate for 42 days while in place, even in obese women according to a recent study *[Dragoman 2013]* and releases less estrogen daily at a steadier rate than pills or patches

**HOW CONTRACEPTIVE VAGINAL RINGS WORK:** ***contraceptive effects similar to combined pills.*** This method suppresses ovulation for 35 days, while in place *[Mulders-2001]*. Also see COCs, p. 92

**COST:** Each ring costs approximately the same as one cycle of pills. It is possible to get some free rings via the website at www.nuvaring.com. Public health programs pay much less for each NuvaRing

**EFFECTIVENESS:** Overall pregnancy rate of 0.3 *[Trussell-2004]* to 0.65 *[Roumen-2001]* per 100 woman-years (all first-year users). There is no information about typical use failure rate, so a typical use failure rate of 9% is used by Trussell in the 18th edition of ***Contraceptive Technology*** (same figure as for combined pills). It is likely that since the method needs to be remembered once per month rather than once per day, that the typical user failure rate would be lower

**ADVANTAGES: No daily fluctuation in hormone levels**

***Menstrual:***
- Withdrawal bleeding occurs in 98.5% of cycles, and bleeding at other times in only 5.5% of cycles *[Dieben-2002]*; much better withdrawal/spotting pattern than COCs probably due to NOT forgetting pills and the steady even blood levels that are achieved
- Irregular bleeding is low in the first cycle of use (6%) and continues to be low throughout subsequent cycles *[Dieben-2002]*

***Sexual/Psychological:*** Decreased fear of pregnancy may increase pleasure from intercourse
***Cancers/tumors and masses:*** No published data; probably similar to COCs
***Other:*** There are only 2 tasks for ring users to remember: insertion and removal once a month so compliance may be easier (92% vs. 75% for pills in one study) *[Bjarnadottir-2002]*

- 85% of women and 71% of partners say they cannot feel it *[Dieben-2002]*
- The lowest serum levels of estrogen and progestin in any combined hormonal method
- Privacy - no visible patch or pill packages. Particularly helpful for some teens
- Little weight gain associated with ring use *[O'Connel-2005]*

## DISADVANTAGES

***Menstrual:*** Withdrawal bleeding continued beyond the ring-free interval in about one quarter of cycles (20% to 27%) *[Roumen-2001]*. However, most of the time it is just spotting. Although not necessary, some women may rinse the ring. Also, ring can be accidentally pulled out by a tampon

***Sexual/Psychological:*** Some women dislike placing/removing objects into/out of vagina Some women or men may feel ring during intercourse. If bothersome, ring may be removed and reinserted within 3 hours

***Cancers/tumors and masses:*** None

***Other***: Adverse events reported by vaginal contraceptive ring users that were judged by the investigators to be possibly device related are headache (6.6%), nausea (2.8%), weight increase (2.2%), dysmenorrhea (1.8%), depression (1.7%), leukorrhea (5.3%), vaginitis (5.0%), and vaginal discomfort (2.2%) *[Roumen-2001]*

**COMPLICATIONS:** Similar to combined pills

## PRESCRIBING PRECAUTIONS

- The CDC Medical Eligibility Criteria for the NuvaRing are the same as for combined pills
- Women who are hesitant about touching their genitalia or who have difficulty inserting or removing ring may not be good candidates
- Women with pronounced pelvic relaxation

## CANDIDATES

- Women wanting to avoid having to do something daily, or at the time of intercourse
- Women wanting regular menstrual periods
- Women satisfied with OCs but willing to try the patch or ring were happier with the ring than their OC *[Creinin-2007]*

***Adolescents:*** Excellent option; requires less discipline than taking pills daily

**INITIATING METHOD:** ***Best approach - teach women to insert and remove ring in office. Ask women if they would like you to insert a ring after you do an exam to demonstrate just how little she will feel the ring***

- A new ring is inserted any time during the first 5 days of a normal menstrual cycle and backup for 7 days is recommended in package insert
- New ring can be inserted at any time in cycle if reasonably certain woman is not pregnant; use backup x 7 days (CDC)
- Provide or recommend EC for when/if needed
- Quick Start of Nuvaring has been studied with high levels of satisfaction by users *[Schafer-2006]*.

**INSTRUCTIONS FOR PATIENT**

- The package insert states that backup must be used during the first 7 days that the first ring is in place
- The NuvaRing is removed at the end of 3 weeks of wear; then, after one ring-free week, the woman inserts a new ring
- The woman's menstrual period (withdrawal bleed) occurs during the ring-free week
- Ring removal during intercourse is not recommended; however, women who want to remove it during intercourse may do so without having to use a backup method as long as it is not removed for longer than 3 hours a day
- Although it is intended to be a once a month method, check for presence frequently, especially after intercourse since 20% of women experience expulsion in the first 3 months
- No special accuracy is required for ring placement; absorption is fine from anywhere in the vagina
- Because the ring is small and flexible, **most women do not notice any pressure or discomfort,** and it is not likely to be uncomfortable for their partners during intercourse
- Always have 2 rings on hand in case one is lost
- Avoid douching with ring in place. Douching is not recommended for any woman
- Tampons, lubricants and vaginal yeast creams can be used with the ring in place
- Rings may be stored at room temperature avoiding extreme heat for up to 4 months. If a woman has more than a 4-month supply of rings, they may be stored in a refrigerator. Rings kept in a refrigerator should not freeze
- A ring that falls into the toilet does float! It can be washed with soap and water and reinserted
- If the ring is left in place longer than three weeks, the user is probably still protected from pregnancy for up to 35 days by the same ring, allowing clinicians flexibility in how often they tell women the ring must be replaced. For example, the ring could be reinserted on the first of the month each month with no hormone-free interval (similar to taking combined pills with no hormone-free days)
- Extended use of the ring has been studied. The number of bleeding and spotting days combined was similar in shorter and extended cycles *[Miller-2005]*. Extended use decrease menstural flow and cramping *[Sulak-2008]*. If breakthrough bleeding occurs, instruct the patient to remove the ring, store it for 4 days, then reinsert *[Sulak-2008]*
- **Dispose of ring with solid waste, preferably in a sealed plastic bag to minimize leakage into waste site**

**FOLLOW UP:** Ask about difficulty during removal or insertion or frequent expulsion. Women may need closer follow-up if they have: genital prolapse, severe constipation, or frequent vaginal infection (i.e. recurrent yeast infection). Otherwise, similar to women on pills.
Offer condoms in large numbers to all women using NuvaRing, both to lower the 9% typical use failure rate and to prevent infections.

**FERTILITY AFTER DISCONTINUATION:** Excellent and immediate. Average return to ovulation: 11 days (range 8-21 d) *[Mulders-2002]*

**Figure 24.9**

## RECOMMENDED ACTIONS AFTER DELAYED INSERTION OR REINSERTION WITH COMBINED VAGINAL RING
### CDC Selected Practice Recommendations (SPR)

**Delayed insertion of a new ring or delayed reinsertion* of a current ring for <48 hours since a ring should have been inserted**

↓

- Insert ring as soon as possible.
- Keep the ring in until the scheduled ring removal day.
- No additional contraceptive protection is needed.
- Emergency contraception is not usually needed but can be considered if delayed insertion or reinsertion occurred earlier in the cycle or in the last week of the previous cycle.

**Delayed insertion of a new ring or delayed reinsertion* for ≥48 hours since a ring should have been inserted**

↓

- Insert ring as soon as possible.
- Keep the ring in until the scheduled ring removal day.
- Use back-up contraception (e.g., condoms) or avoid sexual intercourse until a ring has been worn for 7 consecutive days.
- If the ring removal occurred in the third week of ring use:
  - Omit the hormone-free week by finishing the third week of ring use and starting a new ring immediately.
  - If unable to start a new ring immediately, use back-up contraception (e.g., condoms) or avoid sexual intercourse until a new ring has been worn for 7 consecutive days.
- Emergency contraception should be considered if the delayed insertion or reinsertion occurred within the first week of ring use and unprotected sexual intercourse occurred in the previous 5 days.
- Emergency contraception may also be considered at other times as appropriate.

* If removal takes place but the woman is unsure of how long the ring has been removed, consider the ring to have been removed for ≥48 hours since a ring should have been inserted or reinserted.

*CDC MMWR June 21, 2013, Vol. 62:No. 5*

# CHAPTER 25

# Progestin-Only Contraceptives

www.managingcontraception.com

The progestin-only methods are progestin-only pills, Depo-Provera (Page 139), and Nexplanon or Implanon (Page 148). The LNG IUD is described on Page 97

## LOW DOSE PROGESTIN PILLS - DAILY - often called MINI-PILLS OR POPS

**DESCRIPTION:** Progestin-only pills (POPs) are also known as mini-pills. POPs contain only a progestin and are taken daily with no hormone-free days. POPs have lower progestin doses than combined pills and no estrogen. Each tablet of Micronor and Nor-QD contains 0.35 mg norethindrone.

Usage in US is low, estimated at 0.4% from NSFG data *[Hawks et al. 2012]* and 4% from claims data *[Liang et al. 2012]*

**EFFECTIVENESS** *[Trussell J IN Contraceptive Technology 2011]*

***Perfect use failure rate in first year:*** 0.3% (See Table 12.2, Page 37)

(if 300 women take POPs for 1 year, only 1 will become pregnant in the first year of perfect use)

***Typical use failure rate in first year:*** 9.0%

**HOW POPs or Mini-PILLS WORK:** Primarily by causing a thickened cervical mucus to prevent sperm entry into the upper reproductive track. While ovulation is inhibited so that only 40% of women ovulate normally, this is not nearly good enough to be counted upon. Thickening of cervical mucus happens about 2 to 4 hours AFTER a mini-pill is taken and lasts for about 22 hours. If a woman takes her mini-pill at 10 pm and has sex an hour before or after 10 pm, it is likely NOT to be effective. Mid-day is the time to take mini-pills if a couple is usually going to have sex at night or first thing in the morning. Some POPs in Europe suppress ovulation more than the norethindrone pills used in the US

**COST** *[Trussell, 1995; Smith, 1993]*

- POPs cost more than combined pills both in pharmacies and in sales to public programs

**ADVANTAGES**

***Menstrual:***

- Decreased menstrual blood loss, cramps and pain, amenorrhea (10% of women). Amenorrhea is more likely with punctual dosing
- Decrease in ovulatory pain (Mittelschmerz) in cycles when ovulation suppressed

***Sexual/physiological:***

- May enhance sexual enjoyment due to diminished fear of pregnancy
- No disruption at time of intercourse; facilitates spontaneity

***Cancers, tumors and masses:***

- Possible protection against endometrial cancer

***Other:***

- Rapid return to baseline fertility
- Possible reduction in PID risk due to cervical mucus thickening
- Good option for women who cannot use estrogen but want to take pills
- May be used by smokers over age 35. **Discourage smoking, of course!**
- May be used by breastfeeding women

***Advantages of progestin-only pills over combined pills:***
- To be taken every single day. NO days off.
- Only one "4" in the USMEC: Breast cancer within 5 years
- No thromboembolic complications
- May be used by breastfeeding women

## DISADVANTAGES

***Menstrual:*** Irregular menses ranging from amenorrhea to increased days of spotting and bleeding but with reduced blood loss overall

***Sexual/psychological:***
- Spotting and bleeding may interfere with sexual activity
- Intermittent amenorrhea may raise concerns about pregnancy
- Possible increase in depression, anxiety, irritability, fatigue or other mood changes, but often POPs reduce risk of these disorders

***Cancers, tumors and masses:***
- May be associated with slightly higher risk of persistent ovarian follicles

***Other:***
- Must take pill at same time each day (more than 3-hour delay considered by some clinicians to be equivalent to a "missed pill")
- Effect on cervical mucus decreases after 22 hours and is gone after 27 hours
- No protection against STIs

## COMPLICATIONS

- Allergy to progestin pill is rare
- Amenorrheic, Latina, breast-feeding women who had gestational diabetes may be at higher risk of developing overt diabetes in first year postpartum *[Kjos, 1998]*

## CANDIDATES FOR USE (See 2010 US MEC Medical Eligibility Criteria, Appendix)

- Virtually every woman who can take pills on a daily basis can be a candidate for POPs
- POPs are particularly good for women with contraindications to or side effects from estrogen:
  - Women with personal history of thrombosis
  - Recently postpartum women
  - Women who are exclusively breast-feeding
  - Smokers over age 35
  - Women who had or fear chloasma, worsening migraine headaches, hypertriglyceridemia or other estrogen-related side effects (e.g. nausea)
  - Women with hypertension, coronary artery disease or cerebrovascular disease
  - Women wth lupus

## PRESCRIBING PRECAUTIONS

Progestin-only pills can be used by all women willing and able to take daily pills except:
- Suspected or demonstrated pregnancy (although there are no proven harmful effects for the fetus)
- Current breast cancer or breast cancer less than 5 years ago (US MEC:3)
- Active hepatitis, hepatic failure, jaundice

- Inability to absorb sex steroids from gastrointestinal tract (active colitis, etc.)
- Taking medications that increase hepatic clearance (rifampin, and the anticonvulsants carbamazepine, oxcarbazepine, phenytoin [Dilantin], phenobarbital, primidone, topiramate and felbamate, [not valproic acid], St. Johns Wort or griseofulvin). Efficacy in combination with Orlistat and other fat-binding agents is not well studied

**MEDICAL ELIGIBILITY CHECKLIST: Evidence-based criteria for deciding whether women with 130 different conditions are presented in the appendix, pages A-1 through A-8.** Ask the client the questions below. If she answers YES to a question below, follow the instructions; in some cases she can still use POPs

***1. Do you think you are pregnant?***

☐ No ☐ Yes Assess if pregnant. If she might be pregnant, give her latex male condoms to use until reasonably sure that she is not pregnant. Then she can start POPs

***2. Do you have or have you ever had breast cancer? (See Appendix)***

☐ No ☐ Yes Do not provide POPs. Help her choose a method without hormones. May possibly consider POPs or DMPA if disease-free x 5 years (US MEC:3), but only if there is no better alternative

***3. Do you have jaundice, severe cirrhosis of the liver, acute liver infection or tumor? (Are your eyes or skin unusually yellow?) (See Appendix)***

☐ No ☐ Yes Perform physical exam and arrange lab tests or refer. If she has serious active liver disease (jaundice, painful or enlarged liver, viral hepatitis, liver tumor), may be able to use POPs with more intensive follow-up (US MEC:3)

***4. Do you have vaginal bleeding that is unusual for you? (See Appendix)***

☐ No ☐ Yes If she is not pregnant but has unexplained vaginal bleeding that suggests an underlying medical condition, can provide POPs since neither the underlying condition nor its assessment will be affected. Promptly assess and treat any underlying condition as appropriate, or refer. Reassess POP use based on findings

***5. Are you taking medicine for seizures? Taking rifampin (rifampicin), griseofulvin or aminoglutethimide? St. Johns Wort? (See Appendix)***

☐ No ☐ Yes If she is taking phenytoin, carbamazepine, barbiturate, topiramate, oxycarbamazepine, or primidone for seizures or rifampin, griseofulvin, aminoglutethamide or St. John's Wort, provide condoms or spermicide or help her choose another method that is more effective, such as DMPA. Use of valproic acid does NOT lower the effectiveness of POPs. Discuss ECPs

***6. Do you have problems with severe diarrhea or malabsorption or other bowel disorders? Or are you using medications that block fat absorption?***

☐ No ☐ Yes Help her choose a non-oral method of birth control.

## SPECIAL SITUATIONS

***History of pregnancy while using POPs correctly:***

- Switch to more effective method e.g. IUD, Implanon or DMPA
- Continue POPs but add condoms or other backup with every act of coitus

***Use with a broad-spectrum antibiotic such as tetracycline or erythromycin:***

- Few studies support antibiotic's role in contraceptive failure. See 2010 US Medical Eligibility Criteria for "other antibiotics," US MEC:1, Appendix. Some clinicians encourage backup for first 1-2 weeks, others for full duration of antibiotic use. Explain conflicting advice now being given; let patient decide whether to use backup method.

## INITIATING METHOD

- **A pelvic examination is not necessary prior to initiation of this method** *[Stewart-2001]*
- ***New starts:*** Offer condoms either for back-up for 2 days or for use should patient stop POPs. Also encourage advance obtaining of PLAN B or give her a package of PLAN B
- ***Post-partum:*** May initiate immediately regardless of breast-feeding status (PPFA, UCSF, Grady Memorial Hospital)
  ***Note:*** CDC and IPPF are concerned about theoretical impact of POPs on breast milk production and recommend waiting until 6 weeks to initiate use of DMPA and POPs
- ***After miscarriage or abortion:*** Start immediately
- ***Menstruating women:*** Start on menses if possible. No backup if started within 5 days of LMP. May initiate anytime in cycle if woman is not pregnant, but recommend at least 2 day back-up barrier method
- ***Switching from IUD, COCs, DMPA, to POPs:*** Start immediately. Need for back-up depends on previous method used: **IUD:** start immediately, backup for 7 days; Some clinicians say 48 hours minimum; others say no backup. **COCs:** start immediately if cycle of hormonally active pills completed; backup not necessary if no pill-free interval. **DMPA:** start immediately if switching at or before next DMPA injection due (no backup necessary)

## INSTRUCTIONS FOR PATIENT

- Take one pill daily at same time each day until end of pack. Start next pack the next day
- If at risk for infection, use condoms with every act of intercourse
- If you miss a pill by more than 3 hours from regular time, take the missed pill(s) and use backup for 48 hours. Consider using emergency contraception if sex in past 5 days. Obtain a package of Plan B to have at home in case of a mistake

## FOLLOW-UP

- How many pills do you typically miss or are late taking per week? Per pack?
- Have you missed any pills in last 5 days? (candidate for EC)
- Have you missed any periods or experienced any symptoms of pregnancy?
- What has your menstrual bleeding been like?
- Have you had any increase in headaches, or change in mood or libido?
- Do you plan to have children? OR Do you plan to have more children?
- What are you doing to protect yourself from STIs?
- Offer condoms in large numbers to all women on POPs, both to lower that 9% typical user failure rate and to prevent infection

## PROBLEM MANAGEMENT

- ***Amenorrhea:*** Rule out pregnancy with first episode or whenever symptoms of pregnancy noted. Otherwise, amenorrhea is not harmful when women take progestin-only pills
- ***Irregular bleeding:*** After finding out if missing pills, rule out STIs, pregnancy, cancer. If not at risk and no evidence of underlying pathology, reassure patient.
- ***Heavy bleeding:*** Rule out STIs, pregnancy, cancer. If no evidence of underlying pathology, rule out clinically significant anemia. Trial of 3 days high dose NSAIDS. If fails, may need estrogen-containing contraceptives (addition of physiologic doses ET only may compromise cervical mucus barrier), Mirena IUS or non-hormonal methods of contraception
- ***Abdominal pain:*** Consider pelvic pathology (ectopic pregnancy, torsion, appendicitis, PID) and refer for treatment. If ovarian cyst is cause, it may usually be managed conservatively unless pain is severe. Progestin slows follicular atresia. Recheck in 6 weeks and anytime her symptoms worsen

**FERTILITY AFTER DISCONTINUATION OF METHOD:** Fertility returns to its baseline levels promptly

## DMPA INJECTIONS (DEPO-PROVERA) - EACH 3 MONTHS

**DESCRIPTION:** Every woman's periods change on Depo. Women who would find it unacceptable for their periods to change simply should not start using this method.1 cc of a crystalline suspension of 150 mg depot medroxyprogesterone acetate injected intramuscularly into the deltoid or gluteus maximus muscle every 13 weeks For more information, call 1-800-253-8600.

Depo-Provera Subcutaneous - 104, subcutaneous injections of 104 mg of DMPA facilitate women giving themselves Depo-Provera injections at home. Women receive up to 14 weeks of contraceptive protection from an injection of 104 mg of DMPA SQ

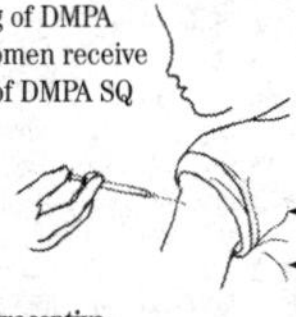

**EFFECTIVENESS** *[Trussell J IN Contraceptive Technology - 2011]*

• Approved labeling indicates each injection effective for up to 13 weeks

***Perfect use failure rate in first year:*** 0.2% (See Table 12.2, Page 37)

***Typical use failure rate in first year:*** 6%

***Continuation at 1 year:*** 23% *[Westfall-1996]* 42% *[Polaneczky-1996]* 56% *[Trussell-2011]* **Contiuation rates for Depo are the lowest of any current contraceptive.**

**Subcutaneous Depo-Provera**

Despite the lower dose of Sub Q DMPA (104 vs 150 mg), no pregnancies occurred among the 44% of study subjects who were overwieght (26%) or obese (18%). In fact, there were no pregnancies at all in 720 women over one year. 55% were amenorrheic at the end of one year. *[Jain J, Jakimiuk AJ et all-2004]*

**HOW DEPO WORKS:** Suppresses ovulation by inhibiting LH and FSH surge, thickens cervical mucus blocking sperm entry into female upper reproductive tract, slows tubal and endometrial mobility, and causes thinning of the endometrium

**COST:** In Washington State, health departments pay $4.75 for 28 days of contraception for a woman receiving Depo-Provera each 3 months. This is 4 times greater than the cost of pills for the same clinics, $1.35 per cycle. *[Margulies - 2001]* In some settings, the co-pay for DMPA is about $60/vial

### ADVANTAGES

***Menstrual:***

- Less menstrual blood loss, anemia, or hemorrhagic corpus luteum cysts
- After 1 year of use, 50% of women develop amenorrhea; 80% develop amenorrhea in 5 years. For this to be an advantage, it must be clearly explained at first and subsequent visits. See discussion of structured counseling on pages 13 and 134
- Decreased menstrual cramps, pain and ovulation pain. May decrease PMS symptoms
- Improvement in endometriosis. ***Depo-Provera Subcutaneous 104*** is also FDA approved for management of endometriosis pain

***Sexual/psychological:***

- Intercourse may be more pleasurable without worry of pregnancy
- Convenient: permits spontaneous sexual activity; requires no action at time of intercourse

***Cancers, tumors, and masses:***

- Decrease blood loss in women with fibroids
- Significant reduction in risk of endometrial cancer
- Possible reduction in risk of ovarian cancer

***Benefits for women with medical problems:***

- Suppresses ovulation, bleeding and menstrual blood loss in anticoagulated women and women with bleeding diathesis; decreases anemia
- Reduces acute sickle cell crises by 70% *[de Abood-1997]*
- Excellent method for women on anticonvulsant drugs; **may actually decrease seizures** and effectiveness not compromised

- Amenorrhea and prolonged effective contraception may be very important for severely developmentally or physically challenged women. One reviewer makes home visits for some wheelchair bound patients who love Depo-Provera

*Other:*

- The drop in teen pregnancies in 1990s, abortions and births, is attributed to Depo-Provera, Norplant, EC, condoms and abstinence promoting programs
- Significantly reduces risk for ectopic pregnancies and slightly decreases risk of PID
- Convenient: single injection provides at least 13 weeks protection
- Most protocols call for administration anytime between 11 and 13 weeks. However, DMPA is usually forgiving of late injections
- Less user-dependent than POPs, COCs
- Good option for women who cannot use estrogen (see CANDIDATES FOR USE)
- Private: no visible clue that patient is using contraception. This may prevent physical abuse of a woman.
- May be used by nursing mothers
- Return to baseline fertility may be delayed, but is excellent

## DISADVANTAGES

*Menstrual:*

- Irregular menses during first several months: many women experience unpredictable spotting and bleeding, occasionally blood loss reported to be heavy but unlikely to cause anemia. After 6-12 months, amenorrhea more likely (50% after 1 year)

***Sexual/psychological:*** Also see weight gain, below

- Spotting and bleeding may interfere with sexual activity
- Amenorrhea may raise patient's fears of pregnancy or myth of "build-up of menses" in uterus if not explained well
- Hypoestrogenism can (infrequently) cause dyspareunia, hot flashes or decreased libido
- Possible increase in depression, anxiety, irritation, PMS, fatigue or other mood changes, but often DMPA reduces risk of these disorders
- Fear of needles may make this an unacceptable choice

***Cancers, tumors, and masses:*** none

*Other:* (See boxed message: Depo Provera & Bones on Page 141)

- No protection against STIs: must use condoms if at risk
- Must return every 11-13 weeks for injection
- No contraceptive requires more return visits than Depo-Provera injections
- Long acting: ***not*** immediately reversible
- Slow to return to baseline fertility: average 10 months from last injection
- After Depo is discontinued there is a great deal of variability in time to ovulation postinjection, with most women resuming ovulation 15 to 49 weeks from last injection. *[Paulen ME, Curtis KM. Contraception 2009]*
- Occasionally, hypoestrogenism ($E_2 < 25$) may develop as a result of FSH suppression. Potential for decreased bone mineral density if used for prolonged period without opportunity for recovery prior to menopause. May have more effect on teen bones. See box on Page 141
- Severe headaches may occur - rarely attributable to DMPA
- Acne, hirsutism may develop
- Possible increase in diabetes risk in amenorrheic breastfeeding women with diagnosis of gestational diabetes during first year postpartum *[Kjos 1999]*
- Metabolic impacts: glucose (slight rise), LDL (slight rise or neutral), HDL (may decrease)
- Other hormone-related Sx: breast tenderness, bloating, hair loss, vasomotor symptoms
- Associated with modest weight gain in most women *[2007]*

## COMPLICATIONS

- Progressive significant weight gain possible. Average of 5.4 lbs in first year and 16.5 lbs after 5 yrs *[Schwallie-1973]* See Page 143: WEIGHT GAIN: A TEACHABLE MOMENT. Adolescent girls who were obese when starting Depo gained significantly more weight (mean 9.4 kg) than obese girls starting OCs (mean 0.2 kg) and controls (mean 3.5 kg) *[Ziegler-2006]*

- If a woman does not gain weight during first year on Depo, that is a good indication that she will not gain weight on Depo in subsequent years
- Worsening depression (rare) (average MMPI does not change in women on DMPA).
- Severe allergic reaction, including anaphylaxis (very rare). May consider having women wait in or near office for 20 minutes after injection. (Reviewers disagree about this recommendation, especially for previous DMPA users). Ask patients to report itching at injection site

**CANDIDATES FOR USE** (See 2010 US MEC on pages A-1 through A-8)

- Women who want intermediate-to-long-term contraception and can return every 11-13 weeks
- Women who do not plan a pregnancy soon after DMPA discontinuation
- Women who want privacy, convenience, and high efficacy
- Women who want or need to avoid estrogen:
  - Women with personal history of thrombosis (US MEC: 2) or strong family history of venous thromboembolism (US MEC: 1)
  - Recently postpartum women (US MEC: 1)
  - Women who are exclusively breast-feeding beyond 6 weeks postpartum (US MEC: 1). There is debate about use of DMPA in breastfeeding women less than 6 weeks PP (see p. 125 under INITIATING METHOD POSTPARTUM)
  - Smokers over age 35 (US MEC: 1)
  - Women who fear chloasma or had vomiting, migraine headaches, hypertriglyceridemia, or other estrogen-related side effects
- Women who use drugs which affect liver clearance (except aminoglutethimide)
- Women with anemia, fibroids, seizure disorder (US MEC 1), sickle cell disease (US MEC: 1), endometriosis, hypertriglyceridemia (US MEC: 2), systemic lupus erythematosus or coagulation disorder (hyper- or hypo-coagulation)
- Physically compromised women for whom bleeding is a nuisance or a problem

***Adolescent women:*** (US MEC: 2) Only 4 things to remember to do each year!

- Extremely effective with long carry-over if patient returns late for reinjection (see Figure 24.1, Page 146); Decreases menstrual cramps and pain
- Does not protect against STIs
- Privacy and confidentiality possible
- For some teens may be only acceptable method
- May be associated with significant weight gain, acne, complexion changes
- Requires periodic reinjections

**Bone Mineral Density (BMD) and Depo-Provera**

Depo-Provera received a black box warning from the FDA in 11/04 due to this issue. ACOG and AAP recommend no limit to use and no BMD testing. Some reviewers of this book think this was too severe a warning. All DMPA users should have the warning clearly explained to them and a discussion of alternatives if they choose to change methods. Women who used DMPA for more than 2 years have significantly reduced bone mineral density (BMD) of lumbar spine and femoral neck. But effect is largely reversible, even after ≥ 4 years of DMPA use, comparable to the effect and reversal seen after lactation *[Petitti-2000]*. **All women using DMPA including teens should be taking in sufficient calcium in diet or be encouraged to take calcium supplements. Also encourage to exercise regularly and avoid smoking.** Longitudinal studies of DMPA use in teens found a significant difference in BMD between DMPA users and non-users due to a decrease in users and an increase in nonusers. By 12 months after discontinuation, BMD of former users was the same as for non-users. *[Scholes-2005]*

**PRESCRIBING PRECAUTIONS: Women unwilling to accept a change in their menstrual periods**

- Pregnancy
- Undiagnosed abnormal vaginal bleeding
- Unable to tolerate injections; afraid of shots
- History of breast cancer, MI or stroke
- Current venous thromboembolism (unless anticoagulated)
- Active viral hepatitis
- Known hypersensitivity to Depo-Provera

**See previous page "Bone Mineral Density and Depo-Provera" about package insert black box warning**

**DRUG INTERACTIONS:** Aminoglutethimide (Cytodren), used to treat Cushings disease, reduces DMPA efficacy

## MEDICAL ELIGIBILITY CHECKLIST

Ask the client the questions below. If she answers NO to ALL the questions, then she CAN use DMPA if she wants. If she answers YES to a question below, follow the instructions

***1. Do you think you are pregnant?***

☐ No ☐ Yes Assess if pregnant. If she might be pregnant, give her condoms or spermicide to use until reasonably sure that she is not pregnant. Then she can start DMPA

***2. Do you plan to become pregnant in the next year?***

☐ No ☐ Yes Use another method with less potential delay in return of fertility

***3. Do you have serious medical problems such as heart attack, severe chest pain, or uncontrolled high blood pressure? Have you ever had such problems? (See Appendix)***

☐ No ☐ Yes In general, do not provide DMPA if she reports heart attack (US MEC:3), stroke (US MEC:3), heart disease due to blocked arteries, severe high blood pressure (systolic $\geq$ 160 or diastolic $\geq$ 100)(US MEC:3), diabetes for more than 20 years (US MEC:3), or damage to vision, kidneys, or nervous system caused by diabetes or by HTN. Help her choose another effective method. All the above conditions receive a "3" in the 2010 CDC Medical Eligibility Criteria

***4. Do you have or have you recently had breast cancer (US MEC: 3 or 4)? (See Appendix)***

☐ No ☐ Yes Do not provide DMPA. Help her choose a method without hormones. If cancer-free for 5 or more years, a woman with a history of breast cancer may possibly use DMPA (US MEC: 3)

***5. Do you have jaundice, cirrhosis of the liver, a liver infection or tumor? (Are her eyes or skin unusually yellow?) (See Appendix)***

☐ No ☐ Yes Perform physical exam or refer. If she has serious liver disease (jaundice, painful or enlarged liver, viral hepatitis, liver tumor), do not provide DMPA. Refer for care. Help her choose a method without hormones

***6. Do you have vaginal bleeding that is unusual for you? (See Appendix)***

☐ No ☐ Yes If she is not pregnant but has unexplained vaginal bleeding that suggest a serious underlying medical condition (US MEC:3), assess and treat any underlying condition as appropriate, or refer. Provide DMPA based on findings

**INITIATING METHOD** (see Figure 25.1, Page 146)

**A pelvic exam is NOT necessary prior to the initiation of this method** *[Stewart-2001]*

***Cycling women:***

- Preferred start time is during first 7 days from the start of menses
- Alternative: inject anytime in the cycle if not pregnant, back-up x 7 days

***Postpartum women:*** May give injection prior to hospital discharge. Special considerations:

- After severe obstetrical blood loss, delay injection until lochia stops
- If woman has history or high risk for severe postpartum depression, observe carefully and delay injection at least 4-6 weeks
- Breast-feeding women: May either start DMPA immediately or wait 4-6 week.

***Women who have spontaneous or therapeutic abortion:*** May initiate immediately.

***Women switching methods:***

- May start anytime patient is known not to be pregnant
- Hormonal method: if she has been using her current method consistently and correctly, may initiate immediately
- If switching from non-hormonal method, offer same options as cycling women

**INSTRUCTIONS FOR PATIENT:** ***Some women may be able to give themselves Depo-Provera injections***

- **Do NOT massage area where shot was given for a few hours** (massaging area may reduce duration of action and thereby effectiveness)
- Expect irregular bleeding/spotting in beginning. Usually decreases over time. Return at any time spotting or bleeding is bothersome. Rx may make bleeding pattern more tolerable
- It is not harmful or dangerous if you do not have periods while you use DMPA

**WEIGHT GAIN: A TEACHABLE MOMENT**

When you see a patient who is very heavy or has gained enough weight to disturb her, you have a teachable moment. BE PREPARED FOR THAT TEACHABLE MOMENT.

***Simple messages to share:***

1. **Eat less (small, frequent meals helps some to lose weight); eat balanced diet with lots of fruits and vegetables and minimal saturated fats, chips, cookies, pasta and other carbohydrates**
2. **Exercise more...and every day**
3. **Find patterns of eating and exercising that you enjoy! You won't do them for long unless you enjoy the process.**
4. **Drinking calories leads as quickly to obesity as eating them**
5. **Call Overeaters Anonymous (OA) - www.overeatersanonymous.org**
6. **Drink 8-10 glasses of water daily. Avoid juice and sweetened drinks.**

- Be sure to take in 1000 mg (women over age 25) to 1200 mg (adolescent women) of calcium every day to build your bones. Take calcium tablets like calcium carbonate or TUMS daily if your diet does not include enough calcium. Calcium is best absorbed when 500 mg is taken late in the day with a glass of orange juice. Get weight bearing and muscle-strengthening exercise at least 3 times a week (preferably 20 minutes daily)
- Return in 11-13 weeks for your next injection. Use abstinence, condoms, and EC, if necessary, if you are late coming for your re-injection (more than 13 weeks)
- Pregnancy is rare; return if you develop pregnancy symptoms other than amenorrhea
- Serious complications with DMPA are rare, but return if you develop severe headaches; heavy bleeding; depression or problems at the shot site (pus, pain, allergic reaction)
- If a woman becomes pregnant when she starts or while using Depo as her contraceptive, there is no increase in birth defects if her pregnancy goes term.

## FOLLOW-UP

- Are you experiencing spotting or irregular bleeding? Have you missed periods or had very light periods? Are you concerned about your pattern of bleeding?
- Did you have pain at the injection site after previous injection?
- Have you felt depressed or had major mood changes?
- Have you gained 5 pounds or more? (See WEIGHT GAIN, A TEACHABLE MOMENT, Page 143) Be sure to weigh patients at each visit. This means at **each and every visit**
- Consider measuring height and calculating a BMI
- Do you have any increase in your headaches?
- Have you had the feeling that you may be pregnant?
- Did you have any problems returning on time for this injection?
- Do you plan to have children? OR Do you plan to have more children?
- **Offer condoms to all women on Depo, both because it has the highest discontinuation rates of all contraceptives and also to prevent STIs.**

### STRUCTURED COUNSELING FOR DEPO-PROVERA PATIENTS WORKS! (Also see p. 8)

- Discontinuation rates for DMPA users at 1 year are high in the absence of structured counseling: 70% in a New York study of low-income women *[Polaneczky-1996]*; 43.4% in a rural Mexican study *[Canto-DeCetina-2001]*
- Importance of focused, structured, repeated counseling at initiation and follow-up visits can't be overstated.
- Structured counseling may include repetition, having patient repeat back instructions, showing videotapes, providing videotapes, audiotapes and written instructions and asking focused questions such as "What has happened to your pattern of bleeding?", "Have your periods become extremely light?", OR "Does your pattern of bleeding bother you?" rather than unfocused questions like "Are you having any problems?"
- **Structured counseling in Mexico lowered DMPA discontinuation associated with three bleeding problems: amenorrhea, irregular bleeding and heavy bleeding, from 32% to 8%. Discontinuation from amenorrhea fell from 17 to 3%; from SPT or BTB from 10 to 3%; and from heavy bleeding from 5 to 2%** *[Canto-DeCetina-2001]*
- **Isn't it fascinating that an effect, such as amenorrhea that might be considered an ADVANTAGE of using Depo-Provera, proved to be the most common reason for the discontinuation of Depo injections. Unless explained well and often, absence of bleeding is seen as a problem by many women.**
- Weight should be taken at each visit and weight control discussed carefully if there has been weight gain (see progressive weight gain Page 140 and WEIGHT GAIN: A TEACHABLE MOMENT Page 143)

## PROBLEM MANAGEMENT

***Allergic reaction or vasovagal reaction:*** In acute setting, provide support as needed. Benadryl may reduce pruritus and swelling. Oxygen and other resuscitation may be needed for severe reactions (extremely rare). Most allergic manifestations subside in 1 week or so. Refer if symptoms severe or do not improve appropriately. Avoid future injections and help her choose a different method. While women have had anaphylactic allergic reactions to Depo-Provera, they are extremely rare.

***Vaginal dryness (dyspareunia) or atrophic vaginitis:*** May be due to hypoestrogenism. Consider measuring $E_2$ levels and giving physiologic replacement dose of estrogen, if needed.

May give estrogen as vaginal cream, ring, tablets or systemic estrogen (tablets or patch) supplementation. Dyspareunia may be relieved with water soluble or silicone lubricants

***Pain or infection at injection site:*** Offer anti-inflammatory medications. Rule out infection or needle damage to nerve, etc. Provide appropriate antibiotics if cellulitis present

***Patient returns early (<11 weeks) wanting reinjection (eg b/c of travel):*** May give DMPA

***Patient returns late (>13 weeks) for reinjection:*** See Figure 25.1 on Page 146

- CDC Selective Practice Guidelines: repeat injection of DMPA can be given up to 2 weeks late without requiring additional contraceptive protection.

***Switching to another method (eg OCs, IUD, etc) from DMPA:*** Initiate new method at any time convenient for patient. Preferred time would be near end of effectiveness of last DMPA injection unless switching to OCs, patch or vaginal rings to control menstrual disorders on DMPA. **Do NOT wait until next menses to start pills.** She may have amenorrhea for a number of months after DMPA

***Transitioning perimenopausal women:*** See Figure 24.2 on Page 147

***Weight gain:*** Advise to watch caloric intake and to increase exercise. Refer to OA, Overeaters Anonymous. **Be ready to discontinue method if weight gain is excessive or unacceptable** (See teachable moment Page 143)

***Heavy bleeding:***

- Rule out pregnancy, cervical infection or neoplasia and other causes
- Rule out anemia - recommend iron rich foods and/or supplements
- May treat with NSAIDs or low dose estrogen supplements:
  - Ibuprofen 800 mg orally every 8 hours for 3 days
  - Mefenamic acid: 500 mg once, then 250 mg every 6 hours for 2-3 days
  - Conjugated equine estrogen (2.5, 1.25 or 0.625 mg) orally once a day up to four times per day for 4-6 days OR ethinyl estradiol x 21 days (expensive)
  - COCs for 1-2 months (in addition to DMPA use)

***Irregular bleeding and spotting:***

- **Reassure that cumulative blood loss is usually less not more**
- Rule out infection or cervical lesions as source
- Reassure that irregular spotting and bleeding is to be expected in first several months
- May use same therapies as outlined in heavy bleeding section above

***Amenorrhea:***

- Reassure her at each visit that this is not a medical problem. Do pregnancy test if she has other symptoms of pregnancy or in some instances, to assure her that she is not pregnant.
- Switch method if patient desires regular menses (consider patch, ring, COCs). Even if she stops DMPA, menses may not return for months

***Depression:***

- Evaluate suicide potential and refer immediately, if indicated
- Explain that DMPA usually does not worsen depression. Start antidepressant therapy, if needed. Discontinue DMPA if you or your patient has any misgivings about continuing its use

## FERTILITY AFTER DISCONTINUATION OF METHOD

- **Because anovulation may last for more than 1 year, women who know they will want to become pregnant within one year of cessation of use would be wise to consider another option, especially women over 35 years of age**
- Fertility returns afer 3 months; however, the conception rates overall are lower than women discontinuing other contraceptive methods. After last shot, 50% of women are pregnant after

**Figure 25.1 Initial Injection or Late Reinjection (more than 4 weeks since scheduled return visit at 13 weeks) of DMPA or Switching From DMPA to COCs or Another Hormonal Method***

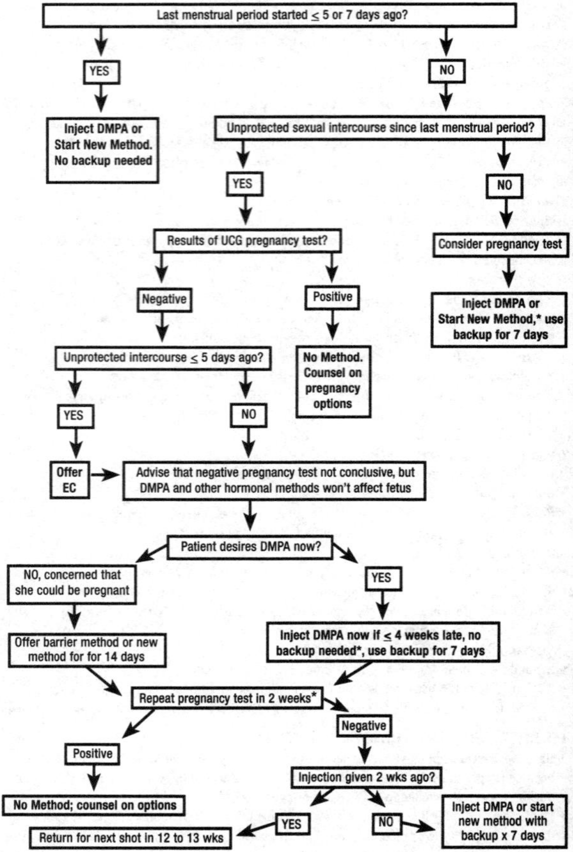




*Steiner MJ, Kwok C, Starback J et al. Contraception 2008 77 (2008) 410-414.*

**Figure 25.2 Making Transition from DMPA to Menopause, With or Without Hormone Replacement Therapy (HRT, EPT, or HT)**

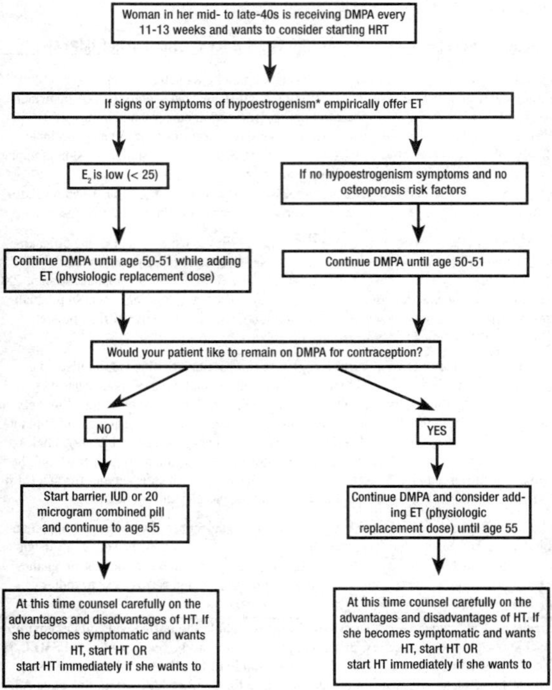


* DMPA can suppress gonadotropins, so measuring FSH or LH may not be informative of menopausal state. DMPA use decreases endogenous estrogen levels. Long-term DMPA users in their 40s may benefit from estrogen supplementation *[Kaunitz, 1998]*. Some researchers recommend that, at age 50, 2 FSH measurements be done at injection visit to assess menopausal status. If 2 consecutive levels are $\geq$ 35-40 m IU/ml, this is suggestive of menopause *[Juliato-2007]*.

6-7 months (compared to 4 months with other methods). (Delay not increased with increased duration of use). More than 90% of women become pregnant within 2 years

- Women who do not want to await spontaneous return of ovulation will require gonadotrophin therapy to induce ovulation. Gonadotropins will not overcome effect of DMPA on cervical mucus

## IMPLANTS: NEXPLANON OR IMPLANON - THE SINGLE ETONOGESTREL IMPLANT

**DESCRIPTION:** Single implant is 4-cm long and 2 mm in diameter (5 mm longer than one Norplant implant), with a membrane of ethylene vinyl acetate (EVA) copolymer and with a core of 68 mg of etonogestrel in EVA (the new name for 3-ketodesogestrel). Initially, progestin is released at rate of 60 µg per day decreasing to 25-30 mcg/day by end of year 3. Implant is effective for at least 3 years. Implant is placed under the skin of upper arm with a 16 gauge disposable, preloaded inserter

- Nexplanon is new version of Implanon that is radioopaque because it has barium sulfate replacing some of the EVA core. The inserter was improved to eliminate failed insertions.

**EFFECTIVENESS:** No pregnancies in earliest studies. Infrequent postmarketing pregnancies. Overall, 82% of women continue to use Implanon for 2 or more years. Women > 30% above ideal body weight excluded from initial studies. However, serum concentration of ENG remains high enough to suppress ovulation (0.3 ng/ml) even in heavier users. No pregnancies occurred in overweight women provided implants in the St Louis CHOICE project. *[Peipert Presentation in San Francisco, CA, March 2014]*

Of 173 classifiable Implanon failures reported to the Therapeutic Goods Administration in Australia, 49% were attributed to non-insertion of the implant, 27% were apparently conceived before the women had Implanon inserted, 11% were ascribed to insertion outside the recommended time in the menstrual cycle, 2% occurred after expulsion of the implant, and 12% were true product failures. In a much larger number of classifiable pregnancies reported to Merck (which may have included most of the Australian pregnancies), half had no implant present, and 38% were true product failures. In both series, a quarter to a third of the true method failures occurred in women taking possibly interacting drugs.

Whether user characteristics, such as body weight, might reduce the efficacy of Implanon is unknown. Serum etonogestrel levels appear inversely related to body weight, although no evidence has been found of a relationship between weight and ovulation or pregnancy rates. The number of obese women included in prospective and retrospective studies was relatively small.

**Drugs that may lower Nexplanon effectiveness include the anticonvulsants phenytoin, carbamazepine, barbiturates, primidone, topiramate, and oxcarbazepine. [USMEC:3] Condoms definitely should be used if Nexplanon is to be effective in a woman using one of these meds either as an anticonvlsant or for another indication. See page A8.**

Implanon is marketed with a duration of action of 3 years. However, pharmacokinetic data from Implanon users show stable serum concentrations of etonogestrel out to 36 months, suggesting that the method is effective for longer than that. Three studies in which a total of 275 women used Implanon for longer than 3 years found no pregnancies during the fourth year of use. (p.195 Contraceptive Implant chapter (20th edition of Contraceptive Technology) Women in the St. Louis CHOICE project are now in their 5th and 6th years of using the same Implanon Implant.

## HOW IMPLANON WORKS:

- Within 24 hours of insertion thick cervical mucus prevents normal sperm transport
- Inhibition of ovulation. No ovulation in first 2 years and only 2 women had 4 ovulatory events in third year of Implanon use. However, they did not get pregnant
- Atrophic endometrium

**COST:** $659.42 - Private Sector

## ADVANTAGES

***Menstrual:*** Decreased menstrual and ovulatory cramping or pain; overall, less bleeding than with Norplant and more amenorrhea (15% at one year). Less anemia. Dysmenorrhea decreases by 48% *[Affandi-1998]*

***Sexual/psychological:***

- Sexual intercourse may be more pleasurable because fear of pregnancy is reduced
- Usage not linked to sexual intercourse—allows spontaneity

***Cancers/tumors and masses:*** None

***Other:***

- High continuation rate in clinical trials. Cyclic headaches may improve
- Single implant is easier and faster to insert and remove than multiple implants. Removal is usually accomplished with only a #11 scalpel and gentle finger pressure with < 1.0 cc ml of local anesthetic (use tuberculin syringe)
- Asymptomatic (usually ) follicular cysts are less common

## DISADVANTAGES

***Menstrual:***

- Unpredictable/irregular menstrual bleeding frequent and may persist but usually is light and well tolerated
- Amenorrhea and oligomenorrhea common

***Sexual/psychological:***

- Irregular bleeding may inhibit sexual intercourse
- Insertion and removal require procedures, for which special training is needed

***Cancers/tumors and masses:*** None

***Other:***

- No STI protection
- Hormonal side effects: headache is most common
- May develop acne (or acne may improve)
- Ovarian cysts; usually resolve without treatment
- Dependent on clinician to remove

## COMPLICATIONS:

- Removal difficulties much less frequent than with Norplant
- Rarely, sonographic or MRI localization is required
- Rare infections

## CANDIDATES FOR USE:

- Implanon is particularly good for women with contraindications to or side effects from estrogen:
  - Women with personal history of thrombosis
  - Recently postpartum women
  - Women who are exclusively breast-feeding as there are no effects on breast milk or breast-feeding infants associated with Implanon use *[Reinprayoon-2000, Taneepanichskul-2005]*

- Smokers over age 35
- Women who had or fear chloasma, worsening migraine headaches, hypertriglyceridemia or other estrogen-related side effects
- Women with hypertension, coronary artery disease or cerebrovascular disease

## PRESCRIBING PRECAUTIONS, MEDICAL ELIGIBILITY CHECKLIST, INITIATING METHOD:

Same precautions as for progestin-only pills

## INITIATING METHOD:

- If inserted within 7 days of LMP, no backup needed. Can be inserted any time of cycle if reasonably certain not pregnant. If later than 7 days from LMP, use backup x 7 days
- If has been on DMPA, insert at time next injection due. No backup needed

**INSTRUCTIONS FOR PATIENT**: Irregular bleeding is to be expected and persists while rod is in place. If your pattern of bleeding is unacceptable, come back because there are several treatments that may make your bleeding pattern more acceptable (Periodic COC, patch, ring use). Amenorrhea more likely than with Norplant, but less likely than with DMPA

**FOLLOW-UP:** Routine GYN follow-up

## PROBLEM MANAGEMENT:

***Amenorrhea:*** Quite common. Pregnancy test if symptoms of pregnancy

***Spotting/breakthrough bleeding:*** to be expected; not harmful. If bothersome may provide several cycles of low-dose pills, patch or rings or NSAIDs

***Arm Pain after insertion***

- Rule out nerve damage or infection
- If due to bruising, advise her to make sure bandage is not too tight
- Apply ice packs for 24 hours
- Take acetaminophen or NSAID

***Infection in insertion area***

- *No abscess:* cellutlitis only. Do not remove, Clean infected area with antiseptic. Oral antibiotics for 7 days. (Recheck in 24-48 hours to make sure improving and at end of therapy)
- *Abscess:* Preload with antibiotics; prepare infected area with antiseptic, make incision, drain pus, and remove implant. Continue antibiotic therapy and wound care

***Difficult to locate rod:*** may be found by ultrasound or MRI. This requires experienced sonographer using tranducer of 10 MHz or greater. Rarely, there may be a failure of provider to insert the rod (implant left in inserter)

**FERTILITY AFTER DISCONTINUATION OF USE**: Return to baseline fertility is rapid and complete; 94% ovulate within 3-6 weeks of removal

## NEXPLANON INSERTION

**Initiating Contraception with Nexplanon**

**IMPORTANT: Rule out pregnancy before inserting the implant.**

Timing of insertion depends on the woman's recent contraceptive history, as follows:

- **No preceding hormonal contraceptive use in the past month**

Nexplanon should be inserted between Day 1 (first day of menstrual bleeding) and Day 5 of the menstrual cycle, even if the woman is still bleeding.

If inserted as recommended, back-up contraception is not necessary. If deviating from the recommended timing of insertion, the woman should be advised to use a barrier method until 7 days after insertion. If intercourse has already occurred, pregnancy should be excluded.

- **Switching contraceptive method to Nexplanon**

**Combination hormonal contraceptives:**
Nexplanon should preferably be inserted on the day after the last active tablet of the previous combined oral contraceptive or on the day of removal of the vaginal ring or transdermal patch. At the latest, Nexplanon should be inserted on the day following the usual tablet-free, ring-free, patch-free or placebo tablet interval of the previous combined hormonal contraceptive. If inserted as recommended, back-up contraception is not necessary. If deviating from the recommended timing of insertion, the woman should be advised to use a barrier method until 7 days after insertion. If intercourse has already occurred, pregnancy should be excluded.

**Progestin-only contraceptives:**
There are several types of progestin-only methods. Nexplanon should be inserted as follows:
- Injectable Contraceptives: Insert Nexplanon on the day the next injection is due.
- Minipill: A woman may switch to Nexplanon on any day of the month. Nexplanon should be inserted within 24 hours after taking the last tablet.
- Contraceptive implant or intrauterine system (IUS): Insert Nexplanon on the same day the previous contraceptive implant or IUS is removed.

If inserted as recommended, back-up contraception is not necessary. If deviating from the recommended timing of insertion, the woman should be advised to use a barrier method until 7 days after insertion. If intercourse has already occurred, pregnancy should be excluded.

**Insertion of Nexplanon**
Successful use and removal of Nexplanon is based on careful subdermal insertion of the single, rod-shaped implant in accordance with the instructions. The implant should be palpable under the skin by both the woman and the healthcare provider after placement.

**All healthcare providers performing insertions and/or removals of Nexplanon should receive instructions and training prior to inserting or removing the implant. For information regarding the insertion and removal of Nexplanon call 1-877-467-5266.**

**Preparation**
**Prior to inserting Nexplanon carefully read the instructions for insertion as well as the full prescribing information.**

Before insertion of Nexplanon, confirm that the woman receiving the implant:
- is not pregnant nor has any other contraindication for the use of Nexplanon
- has undergone a medical history and physical examination, including a gynecologic examination
- understands the benefits and risks of Nexplanon

Insert Nexplanon under aseptic conditions.

The following equipment is needed for the implant insertion:
- An examination table for the woman to lie on
- Sterile surgical drapes, sterile gloves, antiseptic solution, sterile marker (optional)
- Local anesthetic, needles and syringe
- Sterile gauze, adhesive bandage, pressure bandage

**Insertion of Nexplanon**

The basis for successful use and subsequent removal of Nexplanon is a correct and carefully performed subdermal insertion of the single, rod-shaped implant in accordance with the instructions. Both the healthcare provider and the woman should be able to feel the implant under the skin after placement.

**All healthcare providers performing insertions and/or removals of Nexplanon should receive instructions and training prior to inserting or removing the implant. Information concerning the insertion and removal of Nexplanon will be sent upon request free of charge (1-877-467-5266).**

**Preparation**

**Prior to inserting Nexplanon carefully read the instructions for insertion as well as the full prescribing information.**

Before insertion of Nexplanon, the healthcare provider should confirm that:
• The woman is not pregnant nor has any other contraindication for the use of Nexplanon
• The woman has had a medical history and physical examination, including a gynecologic examination, performed
• The woman understands the benefits and risks of Nexplanon
• The woman has received a copy of the Patient Labeling included in packaging
• The woman has reviewed and completed a consent form to be maintained with the woman's chart
• The woman does not have allergies to the antiseptic and anesthetic to be used during insertion.

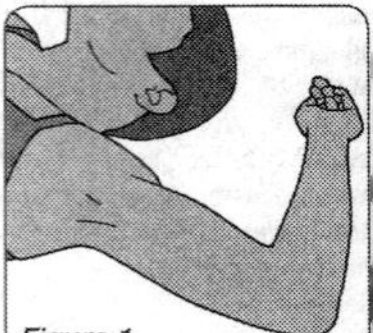

Figure 1

The following equipment is needed for the implant insertion:
• An examination table for the woman to lie on
• Sterile surgical drapes, sterile gloves, antiseptic solution, sterile marker (optional)
• Local anesthetic, needles and syringe
• Sterile gauze, adhesive bandage, pressure bandage

Figure 2

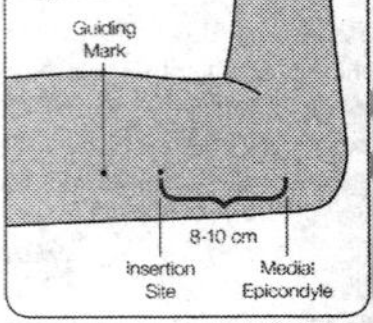


**Insertion Procedure**

**Step 1:** Have the woman lie on her back on the examination table with her non-dominant arm flexed at the elbow and externally rotated so that her wrist is parallel to her ear or her hand is positioned next to her head (Figure 1).

**Step 2:** Identify the insertion site, which is at the inner side of the non-dominant upper arm about 8-10 cm (3-4 inches) above the media epicondyle of the humerus (Figure 2). **The implant should be inserted subdermally just under the skin to avoid the large blood vessels and nerves that lie deeper in the subcutaneous tissue in the sulcus between the triceps and biceps muscles.**

**Step 3:** Make two marks with a sterile marker: first, mark the spot where the etonogestrel implant will be inserted, and second, mark a spot a few centimeters proximal to the first mark (Figure 2). The second mark will later serve as a direction guide during insertion.

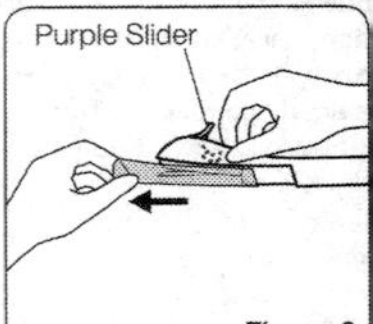


Figure 3

**Step 4:** Clean the insertion site with an antiseptic solution.
**Step 5:** Anesthetize the insertion area (for example, with anesthetic spray or by injecting 2 mL of 1% lidocaine just under the skin along the planned insertion tunnel).
**Step 6:** Remove the sterile preloaded disposable Nexplanon applicator carrying the implant from its blister. The applicator should not be used if sterility is in question.
**Step 7:** Hold the applicator just above the needle at the textured surface area. Remove the transparent protection cap by sliding it horizontally in the direction of the arrow away from the needle (Figure 3). If the cap does not come off easily, the applicator should not be used. You can see the white colored implant by looking into the tip of the needle. **Do not touch the purple slider until you have fully inserted the needle subdermally, as it will retract the needle and prematurely release the implant from the applicator.**
**Step 8:** With your free hand, stretch the skin around the insertion site with thumb and index finger (Figure 4).
**Step 9:** Puncture the skin with the tip of the needle angled about 30° (Figure 5).
**Step 10:** Lower the applicator to a horizontal position. While lifting the skin with the tip of the needle (Figure 6), slide the needle to its full length. You may feel slight resistance but do not exert excessive force. **If the needle is not inserted to its full length, the implant will not be inserted properly.**
**You can best see movement of the needle if you are seated and are looking at the applicator from the side and NOT from above. In this position, you can clearly see the insertion site and the movement of the needle just under the skin.**
**Step 11:** Keep the applicator in the same position with the needle inserted to its full length. If needed, you may use your free hand to keep the applicator in the same position during the following procedure. Unlock the purple slider by pushing it slightly down. Move the slider fully back until it stops (Figure 7). The implant is now in its final subdermal position, and the needle is locked inside the body of the applicator. The applicator can now be removed. **If the applicator is not kept in the same position during this procedure or if the purple slider is not completely moved to the back, the implant will not be inserted properly.**
**Step 12: Always verify the presence of the implant in the woman's arm immediately after insertion by palpation.** By palpating both ends of the implant, you should be able to confirm the presence of the 4 cm rod (Figure 8).

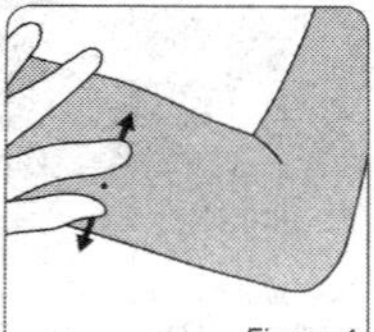

Figure 4

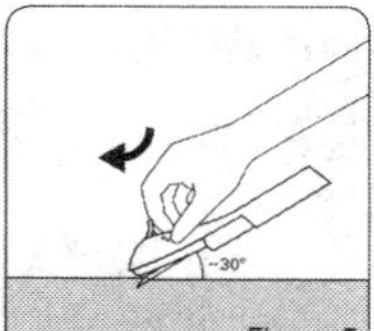


Figure 5

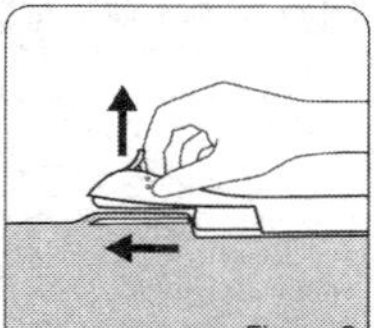

Figure 6

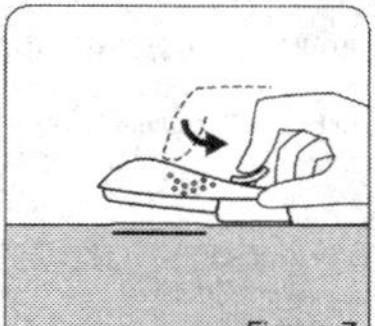

Figure 7

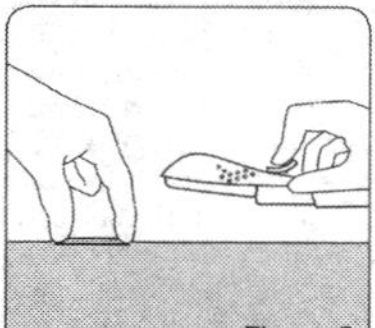

Figure 8

# CHAPTER 26

# Female Sterilization: Tubal Ligation or Occlusion

www.engenderedhealth.org, www.plannedparenthood.org or www.essure.com

➔ **DESCRIPTION:** Surgery to remove (salpingectomy) or to interrupt the patency of fallopian tubes. In 2002 in the USA, 27% of married women reported having had tubal sterilization while 9% of their husbands had a vasectomy *[Mosher-2004]*. Many single women have sterilization operations. Approximately half of sterilizations in the USA are done in the postpartum period within 48 hours of delivery *[Peterson-1998]*.

**EFFECTIVENESS:** Failure rates vary depending on sterilization method and patient's age.

**Table 26.1 Cumulative 10-year failure rates for some methods of voluntary female sterilization methods***

| *Method* | *Failure rate (highest rate)* |
|---|---|
| Postpartum partial salpingectomy | 0.8%* |
| Silastic bands over loop of tube | 1.8%* |
| Interval partial salpingectomy | 2.0%* |
| Bipolar cautery | 2.5%* |
| Spring clip application | 3.7%* |
| Filshie clip (7 years) | 0.9%+ |

For each sterilization method, at least 50% more failures were ascertained AFTER 2 YEARS as had been identified in the 2 years immediately following the sterilization procedure

* *U.S. Collaborative Review of Sterilization. The risk of pregnancy after tubal sterilization. Am J Obstet Gynecol 1996;174:1161-70.*

+ *Filshie clip (0.9% failure rate - 7 years) [Chi-Chen Contraception 1987;35:171-8]*

- Younger women had higher failure rates
- All methods require proper application to maximize effectiveness
- Teaching institution rates(above study) may differ from private settings

**Hysteroscopic tubal occlusion:** 99.74% effective at 5 years (if post-op verified occlusion by hysterosalpingogram)

➔ **HOW FEMALE STERILIZATION WORKS**: Since many of the most lethal ovarian cancers originate in the fimbria of the distal fallopian tubes, serious consideration should be given to removal of fallopian tubes by salingectomy as the tubal sterilization precedure of choice. Interruption of patency of the fallopian tubes preferably in isthmic region thereby preventing fertilization

## LAPAROSCOPIC STERILIZATION: TRANSABDOMINAL

***Bipolar cautery:***

- Apply to area along fallopian tube with no vessels ascending through broad ligament, where the diameter of tube is similar on either side of selected area (at least 2 cm from uterotubal junction). Thoroughly cauterize tissue using bipolar cutting current of 25 Watts passing through jaws of instrument. Bipolar cautery has the highest risk of subsequent fistulization and ectopic pregnancy.

***Silastic band:*** (Fallope Ring, Yoon Band)

- Apply over knuckle of tube at least 3 cm from utero-tubal junction. Loop of banded tube should clearly contain two complete diameters of tube

***Hulka-Clemens clip (spring clip):***

- Spring-loaded clip. Apply to isthmic portion of tube. 1-2 cm distal to cornu at an angle of 90% relative to long axis of tube. Highest failure rate

***Filshie clip:***

- Hinged titanium clip with cured silicone rubber lining. Apply to isthmic portion of tube, 1 to 2 cm from cornu. Should see hook end of clip through filmy mesosalpinx. May apply postpartum with special applicator (0.9% failure vs. 0.4% failure for interval application) *[Penfield--2000]*

## Figure 26.1 Laparoscopic Technique Diagrams

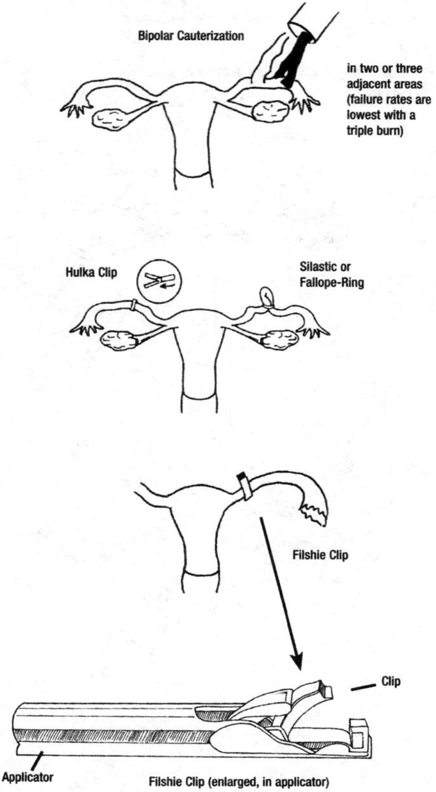

## POSTPARTUM OR INTERVAL MINI-LAPAROTOMY METHODS

***Modified Pomeroy:***

- Ligation at the base of a loop of isthmic portion of tube with plain absorbable catgut suture (2 separate ties) followed by excision of the knuckle of tube. Segment is histologically confirmed to contain tubal ostia.

***Modified Parkland:***

- Excision of segment of isthmic portion of tube after separate ligation of cut ends, no "knukle formed"

***Irving, Uchida and Fimbriectomy are rarely performed***

**Figure 25.2 Postpartum or Mini-Laparotomy Techniques**

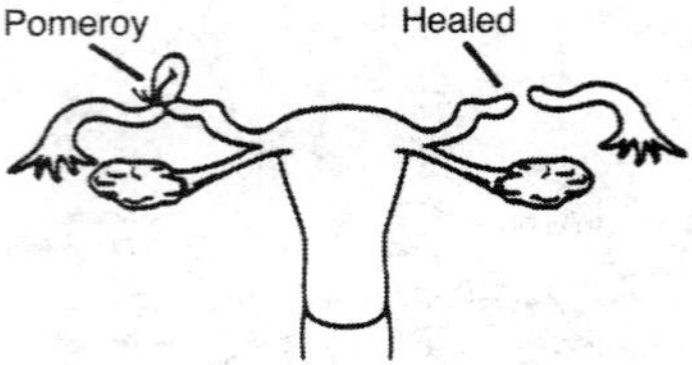


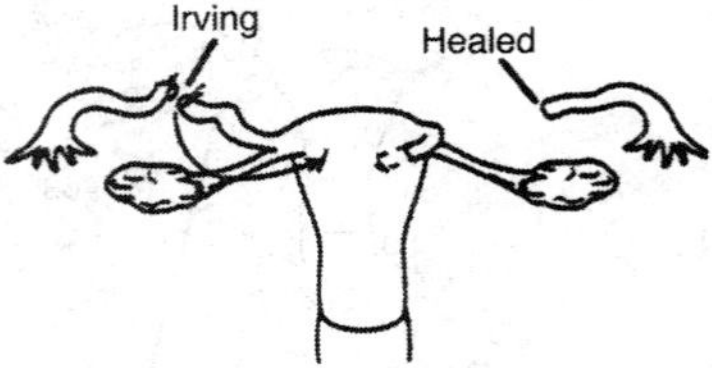

## ADVANTAGES

***Menstrual:*** None

***Sexual/psychological:*** Enhanced enjoyment of sex by reducing worry of pregnancy

***Cancers, tumors, and masses:***

- Decreased risk of ovarian cancer. Women with BRCA 1 mutations who have undergone a tubal ligation have a 60% lower risk of developing invasive ovarian cancer. *[Narod-Lancet 357 (9267): 1467-70, 2001]*. Overall 40% reduction in risk of ovarian cancer. Salpingectomy may be the best procedure to reduce a women's risk to ovarian cancer.

***Other:***

- Permanent and highly effective

## DISADVANTAGES

***Menstrual:***

- Data from 9514 women who underwent tubal sterilization by 6 techniques and followed for up to 5 years suggest no "post-tubal ligation syndrome" and no increases in the amount or duration of menstrual bleeding or menstrual pain. *[Peterson, 2000]*

***Sexual/psychological:***

- Regret may occur especially with young patients; counsel well and offer reversible methods if any hesitancy (see Fig. 26.5, Page 160)

***Cancers, tumors, and masses:*** None

***Other:***

- Requires outpatient surgery (usually with general anesthesia); Expensive in short term
- If failure occurs, higher risk of ectopic pregnancy (30%)
- Not readily reversible
- Does not prevent spread of HIV and STIs

## COMPLICATIONS *[Peterson, 1997]*

| | ***Minilaparotomy*** | ***Laparoscopy*** |
|---|---|---|
| ***Minor*** | 11.6% | 6.0% |
| ***Major*** | 1.5% | 0.9% |

- Minor complications include infection, wound separation
- Major complications include conversion to laparotomy, hemorrhage, viscus injury especially with cautery, anesthetic complications
- Major vessel injury risk with laparoscopy 3-9/10,000 procedures
- Mortality: 1-2/100,000 procedures (leading cause is general anesthesia)

## LONG-TERM RISKS

- Statistically higher risk for subsequent hysterectomy, but only in women who had gynecologic complaints prior to sterilization
- Regret (0.9% - 26.0%) Risk factors include: age under 30, low parity, sterilization at time of cearean delivery, change in marital status, poverty, minority status, misinformation about permanence or risks, hurried decision. If sterilized < 30 years old, 40% requested information on reversal, 20% expressed regret but only 1% had a reversal done *[Schmidt-2000]*. **This issue requires careful counseling**

## CANDIDATES FOR USE

- Woman who is certain she wants no more children
- Woman over age 21 (only required for Medicaid reimbursement, not for medical requirements or for California state funding)
- Woman for whom surgery is considered safe

***Adolescents:*** Not a preferred method, generally higher regret and higher failure rates

## ESSURE: HYSTEROSCOPIC STERILIZATION VIA POLYESTER FIBERS

*www.essure.com*

- Essure insert is 4cm long, 1-2mm wide
- Inner coil stainless steel and polythylene terephthalate (PET) fibers
- Outer coil nickel-titanium alloy
- After placement in proximal tube, PET stimulates benign tissue growth that blocks tubes
- It takes 3 months after procedure for tubes to become occluded
- An hysterosaplingogram (HSG) is needed 3 months after placement to document a) bilateral satisfactory placement AND b) bilateral occlusion.

### Figure 26.3 Essure System Overview: Micro-Insert Design

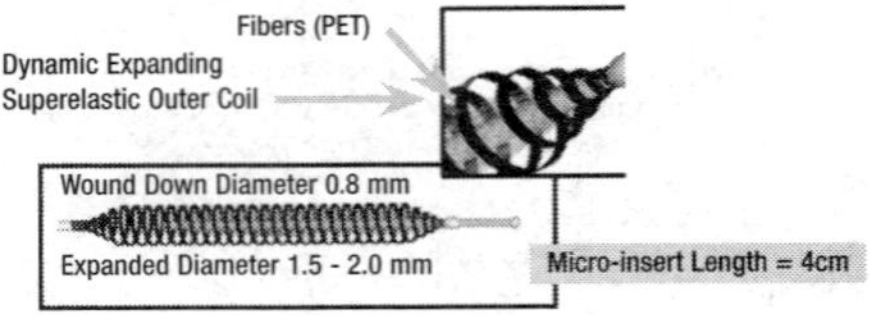


**ADVANTAGES: "The alternative to incision"**

- Provides tubal sterilization in physician's or ambulatory surgery office (average operating time: 13 to 35 minutes)
- No change in a woman's menstrual cycles
- There is no need for conscious sedation or general anesthesia (nonsteriodal premedication is strongly recommended to prevent tubal spasm)
- In clinical trial, (Australia, Europe, and the U.S.) 92% of women returned to work in one day, most resumed normal activities the same day as the procedure
- May be preferred for obese women, women with abdominal adhesions, or women with risk factors for anesthesia
- Successful bilateral placement rates vary from 86% in the first trial to 94.6% in the post-approval study
- If bilateral placement successful, there is a 3% chance that HSG does NOT confirm correct location AND bilateral occlusion. This may be due to perforation (<1%), expulsion (<1%) or continued patency
- Cumulative risk pregnancy 2.6 per 1000 procedures
  -Most common cause of pregnancy: pregnant at time of placement.

**DISADVANTAGES: Requires specialized training and equipment**

- **Hysterosaplingogram must be done at 3 months to confirm blockage. Until that time, couple must use another contraceptive.**
- The option of using transvaginal ultrasound to replace the Essure confirmation test, which was already approved in Europe and Canada, is being currently reviewed by the FDA.
- Procedure designed for interval sterilization. It is not to be used at Cesarean delivery or immediately postpartum *[Bullagh, 2003]*
- Luteal pregnancies occured in 4 of 466 women in spite of negative urine pregnancy tests on the day of the procedure

**ESSURE:** continued

- It may not be possible to visualize both tubal ostia (this occurs about 2% of the time)
- May require more than one operative procedure
- Expulsion of one or both devices (14 of 466 successful procedures or 3.0%)
- Perforation of the uterus occured during 1% of procedures
- This form of sterilization cannot be reversed

**ADIANA: HYSTEROSCOPIC STERILIZATION**

- Used silicone plugs with low-level bipolar radio frequency (RF) energy to block the tubes
- Was marketed in the US from 2009-2012 and then discontinued

## PRESTERILIZATION COUNSELING CHECKLIST*

- Discuss alternative reversible methods and quote their effectiveness. (IUDs and implants are more effective than some forms of tubal sterilization)
- Discuss vasectomy as an alternative
- Insure patient commitment to having no future children, even if something happened to her current family
- Describe details of surgery (informed consent later) and possible intraoperative and long-term complications (risk for ectopic pregnancy)
- Stress that procedure must be considered irreversible and that about 10% of women regret their decision and answer all of her questions
- Discuss that ~ 2% of laparoscopic and transcervical procedures cannot be completed on first attempt. Review the "what if" intended procedure cannot be completed
- Obtain informed consent using locally approved consent forms - No requirement that spouse must be involved

**Adapted from ACOG Technical Bulletin, April 1996.*

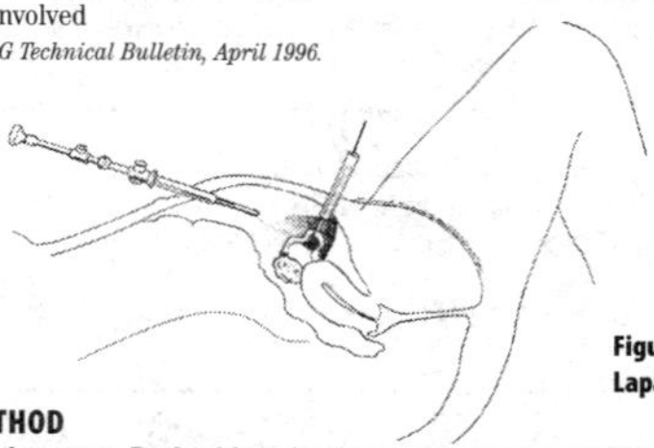

**Figure 26.4 Laparoscopy**

## INITIATING METHOD

- Obtain informed consent. Preferable to involve partner in process, but not necessary
- Any time in cycle with certainty of no conception, otherwise follicular timing preferred. Not true for Essure. With Essure, you want to time when lining will be <u>very</u> thin
- The routine provision of antibiotics is generally NOT recommended *[see ACOG Practice Bulletin No. 23, January, 2001]*

## FOLLOW-UP

- For women having interval occlusion procedure, follow up in two weeks for post-op wound check is typical, but not required. Routine annual gynecology exams
- 3-month follow up visit for Essure (see Page 158)

## MANAGEMENT OF PROBLEMS

- Anesthesia complications, wound infections, intraperitoneal adhesion formation, hydrosalpinx – managed with standard approaches
- Although some women report irregular menses or dysmenorrhea after tubal sterilization, several studies have demonstrated that a syndrome of irregular menses or dysmenorrhea following tubal sterilization does NOT exist *[Peterson-2000]*. These problems are **not** apt to develop at any higher rates in sterilized women. They are most likely age-related and inevitable

## FERTILITY AFTER TUBAL STERILIZATION

- Women must desire to be permanently sterile because reversal is costly and results are unpredictable. In vitro fertilization may be possible, but many cannot afford this procedure and it is not always successful

## Figure 26.5 Sterilization Requested by Young Woman

**Inform her that risk of regret following tubal sterilization is higher in the United States if she is:**

- Young
- Unmarried (single, separated or divorced)
- Unmarried now but is married later on, especially if new husband wants a child with her
- Married now but becomes divorced later
- On Medicaid or has a very low or no income
- African-American or Hispanic
- Close to the end of a pregnancy (postpartum, post-therapeutic abortion or post-miscarriage)
- Thinking that tubal sterilziation is easy to reverse (it is both very expensive and about 60% effective). Essure, the new transcervical sterilization technique, is particularly difficult to reverse. More often now in-vitro fertilization is attempted if pregnancy is desired post BTL. It is very expensive and may not be successful

- Counsel her to consider waiting until her later 20's or early 30's for tubal sterilization
- Offer use of effective long-term contraceptive: Copper T 380 A or Levonorgestrel IUD (Mirena)
- Be sure she knows that the final decision is ***hers*** to make, not yours or her partner's
- Ask if partner is interested in vasectomy

Still wants tubal sterilization

Respect this wish and assist her in accomplishing her goal

Willing to initiate long-term reversible contraceptive

Do all you can to ensure consistent, correct use of reversible method. Remain willing to provide her with sterilization at her request

# CHAPTER 27

## Male Sterilization: Vasectomy

www.engenderedhealth.org or www.plannedparenthood.org

**DESCRIPTION:** Permanent male contraception. Outpatient surgical procedure. No-scalpel technique punctures scrotum, delivers vas; ligates or cauterizes vas. Among married men, ages 15-44, 13.1 % reported vasectomy compared to 21.1% of married women reporting tubal sterilization. Men with higher education and income had greater prevalence vascetomy vs. women with lower education and income having higher prevalence of female sterilization. *[Anderson et al. 2012]*

**EFFECTIVENESS** (See Table 12.2, Page 37)
***Perfect use failure rate in first year:*** 0.10%
***Typical use failure rate in first year:*** 0.15%
*[Trussell J, IN Contraceptive Technology, 2004]*

> Although vasectomy is safer and potentially more effective than tubal sterilization, as of mid-2000, there are only 4 nations in the world where vasectomies exceed tubal sterilizations: Great Britain, the Netherlands, New Zealand and Bhutan.

Recent analysis of the 540 women in the CREST study who were protected by vasectomy found a cumulative failure rate of 9.4 per 1000 procedures at one year (0.9%) and 11.3 at years 2, 3 and 5. *[Jamieson, Costello, Trussell et al-2004]*

**HOW VASECTOMY WORKS:** Interrupts vas deferens preventing passage of sperm into seminal fluid and female reproductive tract

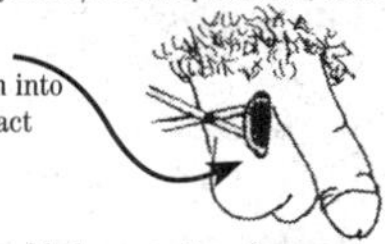

Vas deferens isolated following incision with scapel

**ADVANTAGES**

***Sexual/psychological:***

- Sexual intercourse may be more enjoyable because fear of pregnancy decreased
- Permits man opportunity to take on an important contraceptive role
- No interference during sexual intercourse and no contraceptive burden for female

***Cancers, tumors, and masses:*** None

***Other:***

- Simpler, safer and more effective than female sterilization
- More cost-effective than female sterilization and more convenient
- Shares contraception responsibility with partner
- No supplies or further clinic visits needed after sperm count has been documented to be zero
- Only local anesthesia required

**DISADVANTAGES**

***Sexual/ psychological:***

- Some men resist vasectomy fearing that it will interfere with sexual function (it doesn't) or because they feel contraception is solely the woman's responsibility (it isn't)
- Regret at a later time possible (1% of men request a reversal)
- Will need back-up method until there are no motile sperm. Female partner may still need contraception if she has other partner(s) or if STI protection needed

***Cancers, tumors, and masses:*** None

***Other:***

- Does not reduce risk for STIs; will still need to use condom if at risk
- Short-term post-operative discomfort, bruising, and swelling

## COMPLICATIONS

- Surgically related complaints such as hematoma, bruising, wound infection, or adverse reaction to local anesthesia
- Severe chronic pain (2%) *[Choe, Kirkema - 1996]*. Usually limited to less than 1 year
- Later regret possible

**CANDIDATES FOR USE:** Men who desire a permanent method

## INITIATING METHOD

- Take preoperative history; make general health assessment
- Ask if history of genital infections or anomalies
- Obtain informed consent. In general, try to involve partner
- Carefully counsel, especially about permanence of method
- Advise patient to bathe genital area and upper thighs prior to surgery; wear clean, loose-fitting clothes to facility; no food for 2 hours before procedure

## PRESCRIBING PRECAUTIONS

- Current infection of penis, prostate, or scrotum
- Fear of needles or scalpels (scalpels not required if no-scalpel vasectomy)

## INSTRUCTIONS FOR PATIENT

- Plan to rest for 48 hours and wear scrotal support
- Apply ice pack to incision site to decrease swelling, pain and bruising. Small packages of frozen peas conform well around the scrotum
- Keep area dry for two days – wear snug underwear and pants to provide support where needed
- If any symptoms or signs of infection develop, seek help immediately.
- Return as directed for sperm counts. Results from a new study suggest that azospermia is more likely after 12 weeks (60% azospermia) than after 20 ejaculations (28% azospermic) and that neither endpoint is ideal *[Barone-2003]*. Use other forms of contraception until two consecutive sperm samples show no motile sperm

**FOLLOW-UP:** ***To avoid failure due to LATE recanalization, repeating semen analysis every few years makes sense***

- Have you had your semen tested? If yes, were motile sperm absent?

## PROBLEM MANAGEMENT

***Wound infection:*** Treat with antibiotics. Drain and treat any abscesses
***Hematoma:*** Apply warm moist packs to scrotum. Provide scrotal support
***Granuloma:*** Observe; usually it will resolve itself. Occasionally requires surgery
***Pain at site:*** If no infection, provide scrotal support and analgesics
***Excessive swelling:*** If large and painful, may require surgery. Provide scrotal support if hematoma
***Chronic persistent pain considered to be severe:*** *[2% - Choe, Kirkema - 1996]*. IPPF Handbook states that this pain can often be relieved by vasovasectomy or decompression of the distended vas deferens releasing the sperm into the scrotal cavity *[Evans, Huezo IPPF Handbook - 1997]*

## FERTILITY AFTER VASECTOMY

- Man must accept that vasectomy is irreversible and permanent
- Microsurgical techniques of reversal now result in return of sperm to ejaculate in over 90% of men, but in pregnancy rates of only 50% or above. Reversibility rates decrease as time passed since procedure increases

- Important factors for reversal are
  - skill of microsurgeon
  - length of time since vasectomy
  - presence of antisperm antibodies (man)
  - partner's fertility
  - manner in which vasectomy was performed (amount of vas removed or cauterized)

## Figure 27.1 Vasectomy - No-Scalpel Techniques

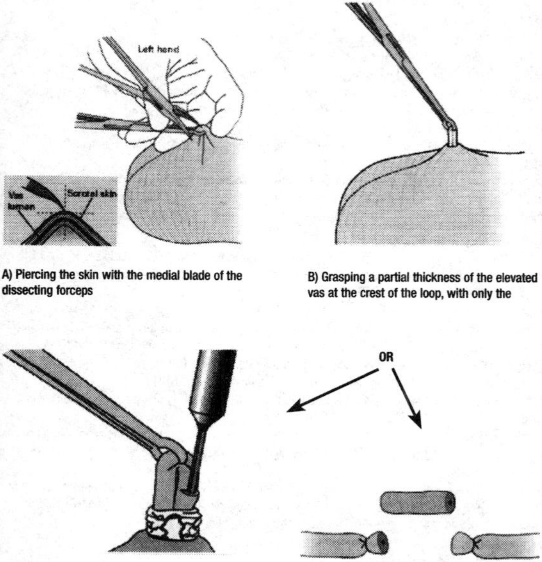


A) Piercing the skin with the medial blade of the dissecting forceps

B) Grasping a partial thickness of the elevated vas at the crest of the loop, with only the

Cautery with a blunt wire inserted into the hemi-transected vas (done in each direction)

Ligation and section

Cornell No-Scalpel Vasectomy Center. No-Scalpel Vasectomy. http://www.vasectomy.com/no-scalpel-vasectomy-diagram.html.2/6/02.

# CHAPTER 28

# Ordering and Stocking Devices: Nexplanon, Mirena/Skyla, ParaGard

www.implanon-usa.com, www.mirena-support.com, www.paragard.com

**ORDERING AND STOCKING DEVICES:** Telephone numbers below are for ordering devices, speaking with customer service, reporting adverse events.

## NEXPLANON

- Call 877-467-5266 to order Nexplanon, www.nexplanon.com
- Nexplanon dispensed by two pharmacies: CuraScript and CVS Caremark
- To set up account, need state license number and DEA number
- Pharmacy verifies that health care provider (HCP) has attended a company sponsored Implanon or Nexplanon training program
- Nexplanon is usually a "medical benefit"; sometimes a pharmacy benefit
- If Nexplanon contaminated prior to insertion or touching the patient, there is no replacement by the company.
- HCPs may complete and fax a benefits search (determine if an individual's insurance covers Implanon) to pharmacy. Search completed within 48-72 hrs. ***Cost*** of implant alone (if no insurance): $659.42 Implanon/Nexplanon. Payment plans available. 6 month plan: $109.00/month. For information, call 1-877-Implanon

## MIRENA/SKYLA

- Call 1-866-647-3646, www.mirenasupport.com, www.mirena-us.com, www.archfoundation.com
- To set up an account, clinician needs license. Bayer verifies that the HCP has been trained. If not, a training kit will be included in the order
- Verify insurance coverage
- Clinicians can order through Caremark/CVS at www.mirena-us.com/hcp/ordering-and-reimbursement/how-do-i-use-it.jsp or by calling 1-866-638-8312. Clinicians fax prescription and Caremark/CVS determines insurance eligibility and calls patient to confirm out-of-pocket costs. The Mirena is shipped to HCP
- If no coverage, patients can pay by credit card with Mirena shipped to HCP.
- Low income patients can apply to the ARCH foundation (1-877-393-9071) or www.archfoundation.com for a subsidized Mirena
- If Mirena is contaminated upon insertion, or removed early for a medical reason, no general replacement policy exists. However, by calling the hotline or their Bayer sales consultant, they will consider each event on a case-by-case basis.
- ***Cost*** (of IUS if no insurance): $843.60 (single payment). Patient may pay by 4 installments or 24 equal payments of $35.15. Call 1-866-638-8312 to take advantage of one of these plans. Mirena will be ordered by health care provider and shipped to the office within 2 to 3 business days.

## PARAGARD

- Call 1-877-727-2427, www.ParaGard.com
- To set up an account, a clinician needs a state license number
- Verify patient insurance coverage prior to insertion
- If no coverage, patients can pay by credit card / ParaGard shipped to HCP
- Replacement policy: If a clinician contaminates the IUD prior to touching the patient (e.g., drops on floor), call the hotline within 7 days AND save the product to ship back to them. They will send a replacement. If the woman has the ParaGard removed for a medical reason within 90 days (and reported within 30 days of removal) they will replace the product if the patient desires. If patient paid for IUD – she will be reimbursed. If she paid and is not satisfied with the IUD, she can get a full refund within the first 150 days
- ***Cost*** (of IUD if no insurance): $ 754.00 or 12 credit card payments

# CHAPTER 29
# HPV Vaccine

www.cdc.gov, www.acog.org, www.gardasil.com, www.cervarix.com

## HPV VACCINE:

- Quadrivalent vaccine (Gardasil) protects against infection with HPV types 6, 11, 16, 18 which account for 70% of HPV-related cervical cancer and 90% of genital warts
- Vaccine prepared from highly purified virus like particles (VLPs) of the major capsid protein of the HPV
- IM injection to deltoid or thigh
- Designed to prevent the following conditions caused by HPV 6,11,16,18 (these conditions may still occur related to other HPV types): cervical dysplasia and cancer, vulvar or vaginal dysplasia and genital warts
- Now offered to males ages 9-26 also for prevention of warts
- 4 Phase 2 and 3 randomized, placebo controlled trials evaluated 20, 451 women ages 16-26. Median duration of follow-up was 4,3,2.4 and 2 years
- Vaccine was found to be highly effective in preventing acquisition of disease
- Vaccine is a preventive tool, not a substitution for cervical cancer screening. These recommendations remain unaffected by the vaccine's approval and use
- Administered in a series of 3 innoculations: initial injection, then 2 months and 4 months after that
- Approved for females ages 9-26: Federal Advisory Committee on Immunization Practices (ACIP) recommends administering to girls between ages 11 and 12; may be given from age 9
- Women with previous HPV infection or abnormal cytology can still be vaccinated and may benefit from protection from strains they may not have yet acquired. Benefits in these women may be more limited and women should be informed of this. Benefits may also decrease in women who have had $\geq 5$ lifetime sexual partners
- Vaccination is not treatment for genital warts
- Immunosuppression is not a contraindication to vaccination; efficacy may be affected
- Currently not recommended to vaccinate women > 26 y/o
- HPV vaccine, Cervarix, also approved for use in females aged 10-25. Protects against HPV types 16, 18

**HAVING VACCINE DOES NOT CHANGE CERVICAL CANCER SCREENING GUIDELINES**

***SEE Prescribing Information for full information***

***Contraindication:*** hypersensitivity to vaccine components. If sensitivity occurs after first dose, do not administer subsequent doses

***Precaution:*** may not result in protection for all recipients

- Not intended to be given to pregnant women, pregnancy category B. Pregnancy registry: 1-800-986-8999
- Adverse events include pain, swelling, erythema, pruritis at injection site

# CHAPTER 30

# Sexually Transmissible Infections (STIs) 2010 CDC Guidelines for Treatment*

**Complete guidelines at www.cdc.gov/std/treatment/2010/default.htm**
**www.hab.hrsa.gov www.aidsinfo.nih.gov**

Since women and men seeking contraceptives are also at risk for STIs, we have included in this book information on the treatment of many of the most important STIs based on the latest abridged CDC recommendations (2010). Please refer to the full document for comprehensive information



## CLINICAL PREVENTION GUIDELINES

- The specific recommendations presented here are taken from that document
- For complete guidelines, go to link above
- A new condom should be used for each act of insertive intercourse (oral, vaginal or anal)

### *Prevention Methods*

- *Male Condoms*
  - Used consistently and correctly, latex condoms are effective in preventing the transmission of HIV infection and can reduce the risk for other STIs
  - Use only water-based lubricants
- *Female Condoms*
  - Laboratory studies indicate that the Reality female condom is an effective mechanical barrier to viruses, including HIV
  - Consider using female condom when male condom cannot be used properly
- *Condoms and Spermicides*
  - Condoms lubricated with spermicides are no more effective than other lubricated condoms in protecting against HIV and STDs
  - Use of condoms with N-9 is not recommended for HIV/STD prevention
  - Condoms with N-9 cost more, have shorter shelf life, associated with UTIs in women

- Vaginal spermicides containing N-9 do not protect against HIV and STDs
- Diaphragm use has been demonstrated to provide some protection against cervical gonorrhea, chlamydia, and trichomoniasis (case control, cross sectional studies)
- Diaphragms are not effective to protect women against HIV infection (Padian 08)

- *Nonbarrier Contraception, Surgical Sterilization, and Hysterectomy*
  - Hormonal contraception (e.g., oral contraceptives, Norplant, and Depo-Provera) offer no protection against HIV or other STDs
  - Women who use hormonal or intrauterine contraception, have been surgically sterilized, or have had hysterectomies should still be counseled on the use of condoms for HIV/STI protection

## SPECIAL POPULATIONS

***Pregnant Women***

- *Recommended Screening Tests*
  - Syphilis: all pregnant women at first prenatal visit; high risk (high areas of syphilis morbidity) retested in early third trimester and at delivery. Some states require all women to be screened at delivery
  - Hepatitis B surface antigen (HbsAg): all pregnant women first visit
  - *Neisseria gonorrhoeae:* first visit for women at risk or living in an area of high prevalence
  - *Chlamydia trachomatis:* all women at first prenatal visit and in the third trimester for women at increased risk (i.e., women aged <25 years and women who have a new or more than one sex partner or whose partner has other partners)
  - HIV screening test: encouraged for all pregnant women as routine prenatal test at the first prenatal visit. If high risk retest in 3rd trimester before 36 weeks
  - Bacterial vaginosis (BV): Only symptomatic women. Current evidence does not support universal testing for BV
  - Papanicolaou (Pap) smear: Test at same frequency as non-pregnant women/mangement differs
  - Hepatitis C antibodies at the first prenatal visit for women at high risk (intravenous drug users, blood transfusions, organ transplant)

- *Other Concerns (Other STI-related Concerns are to Be Considered as Follows:)*
  - HbsAg-positive pregnant women should be reported to the local and/or state health department; household and sexual contacts of HbsAg-positive women should be tested and immunized if negative
  - In the absence of lesions during the third trimester, routine serial culture for herpes simplex virus (HSV) is not indicated for women who have a history of recurrent genital herpes. Prophylactic cesarean section is not indicated for women who do not have active genital lesions at the time of delivery
  - The presence of genital warts is not an indication for cesarean delivery unless size obstructs delivery in labor (rare)

***Adolescents***

- With limited exceptions, all U.S. adolescents can consent to the confidential diagnosis and treatment of STIs. See Table 5.1, Page 16
- All children and adolescents should get HBV vaccine and females 9-26 years old, the HPV vaccine

***Management of Patients Who Have Genital Ulcers***

- In the United States, most young, sexually active patients who have genital ulcers have genital herpes or syphilis, much less common is chancroid, although ulcer may have >one organism. Each disease has been associated with an increased risk for HIV infection
- The evaluation of all patients who have genital ulcers should include a serologic test for syphilis and diagnostic evaluation for herpes; in settings where chancroid is prevalent a test for *Haemophilus ducreyi* should be performed. Specific tests (to be used with clinical assessment) for the evaluation of genital ulcers include the following:
  - Serology, dark-field exam or direct immunofluorescence test for *T. pallidum*
  - Culture or PCR test for HSV and
  - Culture for *Haemophilus ducreyi* in areas of prevalence
- HIV testing should be performed in all persons with an ulcer who are not known to have HIV.

## CHANCROID (SHAN-kroyd)

***Organism:*** *H. ducreyi*

***Presents with:*** ulcers and tender, suppurative inguinal adenopathy

***Diagnosis:*** Culture on special medium of *H. ducreyi*, or if all of the following criteria are met: a) patient has 1 or more painful ulcers; b) no evidence of syphilis on lab exam after at least 7 days; c) the clinical picture is typical of chancroid and d) test for HSV is negative.

***Treatment: Recommended Regimens***

| | |
|---|---|
| Azithromycin | 1 g orally in a single dose, OR |
| Ceftriaxone | 250 mg intramuscularly (IM) in a single dose, OR |
| Ciprofloxacin | 500 mg orally twice a day for 3 days, OR |
| Erythromycin base | 500 mg orally three times a day for 7 days. |

***Follow-up:*** Re-examine in 3-7 days. If no improvement consider whether a) the diagnosis is correct, b) the patient is coinfected with another STI, c)the patient is infected with HIV, d) the treatment was not taken as instructed, or e) the *H. ducreyi* strain causing the infection is resistant to the prescribed antimicrobial.

- *The time required for complete healing:*
  - Depends on the size of the ulcer; large ulcers may require >2 weeks
  - Healing is slower for some uncircumcised men who have ulcers under the foreskin
  - Resolution of fluctuant lymphadenopathy is slower than that of ulcers and may require drainage, even during otherwise successful therapy
  - Although needle aspiration of buboes is a simple procedure, incision and drainage of buboes may be preferred because of less need for subsequent drainage procedures

***Management of Sex Partners:*** Should be examined and treated regardless of symptoms if they had sexual contact within 10 days of the onset of symptoms

***Special Considerations: Pregnancy.*** Ciprofloxacin is contraindicated during pregnancy and lactation. No adverse effects of chancroid on pregnancy outcome or on the fetus have been reported.

## GENITAL HERPES SIMPLEX VIRAL (HSV) INFECTION (Her-pes)

Most persons shed the virus intermittently and are unaware that they are infected and are asymptomatic at the time of transmission.

***Organisms:*** HSV-1 and HSV-2

***Diagnosis:*** See complete *2011 CDC Guidelines* or *Contraceptive Technology (20th Edition)*

***Counseling:*** Counseling of these patients should include the following:

- Patients should be advised to abstain from sexual activity when lesions or prodromal symptoms are present and encouraged to inform their sex partners
- Latex condoms, when used consistently and correctly, might reduce the risk for genital herpes, when the infected areas are covered or protected by the condom
- Sexual transmission of HSV can occur during asymptomatic periods
- Daily use (not episodic) of valacyclovir can reduce transmission
- The risk for neonatal infection should be explained to all patients, including men. Childbearing-aged women who have genital herpes should be advised to inform health-care providers who care for them during pregnancy about the HSV infection
- Patients having a first episode of genital herpes should be advised that a) episodic antiviral therapy during recurrent episodes might shorten the duration of lesions and b) suppressive antiviral therapy can prevent recurrent outbreaks
- Patients may be directed to websites such as: http://www.ashastd.org

***Treatment:*** Although many first-episode cases of genital herpes are caused by HSV-1, clinical recurrences are much less frequent for HSV-1 than HSV-2 genital infection

- ***HSV, Recommended Regimens for First Clinical Infection***

Acyclovir..................................400 mg orally three times a day for 7-10 days, OR
Acyclovir..................................200 mg orally five times a day for 7-10 days, OR
Famciclovir..............................250 mg orally three times a day for 7-10 days, OR
Valacyclovir..............................1.0 g orally twice a day for 7-10 days

- ***HSV, Recommended Regimens for Episodic Recurrent Infection***

Acyclovir..................................400 mg orally three times a day for 5 days, OR
Acyclovir..................................800 mg orally twice a day for 5 days, OR
Acyclovir..................................800 mg orally three times a day for 2 days, OR
Famciclovir..............................125 mg orally twice a day for 5 days, OR
Famciclovir..............................1000 mg orally twice a day for 1 day, OR
Famciclovir..............................500 mg orally once followed by 250 mg twice daily for 2 days, OR
Valacyclovir..............................500 mg orally twice a day for 3 days
Valacyclovir..............................1.0 g orally once a day for 5 days

- ***HSV, Recommended Regimens for Daily Suppressive Therapy***

Acyclovir..................................400 mg orally twice a day, OR
Famciclovir..............................250 mg orally twice a day, OR
Valacyclovir..............................500 mg orally once a day, OR
Valacyclovir..............................1.0 g orally once a day

- Acyclovir, famciclovir and valacyclovir are equally effective for episodic Rx
- Famciclovir somewhat less effective for suppression of viral shedding

***Severe Disease:*** IV therapy should be provided for patients who have severe disease or complications necessitating hospitalization, such as disseminated infection, pneumonitis, hepatitis, or complications of the central nervous system (e.g., meningitis or encephalitis)

- ***HSV, Recommended Regimen for Persons with Severe Disease***

Acyclovir..................................5-10 mg/kg body weight IV every 8 hours for 2-7 days until clinical resolution is attained followed by oral therapy to complete 10 days total therapy

***Special Considerations:***

- *Pregnancy*
  - Available data do not indicate an increased risk for major birth defects in women treated with acyclovir in the first trimester
  - Safety of acyclovir, valacyclovir, and famciclovir Rx in pregnant women not established

- *Perinatal Infection*
  - The risk for transmission to the neonate from an infected mother is high (30% - 50%) among women who acquire genital herpes near the time of delivery and is low (<1%) among women who have a history of recurrent herpes at term and women who acquire genital HSV during the first half of pregnancy
  - Therefore, prevention of neonatal herpes should emphasize prevention of acquisition of genital HSV infection during late pregnancy
  - Susceptible women whose partners have oral or genital HSV infection, or those whose sex partners' infection status is unknown, should be counseled to avoid unprotected genital and oral sexual contact during late pregnancy
  - At the onset of labor, all women should be examined and carefully questioned about whether they have symptoms of HSV. Infants of women who do not have symptoms or signs of HSV infection or its prodrome may be delivered vaginally
  - Cesarean delivery does not completely eliminate the risk for HSV infection in the neonate but is recommended in presence of any lesions (even recurrent)

## GRANULOMA INGUINALE (DONOVANOSIS) (gran-u-LO-ma in-gwi-NAL-e, don-o-van-O-sis)

***Organism:*** Klebsiella granulomatis, formerly known as *Calymmatobacterium granulomatis,* is an intracellular, gram-negative bacterium. It is seen rarely in the USA. Presents as a painless, progressive, vascular, ulcerative lesion without regional lymphadenopathy
***Diagnosis:*** Visualization of Donovan bodies from tissue of lesion or biopsy
***Treatment:*** Appears to halt progressive destruction of tissue. Prolonged duration of therapy often required to enable granulation and re-epithelialization of the ulcers. Therapy should be continued at least 3 weeks and until all lesions have healed completely

- ***Granuloma Inguinale, Recommended Regimens***

Doxycycline..............................100 mg orally twice a day for a minimum of 3 weeks and until all lesions healed.

- ***Granuloma Inguinale, Alternative Regimens: all for at least 3 weeks and until all lesions healed***

Trimethoprim-sulfamethoxazole....................One double-strength tablet orally twice a day for a minimum of 3 weeks, OR
Ciprofloxacin...........................750 mg orally twice a day for a minimum of 3 weeks, OR
Erythromycin base..................500 mg orally four times a day for a minimum of 3 weeks (for use during pregnancy), OR
Azithromycin............................1 g orally per week for at least 3 weeks

NOTE: For any of the above regimens, the addition of an aminoglycoside (gentamicin 1 mg/kg IV every 8 hours) should be considered if lesions do not respond within the first few days of therapy

## LYMPHOGRANULOMA VENEREUM (LGV) (lim-fo-gran-u-LO-ma ve-nar-E-um)

This is most frequently manifested in heterosexuals as unilateral tender inguinal nodes and in women and homosexual men with proctocolitis, or inflammatory involvement or perirectal or perianal fistulas or strictures
***Organism:*** Invasive strains L1, L2, or L3 of *Chlamydia trachomatis*
***Diagnosis:*** Serological and exclusion of other ulcerative lesions or those with lymphadenopathy.

***Treatment:*** Treatment cures infection and prevents ongoing tissue damage, although tissue reaction can result in scarring. Buboes may require aspiration through intact skin or incision and drainage to prevent the formation of inguinal/femoral ulcerations.

- ***LGV, Recommended Regimen***

Doxycycline............................100 mg orally twice a day for 21 days OR

- ***Alternative Regimen***

Erythromycin base..................500 mg orally four times a day for 21 days

## SYPHILIS (SIF-i-lis)

***Organism:*** *Treponema pallidum* (tre-po-NE-ma PAL-e-dum)
***Diagnosis:*** See most recent CDC Guidelines or ***Contraceptive Technology***
***Treatment:***

- Parenteral penicillin G is preferred drug for Rx of all stages of syphilis. The preparation(s) used (i.e., benzathine, aqueous procaine, or aqueous crystalline), the dosage, and the length of Rx depend on the stage and clinical manifestations of disease
- Parenteral penicillin G is the only therapy with documented efficacy for syphilis during pregnancy. Patients who report a penicillin allergy, including pregnant women with syphilis in any stage, should be desensitized and treated with penicillin
- The Jarisch-Herxheimer reaction is an acute febrile reaction often accompanied by headache, myalgia, and other symptoms that might occur within the first 24 hours after any therapy for syphilis; patients should be advised of this possible adverse reaction

### PRIMARY, SECONDARY AND EARLY LATENT SYPHILIS

- ***Recommended Regimen for Adults***

Benzathine penicillin G....... 2.4 million units IM in a single dose

***Management Considerations:*** All patients who have syphilis should be tested for HIV infection. In areas in which the prevalence of HIV is high, patients who have primary syphilis should be retested for HIV after 3 months if the first HIV test result was negative
***Follow-up:*** Serologic test titers may decline more slowly for patients who previously had syphilis. Patients should be reexamined clinically and serologically at both 6 and 12 months
***Management of Sex Partners:*** *Sexual transmission of* T. pallidum *has occurred only when mucocutaneous syphilitic lesions are present;* such manifestations are uncommon after the first year of infection. However, persons exposed sexually to a patient who has syphilis in any stage should be evaluated clinically and serologically
***Special Considerations***

- *Penicillin Allergy:* Nonpregnant penicillin-allergic patients who have primary or secondary syphilis should be treated with one of the following regimens. Close follow-up of such patients is essential. Limited clinical studies suggest that ceftriaxone may be effective for early syphilis. The optimal dose and duration of therapy have not been defined, however, some specialists recommend 1 gm daily IM or IV for 10-14 days

- ***Recommended Regimens***

Doxycycline.............................100 mg orally twice a day for 2 weeks, OR
Tetracycline..............................500 mg orally four times a day for 2 weeks

- Pregnant patients who are allergic to penicillin should be desensitized, if necessary, and treated with penicillin.

**LATENT SYPHILIS:**

See most recent CDC Guidelines

**TERTIARY SYPHILIS:**

See most recent CDC Guidelines

## DISEASES CHARACTERIZED BY URETHRITIS AND CERVICITIS

***Management of Patients Who Have Nongonococcal Urethritis***

***Diagnosis:*** Testing for chlamydia and gonorrhea is strongly recommended because of the increased utility and availability of highly sensitive and specific testing methods and because a specific diagnosis might improve compliance and partner notification

***Treatment:***

- ***Nongonococcal Urethritis, Recommended Regimens***

  Azithromycin............................1 g orally in a single dose, OR
  Doxycycline..............................100 mg orally twice a day for 7 days

- ***Nongonococcal Urethritis, Alternative Regimens***

  Erythromycin base.....................500 mg orally four times a day for 7 days, OR
  Erythromycin ethylsuccinate....800 mg orally four times a day for 7 days, OR
  Ofloxacin.....................................300 mg twice a day for 7 days, OR
  Levofloxacin...............................500 mg orally once daily for 7 days

***Follow-up:*** If symptoms persist, patients should be instructed to return for reevaluation and to abstain from sexual intercourse even if they have completed the prescribed therapy

- Men with documented GC or CT shoud be re-tested 3-6 months after treatment because of high reinfection rates

***Partner Referral:*** Patients should refer all sex partners within the preceding 60 days for evaluation and empiric treatment with a regimen effective against CT.

- ***Recurrent/Persistent Urethritis, Recommended Treatment***

  Retreat with initial regimen if noncompliant or reexposed. Otherwise, do culture for T. vaginalis
  Metronidazole..........................2 g orally in a single dose, OR
  Tinidazole.................................2 g orally in single dose, OR
  Azithromycin............................1 g orally in a single dose (if not used intially)

## CHLAMYDIAL INFECTION IN ADOLESCENTS AND ADULTS

Several important sequelae can result from *Chlamydia trachomatis* (kla-MID-e-a tra-KO-ma-tis) infection in women; the most serious of these include PID, ectopic pregnancy, and infertility. Some women who have apparently uncomplicated cervical infection already have subclinical upper reproductive tract infection. Chlamydial infection is much more common in women under age 25 than in older women. All women ≤ 25 years old should be screened annually.

***Diagnosis:*** See complete *2006 CDC Guidelines*

***Treatment:***

- Treatment of infected patients prevents transmission to sex partners and, for infected pregnant women, might prevent transmission to infants during birth
- Treatment of sex partners helps to prevent reinfection of the index patient and infection of other partners
- Coinfection with *C. trachomatis* often occurs among patients who have gonococcal infection; therefore, presumptive treatment of such patients for chlamydia is appropriate (see GONOCOCCAL INFECTION, Dual Therapy for Gonococcal and Chlamydial Infection, Page 173)
- The following recommended treatment regimens and the alternative regimens cure

infection and usually relieve symptoms:

- ***Chlamydia Infection, Recommended Regimens***

Azithromycin............................1 g orally in a single dose, OR (equally effective)
Doxycycline..............................100 mg orally twice a day for 7 days

- ***Chlamydia Infection, Alternative Regimens***

Erythromycin base....................500 mg orally four times a day for 7 days, OR
Erythromycin ethylsuccinate...800 mg orally four times a day for 7 days, OR
Ofloxacin....................................300 mg orally twice a day for 7 days, OR
Levofloxacin.................................500 mg orally once daily for 7 days

***Follow-up:*** Patients do not need to be retested for chlamydia after completing treatment with doxycycline or azithromycin unless symptoms persist or reinfection is suspected because these therapies are highly efficacious. Rescreening is recommended for chlamydia infection 3 months after treatment due to high prevalence of reinfection.

***Management of Sex Partners:*** Patients should be instructed to refer their sex partners for evaluation, testing, and treatment, if they had sexual contact with the patient during the 60 days preceding onset of symptoms in the patient or diagnosis of chlamydia, and the most recent contact should be tested even if > 60 days ago

***Special Considerations:***

- *Pregnancy:*
  - Doxycycline, ofloxacin and levofloxacin are contraindicated for pregnant women
  - Clinical experience and studies suggest azithromycin is safe and effective
  - Repeat testing, preferably NAAT, 3 weeks after completion of therapy with the following regimens is recommended because sequelae to mom and infant
  - Women <25 years old and those at increased risk (e.g., new partner) should be re-tested in third trimester

- ***Recommended Regimens for Pregnant Women***

Azithromycin...............................1 g orally in single dose OR
Amoxicillin...................................500 mg orally three times a day for 7 days.

- ***Alternative Regimens for Pregnant Women***

Erythromycin base......................500 mg orally four times a day for 7 days, OR
Erythromycin base......................250 mg orally four times a day for 14 days, OR
Erythromycin ethylsuccinate.....800 mg orally four times a day for 7 days, OR
Erythromycin ethylsuccinate.....400 mg orally four times a day for 14 days, OR

NOTE: Erythromycin estolate is contraindicated during pregnancy because of drug-related hepatotoxicity.

## GONOCOCCAL INFECTION

### DUAL THERAPY FOR GONOCOCCAL AND CHLAMYDIAL INFECTIONS

Patients infected with *N. gonorrhoeae* often are coinfected with *C. trachomatis*; this finding led to the recommendation that patients treated for gonococcal infection also be treated routinely with a regimen effective against uncomplicated genital *C. trachomatis* infection. CDC no longer recommends use of fluoroquinolones for treatment of gonococcal infections or PID

***Uncomplicated Gonococcal Infections of the Cervix, Urethra, and Rectum***

- ***Recommended Regimens***

Ceftriaxone...........................250 mg IM in a single dose, AND
TREATMENT FOR CHLAMYDIA
Azithromycin...........................1 g orally in a single dose, if chlamydia not ruled out OR
Doxycycline.............................100 mg orally twice a day for 7 days, if chlamydia not ruled out

***Uncomplicated Gonococcal Infections of the Cervix, Urethra, and Rectum***

- ***Alternative Regimens***

Cefixime..................................400 mg in single dose
PLUS
Azithromycin...........................1 g orally in single dose
OR
Doxycycline ...........................100 mg orally twice daily for 7 days plus test for cure in 1 week

***If patient has severe cephalosporin allergy***

Azithromycin ...........................2 g orally in single dose plus test of cure in 1 week

***Uncomplicated Gonococcal Infection of the Pharynx***

- Gonococcal infections of the pharynx are more difficult to eradicate than infections at urogenital and anorectal sites; are ASx and can be relatively common
- Few antigonococcal regimens can reliably cure such infections >90% of the time
- Although chlamydial coinfection of the pharynx is unusual, coinfection at genital sites sometimes occurs. Therefore, treatment for both gonorrhea and chlamydia is suggested

- ***Recommended Regimen***

Ceftriaxone..............................250 mg IM in a single dose, PLUS
TREATMENT FOR CHLAMYDIA IF CHLAMYDIA INFECTION NOT RULED OUT
Doxycycline..............................100 mg orally twice a day for 7 days OR
Azithromycin...........................1 g orally in single dose

***Management of Sex Partners:*** All sex partners of patients who have *N. gonorrhea* infection should be evaluated and treated for *N. gonorrhea* and *C. trachomatis* infections if their last sexual contact with the patient was within 60 days before onset of symptoms or diagnosis. Most recent partner should be notified even if > 60 days prior

***Special Considerations:***

- Pregnant women should not be treated with quinolones or tetracyclines
- Pregnant women infected with *N. gonorrhoeae* should be treated with a recommended or alternate cephalosporin
- Women who cannot tolerate a cephalosporin should be administered a single 2-g dose of azithromycin
- Either azithromycin or amoxicillin is recommended for treatment of presumptive or diagnosed *C. trachomatis* infection during pregnancy (see CHLAMYDIAL INFECTION, Page 172)

## DISEASES CHARACTERIZED BY VAGINAL DISCHARGE

***Have Vaginal Infections:***

- Vaginitis is usually characterized by a vaginal discharge or vulvar itching and irritation; a vaginal odor may be present
- The three diseases most frequently associated with vaginal discharge are trichomoniasis (caused by *T. vaginalis*), BV (caused by a replacement of the normal vaginal flora by an overgrowth of anaerobic microorganisms and *Gardnerella vaginalis*), and candidiasis (usually caused by *Candida albicans*)
- Mucopurulent cervicitis caused by *C. trachomatis* or *N. gonorrhoeae* can sometimes cause vaginal discharge
- Vaginitis is diagnosed by pH, KOH test, and microscopic examination of fresh samples of the discharge
- The pH of the vaginal secretions can be determined by narrow-range pH paper for the elevated pH typical of BV or trichomoniasis (i.e., pH of >4.5)
- One way to examine the discharge is to dilute a sample in one to two drops of 0.9% normal saline solution on one slide and 10% potassium hydroxide (KOH) solution on a second slide. Always prepare saline slide first
- An amine odor detected immediately after applying KOH suggests BV
- A cover slip is placed on each slide, which is then examined under a microscope at low and high-dry power. The motile *T. vaginalis* or the clue cells of BV usually are identified easily in the saline specimen
- The yeast or pseudohyphae of *Candida* species are more easily identified in the KOH specimen
- The presence of objective signs of vulvar inflammation in the absence of vaginal pathogens, along with a minimal amount of discharge, suggests the possibility of mechanical, chemical, allergic, or other noninfectious irritation of the vulva

## BACTERIAL VAGINOSIS (BV)

- BV is a clinical syndrome resulting from replacement of the normal $H_2O_2$ producing *Lactobacillus* sp. in the vagina with high concentrations of anaerobic bacteria (e.g., *Prevotella* sp. and *Mobiluncus* sp.), *G. vaginalis*, and *Mycoplasma hominis*
- BV is the most prevalent cause of vaginal discharge or malodor
- Most women whose illnesses meet the clinical criteria for BV are asymptomatic
- Treatment of male sex partner has not been beneficial in preventing recurrence

***Diagnostic Considerations:*** BV can be diagnosed by the use of clinical criteria meeting three of the following symptoms or signs:

a. A homogeneous, white, noninflammatory discharge that smoothly coats the vaginal walls
b. The presence of clue cells on microscopic examination
c. A pH of vaginal fluid >4.5
d. A fishy odor of vaginal discharge before or after addition of 10% KOH (i.e., the whiff test)

***Treatment:*** The principal goal of therapy in nonpregnant women is to relieve vaginal symptoms and signs of infection. All women **with** symptoms require treatment, regardless of pregnancy status

- ***BV, Recommended Regimens for Nonpregnant Women***

Metronidazole..................500 mg orally twice a day for 7 days, OR
Clindamycin cream............2%, one full applicator (5 g) intravaginally at bedtime for 7 days OR
Metronidazole gel.............0.75%, one full applicator (5 g) intravaginally, once daily for 5 days OR

- Patients should be advised to avoid consuming alcohol during treatment with metronidazole and for 24 hours thereafter. Clindamycin cream is oil-based and might weaken latex condoms and diaphragms for 5 days after use

- ***BV, Alternative Regimens***

Clindamycin..............................300 mg orally bid x 7 days OR
Clindamycin ovules..................100 mg intravaginally qhs x 3 days OR
Tinidazole..................................2 g orally once daily for 2 days OR
Tinidazole..................................1 g orally once daily for 5 days

- FDA has approved both metronidazole 750-mg extended release tablets once daily for 7 days and a single dose of clindamycin vaginal cream. However, data on the performance of these regimens is limited.

***Follow-up:*** Follow-up visits are unnecessary if symptoms resolve. Recurrence is not unusual
***Management of Sex Partners:*** Routine treatment of sex partners is not recommended
***Special Considerations:***

- *Allergy or Intolerance to the Recommended Therapy:*
  - Clindamycin cream is preferred in case of allergy or intolerance to metronidazole. Metronidazole gel can be considered for patients who do not tolerate systemic metronidazole, but patients allergic to oral metronidazole should not be administered metronidazole vaginally
- *Pregnancy:*
  - BV has been associated with adverse pregnancy outcomes (i.e., premature rupture of the membranes, preterm labor, and preterm birth)
  - Treat all symptomatic pregnant women when diagnosed
  - Treatment of BV in high-risk pregnant women (i.e., those who have previously delivered a premature infant) who are asymptomatic has been evaluated but yielded mixed results
  - Evidence is insufficient to recommend screening for BV in pregnant women at high risk for preterm delivery
  - The recommended regimen is metronidazole 250 mg orally three times a day for 7 days OR metronidazole 500 mg orally twice a day for 7 days OR clindamycin 300 mg orally twice daily for 7 days

## TRICHOMONIASIS

***Diagnosis:***

- Trichomoniasis is caused by the protozoan *T. vaginalis,* easily identified on a wet smear Most men who are infected do not have symptoms of infection, although a minority of men have nongonococcal urethritis
- Many women do have symptoms of infection, characteristically a diffuse, malodorous, yellow-green discharge with vulvar irritation; many women have fewer symptoms

***Treatment:***

- ***Trichomoniasis, Recommended Regimen***

Metronidazole.........................2 g orally in a single dose, OR
Tinidazole................................2 g orally in a single dose

- ***Trichomoniasis, Alternative Regimen***

Metronidazole.........................500 mg twice a day for 7 days

- In randomized clinical trials, the recommended metronidazole and tinidazole regimens have resulted in cure rates of approximately 90% - 95%; ensuring treatment of sex partners might increase the cure rate. Treatment of patients and sex partners results in relief of symptoms, microbiologic cure, and reduction of transmission
- Metronidazole gel is < 50% effective

- Patients should be advised to avoid alcohol through 24 hours after completion of Rx with metronidazole and 72 hours after Rx with tinidazole

***Follow-up:***

- Rescreening 3 months after Rx should be considered in sexually active women
- Infections with strains of *T. vaginalis* that have diminished susceptibility to metronidazole can occur; however, most of these organisms respond to higher doses of metronidazole or tinidazole
- If treatment failure occurs with metronidazole, the patient should be retreated with metronidazole 500 mg twice a day for 7 days or tinidazole
- If treatment failure occurs repeatedly, the patient should be treated with a single, 2g dose of metronidazole or tinidazole once a day for 5 days

***Management of Sex Partners:*** Routine Rx recommended avoid intercourse until Rx is complete and both partners are assymptomatic

***Special Considerations:***

- *Allergy, Intolerance, or Adverse Reactions:* Effective alternatives to therapy with metronidazole or tinidazole are not available. Patients who are allergic to this class of drugs can be managed by desensitization
- *Pregnancy:* Patients may be treated with 2 g of metronidazole in a single dose; see guidelines
- Vaginal trichomoniasis might be associated with adverse pregnancy outcomes, particularly premature rupture of the membranes and preterm delivery
- *HIV Infection:* Patients who have trichomoniasis and also are infected with HIV should receive the same treatment regimen as those who are HIV negative

## VULVOVAGINAL CANDIDIASIS (VVC)

- Vulvovaginal yeast infections are caused by *C. albicans* or, occasionally, by other *Candida* sp. or other yeasts
- An estimated 75% of women will have at least one episode of VVC
- Typical symptoms of VVC include pruritus and vaginal discharge
- Other symptoms may include vaginal soreness, vulvar burning, dyspareunia, and external dysuria
- None of these symptoms is specific for VVC

***Diagnostic Considerations:***

- A diagnosis of *Candida* vaginitis is suggested clinically by pruritus and erythema in the vulvo-vaginal area; a white discharge may occur, as may vulvar edema
- The diagnosis can be made in a woman who has signs and symptoms of vaginitis, and when either a) a wet preparation or Gram stain of vaginal discharge demonstrates yeasts or pseudohyphae or b) a culture or other test yields a positive result for a yeast species
- If culture cannot be done and KOH test is negative, empiric Rx can be considered for symptomatic women
- *Candida* vaginitis is associated with a normal vaginal pH (<4.5)
- Use of 10% KOH in wet preparations improves the visualization of yeast and mycelia by disrupting cellular material that might obscure the yeast or pseudohyphae
- Identifying *Candida* by culture in the absence of symptoms should not lead to treatment because 10%-20% of women usually harbor *Candida* sp. and other yeasts in the vagina. VVC can occur concomitantly with STIs

***Treatment:*** Topical formulations effectively treat VVC. The topically applied azole drugs are more effective than nystatin. Treatment with azoles results in relief of symptoms and negative cultures among 80%-90% of patients who complete therapy

- ***VVC, Recommended Regimens***
- *Intravaginal agents:*

Butoconazole*..........................2% cream 5 g intravaginally for 3 days, **OR**
Butoconazole..........................2% cream 5g (butoconazole 1-sustained release), single vaginal application
Clotrimazole*..........................1% cream 5 g intravaginally for 7-14 days, **OR**
Miconazole*..............................2% cream 5 g intravaginally for 7 days, **OR**
Miconazole*..............................4% cream 5 g intravaginally for 3 days, **OR**
Miconazole*..............................200-mg vaginal suppository, one suppository for 3 days, **OR**
Miconazole*..............................100-mg vaginal suppository, one suppository for 7 days, **OR**
Miconazole*..............................1200-mg vaginal suppository, one time dose, **OR**
Nystatin...................................100,000-u vaginal tablet, one tablet for 14 days, **OR**
Tioconazole*............................6.5% ointment 5 g intravaginally in a single application, **OR**
Terconazole..............................0.4% cream 5 g intravaginally for 7 days, **OR**
Terconazole..............................0.8% cream 5 g intravaginally for 3 days, **OR**
Terconazole..............................80-mg vaginal suppository, one suppository for 3 days, **OR**

- *Oral agent:*

Fluconazole..............................150-mg oral tablet, one tablet in single dose.

* *Over-the-counter preparations*

These creams and suppositories are oil-based and may weaken latex condoms and diaphragms

***Follow-up:*** Patients should be instructed to return for follow-up visits only if symptoms persist or recur

***Management of Sex Partners:*** None; VVC usually is not acquired through sexual intercourse

***Special Considerations:***

- *Pregnancy:* VVC often occurs during pregnancy. Only topical azole therapies applied for 7 days should be used to treat pregnant women.
- *HIV Infection:* Based on available evidence, therapy is same as seronegative women

## PELVIC INFLAMMATORY DISEASE (PID) (see Table 13.1, Page 36)

- PID comprises a spectrum of inflammatory disorders of the upper female genital tract, including any combination of endometritis, salpingitis, tuboovarian abscess, and pelvic peritonitis
- Sexually transmitted organisms, especially *N. gonorrhoeae* and *C. trachomatis*, are implicated in most cases; however, microorganisms that can be part of the vaginal flora (e.g., anaerobes, *G. vaginalis*, *H. influenzae*, enteric gram negative rods, and *Streptococcus agalactiae*) also can cause PID
- In addition, CMV, *M. hominis* and *U. urealyticum* may also be etiologic agents

***Diagnostic Considerations:*** See complete *CDC Guidelines (www.cdc.gov)*. Empiric treatment should be initiated in sexually active young women and others at risk for STIs if they are experiencing pelvic or lower abdominal pain, if no other cause can be identified and if **ONE** of the following minimum criteria are present on pelvic exam:

- cervical motion tenderness **OR**
- uterine tenderness **OR**
- adenexal tenderness

***Treatment:*** Must provide empiric, broad-spectrum coverage of likely pathogens
Antimicrobial coverage should include *N. gonorrhea*, *C. trachomatis*

- Suggested *criteria for **HOSPITALIZATION** decision based on discretion of HCP*
- Surgical emergencies such as appendicitis cannot be excluded
  - Patient is pregnant
  - Patient does not respond clinically to oral antimicrobial therapy
  - Patient is unable to follow or tolerate an outpatient oral regimen
  - Patient has severe illness, nausea and vomiting, or high fever
  - Patient has a tuboovarian abscess

---

- ***PID, Parenteral Regimen A***

Cefotetan................................2 g IV every 12 hours, **OR**
Cefoxitin..................................2 g IV every 6 hours, **PLUS**
Doxycycline.............................100 mg IV or orally every 12 hours

---

- Because of pain associated with infusion, doxycycline should be administered orally when possible, even when the patient is hospitalized
- Both oral and IV administration of doxycycline provide similar bioavailability but oral treatment should continue through 14 days
- When tuboovarian abscess is present, many health-care providers use clindamycin or metronidazole with doxycycline for continued therapy rather than doxycycline alone, because it provides more effective anaerobic coverage

---

- ***PID, Parenteral Regimen B***

Clindamycin............................900 mg IV every 8 hours, **PLUS**
Gentamicin..............................loading dose IV or IM (2 mg/kg of body weight) followed by a maintenance dose (1.5 mg/kg) every 8 hours. Single daily dosing (3-5 mg/kg) may be substituted.

---

- Although use of a single daily dose of gentamicin has not been evaluated for the treatment of PID, it is efficacious in analogous situations
- Parenteral therapy may be discontinued 24 hours after a patient improves clinically, and continuing oral therapy should consist of doxycycline 100 mg orally twice a day or clindamycin 450 mg orally four times a day to complete a total of 14 days of therapy
- When tuboovarian abscess is present, many healthcare providers use clindamycin for continued therapy rather than doxycycline because clindamycin provides more effective anaerobic coverage

---

- ***PID, Alternative Parenteral Regimens:*** Limited data support the use of other parenteral regimens, but the following has been investigated in at least one clinical trial, and it has broad-spectrum coverage.

Ampicillin/Sulbactam............3 g IV every 6 hours, PLUS doxycycline 100 mg IV / orally every 12 hours **OR**

---

***Oral Treatment:*** Can be considered for mild to moderately severe acute PID. Patients who do not respond to oral therapy within 72 hours should be reevaluated to confirm the diagnosis and be administered parenteral therapy on either an outpatient or inpatient basis.

---

• ***PID, Recommended Oral Regimen***

Ceftriaxone..............................250 mg IM once, **OR**

Cefoxitin..................................2 g IM plus probenecid, 1 g orally in a single dose concurrently once, **OR**

Other parenteral third-generation cephalosporin (e.g.,ceftizoxime or cefotaxime), **PLUS**

Doxycycline............................100 mg orally twice a day for 14 days with or without metronidazole 500 mg orally twice daily for 14 days.

• ***PID, Alternative Oral Regimens:*** If parenteral cephalosporin therapy is not feasible, use of fluoroquinolones (levofloxacin 500 mg orally once daily or ofloxacin 400 mg twice daily for 14 days) with or without metronidazole (500 mg orally twice daily for 14 days) may be considered if the community prevalence and individual risk of gonorrhea is low. Tests for gonorrhea must be performed prior to instituting therapy and the patient managed as follows if the test is positive:

- If NAAT test is positive, parenteral cephalosporin is recommended
- If culture for gonorrhea is positive, treatment should be based on results of antimicrobial susceptibility. If isolate is QRNG, or antimicrobial suseptibility can't be assessed, parenteral cephalosporin is recommended

***Follow-up:***

- Patients receiving oral or parenteral Rx should demonstrate substantial clinical improvement (i.e., defervescence; reduction in direct or rebound abdominal tenderness; and reduction in uterine, adnexal, and Cx motion tenderness) within 3 days after initiation of Rx
- Patients who do not improve within 3 days usually require additional diagnostic tests, hospitalization or surgical intervention

***Special Considerations:***

- *Pregnancy:* Pregnant women who have suspected PID should be hospitalized and treated with parenteral antibiotics.

## HUMAN PAPILLOMAVIRUS INFECTION (HPV)

***Genital Warts: Vaccine now available. See Page 165***

- More than 40 types of HPV can infect the genital tract. Most HPV infections are asymptomatic, subclinical, or unrecognized. Visible genital warts usually are caused by HPV types 6 or 11. Oncogenic HPV types in the anogenital region (i.e., types 16 and 18) have been strongly associated with cervical and oropharyngeal cancers.

***Prevention:*** Two HPV vaccines are available: Cervarix against types 16 and 18, and Gardasil against types 6, 11, 16 and 18. Both may be used in girls ages 9-26, and Gardasil can be used in males to provent warts.

***Treatment:***

- The primary goal of treating visible genital warts is the removal of symptomatic warts
- Treatment can induce wart-free periods in most patients. Genital warts often are asymptomatic
- **No evidence indicates that currently available treatments eradicate or affect the natural history of HPV infection.** The removal of warts may or may not decrease infectivity
- If left untreated, visible genital warts may resolve on their own, remain unchanged, or increase in size or number. No evidence indicates that presence of visible warts or their treatment is associated with the development of cervical cancer

***Regimens:***

- Treatment of genital warts should be guided by the patient's preference, the available resources, and the experience of the health-care provider.

- None of the available treatments is superior to other treatments, and no single treatment is ideal for all circumstances. The treatment modality should be changed if a patient has not improved substantially. The majority respond within 3 months of therapy

---

- ***External Genital Warts, Recommended Treatments:***
- *Patient-Applied*

Podofilox................................0.5% solution or gel OR
Sinecatechins..........................15% ointment OR
Imiquimod..............................5% cream

---

- Patients may apply **podofilox** solution with a cotton swab, or podofilox gel with a finger, to visible genital warts twice a day for 3 days, followed by 4 days of no therapy
- This cycle may be repeated as necessary for a total of four cycles
- The total wart area treated should not exceed 10 $cm^2$, and a total volume of podofilox should not exceed 0.5 mL per day
- If possible, the health-care provider should apply the initial treatment to demonstrate the proper application technique and identify which warts should be treated.
- The safety of podofilox during pregnancy has not been established.
- Patients should apply **imiquimod** cream with a finger at bedtime, three times a week for as long as 16 weeks
- The treatment area should be washed with mild soap and water 6-10 hours after the application
- The safety of imiquimod during pregnancy has not been established
- Sinecatechin ointment should be applied three times daily using a finger to ensure covering with a think layer of ointment until complete clearance of warts, but no longer than 16 weeks. Should not be washed off AND sex should be avoided while ointment on skin. Safety in pregnancy is unknown.

- *Provider-Administered:*
  - Cryotherapy with liquid nitrogen or cryoprobe. Repeat applications every 1 to 2 weeks
  - Trichloroacetic acid (TCA) or BCA 80%-90%. May place petroleum jelly around wart to reduce spread of medication to normal mucosa. Apply a small amount only to warts and allow to dry, at which time a white "frosting" develops; powder with talc or $NaHCO_3$ to remove acid if an excess amount is applied. Repeat weekly if necessary. **OR**
  - Podophyllin resin 10%-25%
- A small amount should be applied to each wart and allowed to air dry
- To avoid the possibility of complications associated with systemic absorption and toxicity, application should be limited to <0.5 mL of podophyllin or <10 $cm^2$ of warts per session and no open wounds should exist nearby
- The preparation should be thoroughly washed off 1-4 hours after application to reduce local irritation. Repeat weekly if necessary
- *The safety of podophyllin during pregnancy has not been established*
- *Surgical removal* by tangential scissor excision, tangential shave excision, curettage, or electrosurgery

---

- ***External Genital Warts, Alternative Treatments (Provider administered)***

Intra-lesional interferon **OR** photodynamic therapy **OR** topical cidofovir

---

- ***Cervical Warts***

For women who have exophytic cervical warts, high-grade squamous intraepithelial lesions

(SIL) must be excluded by biopsy before treatment is begun. Management of exophytic cervical warts should include consultation with an expert

---

• ***Vaginal Warts, Recommended Treatment***
*Cryotherapy with liquid nitrogen.* The use of a cryoprobe in the vagina is not recommended because of the risk for vaginal perforation and fistula formation. **OR**
*TCA or BCA 80%-90%* applied only to warts. Repeat weekly if necessary.

---

• ***Urethral Meatus Warts, Recommended Treatment***
*Cryotherapy* with liquid nitrogen **OR**
*Podophyllin 10%-25%* in tincture of benzoin. The treatment area must be dry before contact with podophyllin. Podophyllin may be applied weekly if necessary. *The safety of podophyllin during pregnancy has not been established.*

---

• ***Anal Warts, Recommended Treatment***
*Cryotherapy* with liquid nitrogen **OR**
*TCA or BCA 80%-90%* applied to warts. Apply a small amount only to warts and allow to dry, at which time a white "frosting" develops; powder with talc or sodium bicarbonate (i.e., baking soda) to remove acid if an excess amount is applied. Repeat weekly if necessary. May place petroleum jelly around wart to reduce spread of medication to normal mucosa **OR**
*Surgical removal*
- Management of warts on rectal mucosa should be referred to an expert

---

***Management of Sex Partners:*** None. Examination of sex partners is not necessary for the management of genital warts, however both partners should be tested for other STIs
***Special Considerations:***
- *Pregnancy:* Imiquimod, sinecatechins, podophyllin, and podofilox should not be used during pregnancy. Genital warts can proliferate and become friable during pregnancy, removal can be considered, but resolution may be incomplete. HPV types 6 and 11 can cause respiratory papillomatosis in infants and children. Vaginal delivery not contraindicated unless lesion size obstructive in labor (rare) or would result in excessive bleeding. The route of transmission (i.e., transplacental, perinatal, or postnatal) is not completely understood

## VACCINE-PREVENTABLE STIs

One of the most effective means of preventing the transmission of STIs is preexposure immunization. Currently licensed vaccines for the prevention of STIs include those for hepatitis A and hepatitis B. Clinical development and trials are underway for vaccines against a number of other STIs, including HIV and HSV. As more vaccines become available, immunization possibly will become one of the most widespread methods used to prevent STIs. Each person being evaluated for an STI should receive Hep B vaccine unless already vaccinated.

## ECTOPARASITIC INFECTIONS

### PEDICULOSIS PUBIS

Patients who have pediculosis pubis (i.e., pubic lice) usually seek medical attention because of pruritus. Such patients also usually notice lice or nits on their pubic hair. Usually sexually transmitted

***Treatment:***

- ***Pediculosis Pubis, Recommended Regimens***

Permethrin..........................1% creme rinse applied to affected areas and washed off after 10 minutes **OR**

Pyrethrins with piperonyl butoxide applied to the affected area and washed off after 10 minutes.

*See 2006 guidelines for alternative regimens*

***Other Management Considerations:***

- The recommended regimens should not be applied to the eyes. Pediculosis of the eyelashes should be treated by applying occlusive ophthalmic ointment to the eyelid margins twice a day for 10 days
- Bedding and clothing should be decontaminated (either machine-washed and machine-dried using the heat cycle or drycleaned) or removed from body contact for at least 72 hrs
- Fumigation of living areas is not necessary

***Follow-up:*** Patients should be evaluated after 1 week if symptoms persist. Retreatment may be necessary if lice are found or if eggs are observed at the hairskin junction. Patients who do not respond to one of the recommended regimens should be retreated with an alternative regimen

***Management of Sex Partners:*** Sex partners within the last month should be treated

***Special Considerations:***

- *Pregnancy:* Pregnant and lactating women should be treated with either permethrin or pyrethrins with piperonyl butoxide. Lindane and ivermectin contraindicated.

## SCABIES

- Predominant symptoms is pruritus; sensitization takes several weeks to develop; pruritus might occur within 24 hours after a subsequent reinfestation
- Scabies in adults may be sexually transmitted, although scabies in children usually is not

- ***Scabies, Recommended Regimen***

Permethrin cream..................(5%) applied to all areas of the body from the neck down and washed off after 8-14 hours. **OR**

Ivermectin................................200 mcg/kg orally, repeated in 2 weeks

- ***Scabies, Alternative Regimens***

Lindane...................................(1%) 1 oz. of lotion or 30 g of cream applied thinly to all areas of the body from the neck down and thoroughly washed off after 8 hours

- Lindane should not be used immediately after a bath, and it should not be used by a) persons who have extensive dermatitis, b) pregnant or lactating women, and c) children aged <2 years. Not first-line because of toxicity, d) as first-line therapy

***Other Management Considerations:*** Bedding and clothing should be decontaminated (i.e., either machine-washed or machine-dried using the hot cycle or dry-cleaned) or removed from body contact for at least 72 hours. Fumigation of living areas is unnecessary

***Follow-up:*** Pruritus may persist for several weeks. Some experts recommend retreatment after 1-2 weeks for patients who are still symptomatic; other experts recommend retreatment only if live mites are observed. Patients who do not respond should be retreated with an alternative regimen

***Management of Sex Partners and Household Contacts:*** Both sexual and close personal or household contacts within the preceding month should be examined and treated

## SEXUAL ASSAULT AND STIs: Adults and Adolescents

***Evaluation for Sexually Transmitted Infections***

- *Initial Examination* - (See Page 186 and full CDC Guidelines)
- *Follow-up Examination after Assault*
  - Examination for STIs should be repeated 2 weeks after assault (see inside back cover)
  - Serologic tests for syphilis and HIV infection should be repeated 6, 12, and 24 weeks after the assault if initial test results were negative
- Prophylaxis: Many experts recommend routine preventive therapy after a sexual assault. The prophylactic regimen suggested is on inside back cover
- An empiric antimicrobial regimen for chlamydia, gonorrhea, and trichomonas, should be administered, as well as post-exposure Hep B vaccine without HBIG. Following doses are at 1-2 and 4-6 months after first dose. (See inside back cover)

***Other Management Considerations:***

At the initial examination and, if indicated, at follow-up, patients should be counseled about:

- Risk for pregnancy and possible use of emergency contraception
- Symptoms of STIs and the need for immediate examination if symptoms occur
- Abstinence from sexual intercourse until STI prophylactic treatment is completed

***Risk for Acquiring HIV Infection:***

- Although HIV antibody seroconversion has been reported among persons whose only known risk factor was sexual assault or sexual abuse, the risk for acquiring HIV infection through sexual assault is low and depends on many factors
- These factors may include the type of sexual intercourse (i.e., oral, vaginal, or anal); presence of oral, vaginal or anal trauma; site of exposure to ejaculate; viral load in ejaculate; and presence of an STI

## HIV INFECTION

OraQuick, a rapid test (40-60 minutes) was approved by the FDA in November, 2002.
For entire guidelines see www.aidsinfo.nih.gov

Proper management of HIV infection involves a complex array of behavioral, psychosocial, and medical services. This information should not be a substitute for referral to a health-care provider or facility experienced in caring for HIV-infected patients. Hotlines:

CDC AIDS Treatment Information Service.........1-800-HIV-0440 (1-800-448-0440)
e-mail to: atis@hivatis.org & www.hivatis.org
CDC AIDS Clinical Trials Information Service...1-800-TRIALS-A (1-800-874-2572)
e-mailto: actis@actis.org International....1-301-519-0459

*For general information and referrals to local facilities:*

CDC National AIDS Hotline.................................1-800-342-AIDS (1-800-342-2437)
Spanish.............................................................1-800-344-7432
CDC National AIDS Clearinghouse......................1-800-458-5231
CDC Division of HIV/AIDS Prevention................www.cdc.gov/hiv
Post exposure prophylaxis PEP...........................1-888-HIV-4911

***Pregnancy***: All pregnant women should be offered HIV testing as early in pregnancy as possible. Birthing facilities delivering women who may not have had prenatal HIV testing should make rapid HIV testing available 24/7. This recommendation is particularly important because of the available treatments for reducing the likelihood of perinatal transmission and maintaining the health of the woman. HIV-infected women should be informed specifically about the risk for perinatal infection. Current evidence indicates that 15%-25% of infants born to untreated HIV-infected mothers are infected with HIV; the virus also can be transmitted from an infected mother by breastfeeding. Zidovudine (ZDV) reduces the risk for HIV transmission to the infant from approximately 25% to <2% through use of antiretroviral regimens and obstetric intervention and by avoiding breastfeeding. Therefore, **ZDV TREATMENT SHOULD BE OFFERED TO ALL HIV-INFECTED PREGNANT WOMEN.** Most women in the U.S. now receive triple therapy during pregnancy not just ZDV. In the United States, HIV-infected women should be advised not to breast-feed their infants. In other countries, the reduced risk of death from malnutrition, diarrheal disease, or other infections may outweigh the risk of contracting HIV.

Insufficient information is available regarding the safety of ZDV or other antiretroviral drugs during early pregnancy; however, on the basis of the ACTG-076 protocol, ZDV is indicated for the prevention of maternal-fetal HIV transmission as part of a regimen that includes oral ZDV at 14-34 weeks of gestation, intravenous (IV) ZDV during labor, and ZDV syrup to the neonate after birth.

# EVALUATION & MANAGEMENT OF SEXUAL ASSAULT

**National Domestic Violence Hotline: 1-800-799-SAFE • www.ndvh.org**

**Engage Rape Crisis Services.** Have trained provider do the examination whenever possible. See SANE (Sexual Assault Nurse Evaluation), www.sane-sart.com

↓

**Legal:** Report to authorities if required by your state. Contact child protective services if victim is a minor

↓

**Obtain informed consent before history, physical and treatment**

↓

**History:** circumstances of assault, whether victim had loss of consciousness (may want to test for rohypnol), date/time/location, use of weapons etc, specifics re: oral, vaginal or anal contact, penetration, ejaculation or condom use, areas of trauma, bleeding by victim or assailant, recent consensual sexual activity before or after assault including condom use, LMP, contraceptive use, use of drugs or alcohol, whether victim showered, changed clothing etc.

↓

**Physical exam:** document any trauma with photographs (and patient's consent). Woods lamp (UV) may help identify semen or other debris. Colposcopy helps detect milder trauma. **Forensic exam** done with a special "evidence collection kit" includes victim's clothing, swabs of buccal mucosa, vagina, rectum, combed (and pulled) specimens form scalp and pubic hair, fingernail scrapings and clippings, blood sample etc. Assure proper chain of evidence to legal authorities. PE may also include specimens for DNA, acid phosphatase, pregnancy, HIV, Hep B, syphilis, sperm, BV, Trich, GC/CT and Herpes.

↓

**Treatment:** Offer emergency contraception. Empiric RX for STIs: ceftriaxone 250mg IM plus azithromycin 1g PO or doxycycline 100mg PO BID x 7 days. Metronidazole 2g PO x 1 dose. HEP B vaccine if not immune and consider anti-retrovirals to decrease risk of HIV infection. Advise to abstain from intercourse until prophylaxis therapy completed and consider condom use until follow-up serologic testing complete (6 months)

↓

**Follow-up:** Medical visit in 2 weeks. Ongoing psychosocial support and advocate services should be assessed. Do pregnancy test. Test for GC, CT, Trich and BV if woman declined prophylaxis or developed new symptoms or requests it. Follow-up tests for HIV and RPR at 6 weeks, 3 and 6 months. Follow up doses of Hep B vaccine.

## U.S. MEDICAL ELIGIBILITY CRITERIA FOR CONTRACEPTIVE USE (2010)

The table on the following pages summarizes the latest CDC medical eligibility criteria for starting contraceptives. These criteria are also the basis for the checklists throughout *Managing Contraception*. These criteria are mostly evidence-based. Please visit the CDC website to view the full document. There you will find more information on the evidence supporting category assignment as well as references.

### CDC categories for temporary methods:

**CDC 1** **Can use** the method. No restriction on use.

**CDC 2** **Can use the method.** Advantages generally outweigh theoretical or proven risks.

**CDC 3** **Should not use** the method unless clinician makes clinical judgment that the patient can safely use it. Theoretical or proven risks usually outweigh the advantages of method.

**CDC 4** **Should not use the method.** Condition represents an unacceptable health risk if method is used.

Simplified 2-category system for temporary methods

To make clinical judgment, the CDC 4-category classification system can be simplified into a 2-category system.

| CDC Category | With Clinical Judgment | With Limited Clinical Judgment |
|---|---|---|
| 1 | Use the method in any circumstances | Use the method |
| 2 | Generally use the method | |
| 3 | Use of the method not usually recommended unless other, more appropriate methods are not available or acceptable | Do not use the method |
| 4 | Method not to be used | |

NOTE: In the pages that follow, Category 3 and 4 conditions are shaded to indicate the method should not be provided where clinical judgment is limited.

**To download most recent CDC Medical Eligibility Criteria go to: www.cdc.gov**

## Conditions that Expose a Woman to Increased Risk for Adverse Health Events as a Result of Unintended Pregnancy (§)

For women with conditions that may make unintended pregnancy an unacceptable health risk, long-acting, highly effective contraceptive methods may be the best choice. Women with these conditions should be advised that **sole use of barrier methods for contraception and behavior-based methods of contraception may not be the most appropriate choice** because of their relatively higher typical-use rates of failure. Conditions included in the U.S. MEC for which unintended pregnancy presents an unacceptable health risk are identified throughout the document with the symbol, section symbol (§) (See below for complete list).

| CONDITION (§): |
|---|
| Breast cancer |
| Complicated valvular heart disease |
| Diabetes: *insulin-dependent; with nephropathy/retinopathy/neuropathy or other vascular disease; or of >20 years' duration* |
| Endometrial or ovarian cancer |
| Epilepsy |
| High blood pressure (systolic >160 mm Hg or diastolic >100 mm Hg) |
| History of bariatric surgery within the past 2 years |
| HIV/AIDS* |
| Ischemic heart disease |
| Malignant gestational trophoblastic disease |
| Malignant liver tumors (hepatoma) and hepatocellular carcinoma of the liver |
| Peripartum cardiomyopathy |
| Schistosomiasis with fibrosis of the liver |
| Severe (decompensated) cirrhosis |
| Sickle cell disease |
| Solid organ transplantation within the past 2 years |
| Sexually transmitted infections* |
| Stroke |
| Systemic lupus erythematosus |
| Thrombogenic mutations |
| Tuberculosis |

**Dual protection is strongly recommended against HIV/AIDS and other STIs when a risk for STI/HIV transmission exists. This can be achieved through the simultaneous use of condoms with other methods or the consistent and correct use of condoms alone.*

# CDC MEDICAL ELIGIBILITY CRITERIA FOR STARTING CONTRACEPTIVE METHODS (2010)

| CONDITION | Combined Hormonal Contraceptives (CHCs) COCs, Patch (P), Ring (R) | Progestin-Only OCs | Depo-Provera NET EN | LNG/ETG Implants | LNG IUD | TCu-380A IUD | |
|---|---|---|---|---|---|---|---|
| **PERSONAL CHARACTERISTICS & REPRODUCTIVE HISTORY** | | | | | | | |
| **Pregnant** | NA | NA | NA | NA | | | |
| **Age** | Menarche to < 40=1 | Menarche to < 18=1 | Menarche to < 18=2 | Menarche to < 18=1 | Menarche < 20 = 2 | Menarche < 20 = 2 | ← A |
| | ≥ 40=2 | 18-45=1 | 18-45=1 | 18-45=1 | ≥ 20=1 | ≥ 20=1 | |
| | | > 45=1 | > 45=2 | > 45=1 | | | |
| **Parity** a) nulliparous | 1 | 1 | 1 | 1 | 2 | 2 | |
| b) parous | 1 | 1 | 1 | 1 | 1 | 1 | |
| **Breastfeeding*** < 1 month PP | 3 | 2 | 2 | 2 | | | ← B |
| 1 month or more PP | 2 | 1 | 1 | 1 | | | ← C |
| **Non-breastfeeding*** < 21 days | 4 | 1 | 1 | 1 | | | |
| 21-42 days | | | | | | | |
| (i) with other risk factors for VTE | 3 | 1 | 1 | 1 | | | |
| (ii) without other risk factors for VTE | 2 | 1 | 1 | 1 | | | |
| > 42 days | 1 | 1 | 1 | 1 | | | |
| **Postpartum breastfeeding or non-breastfeeding** <10 mins after placental delivery | | | | | 2 | 1 | |
| 10 min to < 4 weeks | | | | | 2 | 2 | |
| ≥ 4 weeks | | | | | 1 | 1 | |
| Puerperal Sepsis | | | | | 4 | 4 | |
| **Post-abortion** 1st trimester | 1 | 1 | 1 | 1 | 1 | 1 | |
| 2nd trimester | 1 | 1 | 1 | 1 | 2 | 2 | |
| Immediate post septic AB | 1 | 1 | 1 | 1 | 4 | 4 | ← D |
| **Past ectopic pregnancy** | 1 | 2 | 1 | 1 | 1 | 1 | |
| **History of pelvic surgery** | 1 | 1 | 1 | 1 | 1 | 1 | |

**To download most recent CDC Medical Eligibility Criteria go to: www.cdc.gov**

**A** It is not known whether DMPA use among adolescents affects peak bone mass levels or whether adult women with long duration of DMPA use can regain BMD to baseline levels before entering menopause.

**B** Adverse outcomes in infants exposed to estrogen in breast milk have not been demonstrated. Theoretical concerns of CHC on milk production are greater early postpartum.

**C** Direct evidence demonstrates no negative effect of POCs on BF performance or health of infant.

**D** IUD expulsion risk greater when inserted immediately after second trimester abortion.

§ Condition exposes woman to increased risk with unintended pregnancy

| CONDITION | CHCs | POPs | DMPA | LNG/ETG | LNGIUD | TCuIUD | |
|---|---|---|---|---|---|---|---|
| **Smoking:** Less than age 35 | 2 | 1 | 1 | 1 | 1 | 1 | |
| Age ≥ 35 < 15 cigarettes/day | 3 | 1 | 1 | 1 | 1 | 1 | |
| Age ≥ 35 ≥ 15 cigarettes/day | 4 | 1 | 1 | 1 | 1 | 1 | |
| **Obesity** ≥ 30 kg/m² BMI | 2 | 1 | 1 | 1 | 1 | 1 | |
| Menarche to <18 years & ≥ 30 kg/m² BMI | 2 | 1 | 2 | 1 | 1 | 1 | |
| **History of bariatric surgery §** | | | | | | | ← A |
| a) Restrictive procedures: decrease storage capacity of the stomach | 1 | 1 | 1 | 1 | 1 | 1 | ← B |
| b) Malabsorptive procedures: decrease absorption of nutrients and calories by shortening small intestine | COCs: 3 P/R: 1 | 3 | 1 | 1 | 1 | 1 | |
| **CARDIOVASCULAR DISEASE** | | | | | | | ← C |
| **Multiple risk factors for CAD** (older age, smoking, diabetes, HBP) | 3 or 4 | 2 | 3 | 2 | 2 | 1 | |
| **HBP** - alone; no other CV risk factors | | | | | | | |
| HBP adequately controlled | 3 | 1 | 2 | 1 | 1 | 1 | |
| BP systolic 140-159 or Diastolic 90-99 | 3 | 1 | 2 | 1 | 1 | 1 | |
| BP systolic > 160 or Diastolic 100 | 4 | 2 | 3 | 2 | 2 | 1 | |
| Vascular disease | 4 | 2 | 3 | 2 | 2 | 1 | |
| **HBP during pregnancy, BP now normal** | 2 | 1 | 1 | 1 | 1 | 1 | |
| **Deep vein thrombosis/pulmonary embolism** | | | | | | | |
| a) History of DVT/PE/not on AC/low risk/no risk factors | 3 | 2 | 2 | 2 | 2 | 1 | ← D |
| b) History DVT/PE - not on AC/high risk | 4 | 2 | 2 | 2 | 2 | 1 | |
| c) Acute DVT/PE | 4 | 2 | 2 | 2 | 2 | 2 | ← E |
| d) DVT/PE on AC at least 3 months | | | | | | | |
| low risk recurrence | 3 | 2 | 2 | 2 | 2 | 2 | |
| high risk recurrence | 4 | 2 | 2 | 2 | 2 | 2 | |
| e) Family History (first-degree relatives) | 2 | 1 | 1 | 1 | 1 | 1 | |
| f) Major surgery with prolonged immobilization | 4 | 2 | 2 | 2 | 2 | 1 | |
| g) Major surgery without prolonged immobilizaton | 2 | 1 | 1 | 1 | 1 | 1 | |
| h) Minor surgery without immobilization | 1 | 1 | 1 | 1 | 1 | 1 | ← F |
| **KNOWN THROMBOGENIC MUTATIONS §** | 4 | 2 | 2 | 2 | 2 | 1 | |
| (e.g. Factor V Leiden, Prothrombin mutation, Protein S, Protein C and Antithrombin deficiencies) | | | | | | | ← G |
| **Superficial venous thrombosis** | | | | | | | |
| a) varicose veins | 1 | 1 | 1 | 1 | 1 | 1 | |
| b) superficial thrombophlebitis | 2 | 1 | 1 | 1 | 1 | 1 | |

**A** Vertical banded gastroplasty, laparoscopic adjustable gastric band, laparoscopic sleeve gastrectomy

**B** Roux-en-Y gastric bypass, biliopancreateic diversion (P= Patch; R= Ring)

**C** When multiple major risk factors exist, risk of CV disease may increase substantially. Some POCs may increase risk of thrombosis although this risk is substantially less than with COCs.

**D** High risk factors for recurrence: History of estrogen-associated DVT/PE, pregnancy-associated DVT/PE, idiopathic DVT/PE, known thrombophilia including antiphospholipid syndrome, active cancer (metastatic, on therapy, or within 6 mos after clinical remission) excluding non-melanoma skin cancer, history of recurrent DVT

**E** Limited evidence shows IM injections of DMPA in women on AC is not a significant risk for hematoma nor increased risk for heavy or irregular vaginal bleeding

**F** Routine screening not appropriate because of rarity of conditions and high-cost of screening

**G** Varicose Veins are not risk factors for DVT/PE

# CDC MEDICAL ELIGIBILITY CRITERIA FOR STARTING CONTRACEPTIVE METHODS (2010) - CONTINUED

| CONDITION | Combined Hormonal Contraceptives (CHCs) COCs, Patch (P), Ring (R) | Progestin-Only OCs | Depo-Provera NET EN | LNG/ETG Implants | LNG IUD | TCu-380A IUD | |
|---|---|---|---|---|---|---|---|
| Current & history of ischemic heart disease § | 4 | I-2/C-3 | 3 | I-2/C-3 | I-2/C-3 | 2 | |
| Stroke (history of CVA) | 4 | I-2/C-3 | 3 | I-2/C-3 | 2 | 1 | |
| Known hyperlipidemia (screening NOT necessary) | 2 or 3 | 2 | 2 | 2 | 2 | 1 | ← A, B |
| Valvular heart disease uncomplicated | 2 | 1 | 1 | 1 | 1 | 1 | ← C |
| Valvular heart disease complicated | 4 | 1 | 1 | 1 | 1 | 1 | ← D |
| Peripartum cardiomyopathy § a) Normal or mildly impaired cardiac function New York Heart Association Functional Class I or II | | | | | | | ← E |
| < 6 months | 4 | 1 | 1 | 1 | 2 | 2 | |
| ≥ 6 months | 3 | 1 | 1 | 1 | 2 | 2 | |
| b) Moderately or severely impaired cardiac function New York Heart Association Functional Class III or IV | 4 | 2 | 2 | 2 | 2 | 2 | ← F |
| **RHEUMATIC DISEASES** | | | | | | | |
| Systemic lupus erythematosus (SLE) § | | | | | | | ← G |
| a) Positive (or unknown) antiphospholipid antibodies | 4 | 3 | 3 | 3 | 3 | 1 | |
| b) Severe thrombocytopenia | 2 | 2 | I-3/C-2 | 2 | 2 | I-3/C-2 | |
| c) Immunosuppressive treatment | 2 | 2 | 2 | 2 | 2 | I-2/C-1 | |
| d) None of the above | 2 | 2 | 2 | 2 | 2 | 1 | |
| Rheumatoid arthritis | | | | | | | |
| a) On immunosuppressive therapy | 2 | 1 | I-2/C-3 | 1 | I-2/C-1 | I-2/C-1 | ← H |
| b) Not on immunosuppresive therapy | 2 | 1 | 2 | 1 | 1 | 1 | |
| **NEUROLOGIC CONDITIONS** | | | | | | | |
| Headaches: *assumes no other risk factors for stroke (age, HTN, smoking)* | | | | | | | |
| a) non-migraine (mild or severe) | I-1/C-2 | I-1/C-1 | 1 | 1 | 1 | 1 | |
| b) migraine < 35; no aura | I-2/C-3 | I-1/C-2 | 2 | 2 | 1 | 2 | |
| c) migraine ≥ 35; no aura | I-3/C-4 | I-1/C-2 | 2 | 2 | 1 | 2 | |
| d) migraine with aura (any age) | 4 | I-2/C-3 | I-2/C-3 | I-2/C-3 | I-2/C-3 | 1 | ← I |
| Epilepsy § | 1 | 1 | 1 | 1 | 1 | 1 | |
| Depressive Disorders | 1 | 1 | 1 | 1 | 1 | 1 | |

**A** Routine screening not appropriate. Assess risk based on type, severity and presence of other CV risk factors.

**B** 2 or 3 based on the type, severity, and the presence of other CV risk factors.

**C** Not necessary to use prophylactic antibiotics to prevent endocarditis with IUD insertion or removal

**D** E.G. Pulmonary hypertension, risk for atrial fibrilation, history of subacute bacterial endocarditis (SBE)

**E** Patients with no limitation of activities or patients with slight, mild limitation of activity.

**F** Patients with marked limitation of activity or patients who should be at complete rest.

**G** Classifications based on no other CV risk factors. SLE increases risk for CVD and VTE/PE.

**H** DMPA use among women on long-term corticosteroid therapy with a history of, or risk factors for, nontraumatic fractures is classified as Category 3.

**I** Among women with migraines, women who also have focal neurologic symptoms have a higher risk of stroke than those without focal neurologic symptoms. In addition, among women with migraines, those who use COCs have a 2 to 4-fold increased risk of stroke compared with women who do not use COCs.

§ Condition exposes woman to increased risk with unintended pregnancy. I=Initiation/C=Continuation

| CONDITION | CHCs | POPs | DMPA | LNG/ETG | LNGIUD | TCuIUD | |
|---|---|---|---|---|---|---|---|
| **REPRODUCTIVE TRACT INFECTIONS & DISORDERS** | | | | | | | |
| Irregular without heavy bleeding | 1 | 2 | 2 | 2 | 1 | 1 | |
| Heavy or prolonged vaginal bleeding (regular or irregular) | 1 | 2 | 2 | 2 | I-1/C-2 | 2 | |
| Unexplained vaginal bleeding. Suspicious for serious underlying condition. Before evaluation | 2 | 2 | 3 | 3 | I-4/C-2 | I-4/C-2 | |
| Endometriosis | 1 | 1 | 1 | 1 | 1 | 2 | |
| Benign ovarian tumors (including cysts) | 1 | 1 | 1 | 1 | 1 | 1 | |
| Severe dysmenorrhea | 1 | 1 | 1 | 1 | 1 | 2 | |
| Benign gestational trophoblastic disease | 1 | 1 | 1 | 1 | 3 | 3 | |
| Malignant gestational trophoblastic disease § | 1 | 1 | 1 | 1 | 4 | 4 | |
| Cervical ectropion | 1 | 1 | 1 | 1 | 1 | 1 | |
| Cervical intraepithelial neoplasia (CIN) | 2 | 1 | 2 | 2 | 2 | 1 | ← A |
| Cervical cancer (awaiting treatment) | 2 | 1 | 2 | 2 | I-4/C-2 | I-4/C-2 | |
| Undiagnosed breast mass | 2 | 2 | 2 | 2 | 2 | 1 | |
| Benign breast disease | 1 | 1 | 1 | 1 | 1 | 1 | |
| Family history of breast cancer | 1 | 1 | 1 | 1 | 1 | 1 | |
| Breast cancer (current) § | 4 | 4 | 4 | 4 | 4 | 1 | ← B |
| Past breast cancer; No current disease for 5 years § | 3 | 3 | 3 | 3 | 3 | 1 | |
| **Endometrial hyperplasia** | 1 | 1 | 1 | 1 | 1 | 1 | |
| Endometrial cancer § | 1 | 1 | 1 | 1 | I-4/C-2 | I-4/C-2 | |
| Ovarian cancer § | 1 | 1 | 1 | 1 | 1 | 1 | |
| Uterine fibroids | 1 | 1 | 1 | 1 | 2 | 2 | |
| Anatomical abnormalities | | | | | | | |
| distorted uterine cavity | | | | | 4 | 4 | |
| no distorted uterine cavity | | | | | 2 | 2 | |
| Past history PID (no current STI risk factors) with subsequent pregnancy | 1 | 1 | 1 | 1 | 1 | 1 | ← C, D |
| Past history PID (no current STI risk factors) without subsequent pregnancy | 1 | 1 | 1 | 1 | 2 | 2 | |
| Current PID (or within last 3 months) | 1 | 1 | 1 | 1 | I-4/C-2 | I-4/C-2 | |
| **STIs** | | | | | | | |
| a) Current purulent cervicitis or chlamydial infection or gonorrhea | 1 | 1 | 1 | 1 | I-4/C-2 | I-4/C-2 | ← E |
| b) Other STIs (excluding HIV & hepatitis) | 1 | 1 | 1 | 1 | 2 | 2 | |
| c) Vaginitis (including trichomonas vaginalis & bacterial vaginosis) | 1 | 1 | 1 | 1 | 2 | 2 | |
| d) Increased risk of STIs | 1 | 1 | 1 | 1 | I-2/3 C-2 | I-2/3 C-2 | |

**A** There is some concern that COCs and DMPA increase risk of CIN to invasive disease with long-term use (≥ 5 years)

**B** Breast cancer is hormonally sensitive, and the prognosis of women may worsen with hormonal methods

**C** In women at low risk of STIs, IUD insertion poses little risk of PID.

**D** Treat the PID using appropriate antibiotics. IUD usually need not be removed. Continued use depends on woman's informed choice and current risk factors for STIs and PID. Evidence shows clinical course did not differ whether IUD pulled or left in place.

**E** If a woman has a very high risk of exposure to infection (Category 3)

* Initiation: 2 and Continuation: 3 expressed as I-2/C-3

** If distinction is made between levels of severity of a condition it is expressed as 2 or 3

§ Condition exposes woman to increased risk with unintended pregnancy

## CDC MEDICAL ELIGIBILITY CRITERIA FOR STARTING CONTRACEPTIVE METHODS (2010) - CONTINUED

| CONDITION | Combined Hormonal Contraceptives (CHCs) COCs, Patch (P), Ring (R) | Progestin-Only OCs | Depo-Provera NET EN | LNG/ETG Implants | LNG IUD | TCu-380A IUD | |
|---|---|---|---|---|---|---|---|
| **HIV/AIDS** | | | | | | | |
| High risk of HIV | 1 | 1 | 1 | 1 | 2 | 2 | ← A |
| HIV-positive § | 1 | 1 | 1 | 1 | 2 | 2 | |
| AIDS § | 1 | 1 | 1 | 1 | I-3/C-2 | I-3/C-2 | |
| Clinically well on ARV therapy | if on treatment see drug interactions below | | | | 2 | 2 | |
| **DRUG INTERACTIONS: ANTIRETROVIRAL THERAPY** (for information on specific drugs go to www.cdc.gov) | | | | | | | |
| a) Nucleoside reverse transcriptase inhibitors (NRTIs) | 1 | 1 | 1 | 1 | I-2 or 3 C-2 | I-2 or 3 C-2 | |
| b) Non-nucleoside reverse transcriptase inhibitors (NNRTIs) | 2 | 2 | 1 | 2 | I-2 or 3 C-2 | I-2 or 3 C-2 | |
| c) Ritonavir-boosted protease inhibitors | 3 | 3 | 1 | 2 | I-2 or 3/C-2 | I-2 or 3/C-2 | |
| **ENDOCRINE CONDITIONS** | | | | | | | |
| History gestational diabetes | 1 | 1 | 1 | 1 | 1 | 1 | ← B |
| Non-insulin dependent diabetes (non-vascular disease) | 2 | 2 | 2 | 2 | 2 | 1 | |
| Insulin dependent diabetes § (non-vascular disease) | 2 | 2 | 2 | 2 | 2 | 1 | |
| Diabetic nephropathy/retinopathy/neuropathy § | I-3/C-4 | 2 | 3 | 2 | 2 | 1 | ← C |
| Other vascular disease; diabetes of > 20 years § | I-3/C-4 | 2 | 3 | 2 | 2 | 1 | |
| Thyroid: simple goiter | 1 | 1 | 1 | 1 | 1 | 1 | |
| Hyperthyroid | 1 | 1 | 1 | 1 | 1 | 1 | |
| Hypothyroid | 1 | 1 | 1 | 1 | 1 | 1 | |

**To download most recent CDC Medical Eligibility Criteria go to: www.cdc.gov**

**A** Women at high risk of HIV are also at high risk of other STIs

**B** Limited evidence inconsistent about development of NIDDM among users of POCs with history of gestational diabetes.

**C** There is concern about the possible negative effect of DMPA on lipid metabolism, possibly affecting the progression of nephropathy, retinopathy or other vascular disease. Categories should be assessed according to severity of condition.

§ Condition exposes woman to increased risk with unintended pregnancy

I=Initiation/C=Continuation

| CONDITION | CHCs | POPs | DMPA | LNG/ETG | LNGIUD | TCuIUD | |
|---|---|---|---|---|---|---|---|
| **GASTROINTESTINAL CONDITIONS** | | | | | | | |
| Inflammatory bowel disease (IBD) (ulcerative colitis, Crohn disease) | I-2/C-3 § | 2 | 2 | 1 | 1 | 1 | ← A |
| Symptomatic gall bladder disease post cholecystectomy | 2 | 2 | 2 | 2 | 2 | 1 | |
| Symptomatic gall bladder disease medically treated | 3 | 2 | 2 | 2 | 2 | 1 | |
| Symptomatic gall bladder disease - current | 3 | 2 | 2 | 2 | 2 | 1 | ← B |
| Assymptomatic gall bladder disease | 2 | 2 | 2 | 2 | 2 | 1 | |
| History of pregnancy-related cholestasis | 2 | 1 | 1 | 1 | 2 | 1 | |
| Past COC-related cholestasis | 3 | 2 | 2 | 2 | 2 | 1 | |
| Viral hepatitis active | I-3/4 C-2 | 1 | 1 | 1 | 1 | 1 | |
| Viral hepatitis carrier or chronic | 1 | 1 | 1 | 1 | 1 | 1 | |
| Cirrhosis: mild compensated | 1 | 1 | 1 | 1 | 1 | 1 | |
| Cirrhosis: severe (decompensated) § | 4 | 3 | 3 | 3 | 3 | 1 | ← C |
| Benign hepatic adenoma § | 4 | 3 | 3 | 3 | 3 | 1 | |
| Malignant liver tumor (hepatoma) § | 4 | 3 | 3 | 3 | 3 | 1 | |
| **ANEMIAS** | | | | | | | |
| Thalassemia | 1 | 1 | 1 | 1 | 1 | 2 | |
| Sickle cell disease § | 2 | 1 | 1 | 1 | 1 | 2 | |
| Iron deficiency anemia | 1 | 1 | 1 | 1 | 1 | 2 | |
| **SOLID ORGAN TRANSPLANTATION** § | | | | | | | |
| a) Complicated: graft failure (acute or chronic), rejection, cardiac allograft vasculopathy | 4 | 2 | 2 | 2 | I-3/C-2 | I-3/C-2 | |
| b) Uncomplicated | 2 | 2 | 2 | 2 | 2 | 2 | ← D |
| **DRUG INTERACTIONS** | | | | | | | |
| Griseofulvin | 2 | 2 | 1 | 2 | 1 | 1 | |
| ANTICONVULSANT THERAPY | | | | | | | ← E |
| a) Certain anticonvulsants: Phenytoin, barbiturates carbamazepine, primadone, topiramate, oxycarbazepine | 3 | 3 | 2 | 3 | 1 | 1 | |
| b) Lamotrigine | 3 | 1 | 1 | 1 | 1 | 1 | ← F |
| ANTIMICROBIAL THERAPY | | | | | | | |
| a) Broad spectrum antibiotics, anti-fungals, anti-parasitics | 1 | 1 | 1 | 1 | 1 | 1 | |
| b) Rifampicin or Risabutin | 3 | 3 | 1 | 2 | 1 | 1 | |

**A** For women with mild IBD, with no other risk factors for VTE, the benefits of COC/P/R use generally outweigh the risks. However, for women with IBD with increased risk for VTE (e.g. those with active or extensive disease, surgery, immobilization, corticosteroid use, vitamin deficiencies, fluid depletion), the risks for COC/P/R use generally outweigh the benefits.

**B** COCs may cause small increased risk of gall bladder disease. There is also concern that COCs may worsen existing gallbladder disease.

**C** COCs are metabolized by liver and use may adversely affect women whose liver function is already compromised. There is concern about the hormonal load associated with POC use, but it is less than for COCs.

**D** Women with Budd-Chiari syndrome should not use COC/P/R because of the increased risk for thrombosis.

**E** Although the interaction between commonly used liver enzyme inducers and COCs is not harmful to women, it is likely to reduce the efficacy of COCs. Use of other contraceptives should be encouraged for women who are long-term users of any of these drugs. Whether increasing the hormone dose of COCs is of benefit remains unclear.

**F** Lomotrigine levels decrease significantly with COC use. In women using lomotrigine and another anti-convulsant okay to use COCs.

I=Initiation/C=Continuation § Condition exposes woman to increased risk with unintended pregnancy

# HISTORY OF CONTRACEPTION AND POPULATION GROWTH

2050 - 10 billion

| | |
|---|---|
| 2050 | Year when some demographers think population growth will cease at 10 billion |
| 2014 | World population 7.24 billion (United Nations) |
| 2005 | Subcutaneous Depo-Provera and Implanon approved |
| 2003 | Seasonale, first extended-use pill (0.15 mg LNG, 0.03 mg EE), approved and marketed |
| 2001 | Ortho Evra Patch and NuvaRing approved |
| 2000 | RU486 (mifepristone), Lunelle and Mirena approved by FDA |
| 1999 | World population hits 6 billion (this billion took 12 years) |
| 1997 | FDA approves Emergency Contraceptive Pills |
| 1994 | Plastic (polyurethane) condom for men (Avanti) |
| 1993 | FDA approves polyurethane (plastic) female condom (Reality) |
| 1992 | FDA approves Depo-Provera (DMPA) injections |
| 1988 | Copper T 380-A IUD marketing begins, 5 years after FDA approval |
| 1987 | World population reaches 5 billion (this billion took 12 years) |
| 1983 | FDA approves Copper T 380-A and the Today sponge |
| 1982 | Baulieu describes medical abortion using mifepristone |
| 1981 | First documented case of HIV/AIDS |
| 1981 | Garret Hardin writes "nobody ever dies of overpopulation" after 500,000 die from flooding of an overcrowded East Bengal River delta |
| 1975 | World population reaches 4 billion (this billion took 15 years) |
| 1974 | Al Yuzpe describes emergency contraception using Ovral pills |
| 1973 | FDA approved progestin-only pills (minipills) |
| 1973 | U.S. Supreme Court abortion decision (Roe v Wade & Doe v Bolton) |
| 1965 | U.S. Supreme Court overturns anti-birth control laws in most states (Griswold v. CT) |
| 1965 | U.S. Agency of International Development initiates Population Program |
| 1960 | Food and Drug Administration approves combined oral contraceptives |
| 1960 | World population reaches 3 billion (this billion took 30 years) |
| 1942 | American Birth Control League renamed Planned Parenthood |
| 1937 | AMA ends longstanding opposition to contraception |
| 1936 | German gynecologist Friedrich Wilde describes first cervical cap (fitted from a wax impression) |
| 1930-31 | Knaus (Austria) and Ogino (Japan) develop rhythm method |
| 1930 | World population now 2 billion (this billion took 100 years) |
| 1930 | Pope Pius XI virulently attacks both contraception and abortion |
| 1927 | Novak (Hopkins) describes suction as means of performing an abortion |
| 1918 | N.Y. court approves condoms to prevent disease only |
| 1916 | Margaret Sanger opens first Amercian birth control clinic in Brooklyn, NY |
| 1914 | Margaret Sanger coins word "birth control" |
| 1912 | Sadie Sachs post-abortion death affects Margaret Sanger profoundly |
| 1909 | German surgeon Richard Richter reports success with silkworm-gut shaped into a ring |
| 1893 | First vasectomy by Harrison in London |
| 1882 | First contraceptive clinic established in Amsterdam |
| 1880 | First tubal ligation |
| 1873 | Comstock Act: classifies birth control devices and information as obscene |
| 1839 | Charles Goodyear discovers vulcanization technology; quickly leads to rubber condoms |
| 1830 | World population reaches 1 billion (this billion took 100,000 to 6 million years) |
| 1798 | Thomas Robert Malthus proposes dismal theory that population growth eventually will exceed the ability of the earth to provide food |
| Late 1770s | Casanova popularizes condoms for infection control and contraception |
| 1 AD | World population reaches 250 million, abstinence (particularly postpartum), withdrawal, lactation, stones in camels, lemons for mechanical and spermicidal effect, abortion using molokeeia (same stem used today), homosexuality and polygamy |

2014 - 7.24 billion

1999 - 6 billion (10/12/99!!)

1987 - 5 billion

1975 - 4 billion

1960 - 3 billion

1930 - 2 billion

1800 - 1 billion

1 AD - 250 million

Amba J, Chandra A, Mosher V D et al. Fertility, family planning, and women's health: New data from 1995 NSFG. Vital Health Stat 1997; 23:62-63.

American College of Obstetrics and Gynecologists (ACOG). Emergency oral contraception. ACOG Practice Patterns 1996 (Dec. no. 3).

Anderson FD, Hait H, the Seasonale-301 Study Group. A multicenter, randomized study of an extended cycle oral contraceptive. Contraception 2003; 68; 89-96.

Anderson JE et al. Contraceptive Sterilization Among Married Adults: National Data on who Chooses Vasectomy and Tubal Sterilization. Contraception 85(2012):552-7

Anderson, et al, Contraception 49, 1994: 56.

Arevalo N, Jennings V, Nikula M. Efficacy of the new TwoDay method of family planning. Fertil Steril. 2004; 82:885-892.

Arevalo N, Jennings V, Sinai I. Efficacy of a new method of family planning: the Standard Days Method. Contraception. 2001; 65:333-338.

Artz, L, Demand M, Pulley LV, Posner SF, Macaluso M. Predictors of difficulty inserting the female condom. Contraception 65, 2002:151-157.

Association for Voluntary Surgical Contraception. Postpartum IUD insertion: Clinical and programatic guidelines (monograph) 1994 (AVSC has changed name to Engender Health).

Audet MC, Moreau M, Koltun WD, Waldbaum AS, Shangold G, Fisher AC, Creasy MD. Evaluation of contraceptive efficacy and cycle control of a transdermal contraceptive patch vs. an oral contraceptive: a randomized controlled trial. JAMA. 285; 2001:2347-2354.

A van Hylckamu Vlieg et al. The VTE risk of OCs, effects of oestrogendose and progestin type: results of the MEGA case-control study. BMJ 2009; 339: b2921.

Backman T, Huhtala S, Luoto R, Tuominen J, Rauramo I, Koskenvuo M. Advance Information Improves User Satisfaction with the Levonorgestrel Intrauterine System. Obstetrics and Gynecology. 99, 2002: 608-13.

Ballagh SA. Sterilization in the office: the concept is now a reality. Contraceptive Technology Reports. February, 2003 supplement to the newsletter, Contraceptive Technology Update.

Bonny AE, Ziegler J, Harvey R et al. Weight gain in obese and non-obese adolescent girls initiating depot medroxyprogesterone, OCPs and no hormonal method. Arch Pedi Adol Med. 160(1):40-5. 2006.

Barone MA, Nazerali H, Cortez M, et al. A prospective study of time and number of ejaculations to azoospermia after vasectomy by ligation and excision. J Urology 2003; 170:892-896.

Bartlett LA, et al. Risk factors for legal induced abortion related mortality risk by pregnancy outcome, U.S. 1991-1999. Obstet-Gynecol 2004; 103(4): 729-739.

Berel V, Hermon C, Kay C, Hannaford P, Darby S, Reeves G. Mortality associated with oral contraceptive use: 25 year follow-up of cohort of 46,000 women from Royal College of General Practitioners' oral contraceptive study; Br Med J 1999: 918:96-100.

Berga SL, Marcus MD, Loucks TL, Hlastala S, Ringham R, Krohn MA. Recovery of ovarian activity in women with functional hypothalamic amenorrhea who were treated with cognitive behavioral therapy. Fertil Steril 2003; 80:976-981.

Berlex Laboratories, Inc. YASMIN prescribing information: Physician Labeling and Patient Instructions; June, 2001.

Bjarnadottir R, Tuppurainen M, Killick S. Comparison of cycle control with a combined contraceptive vaginal ring and oral levonorgestrel/ethinyl estradiol. American Journal of Obstetrics and Gynecology. March 2002;186:389-95.

Brache V, Alvarez-Sanchez F, Faundes A, Tejada AS, Cochon L. Ovarian endocrine function through five years of continuous treatment with Norplant subdermal contraceptive implants. Contraception 1990;41:169.

Bradner, C.H., et al. Older, but Not Wiser: How Men Get Information About AIDS and Sexually Transmitted Diseases After High School. *Family Planning Perspectives* 2000; January/February.

Briggs GG, Freeman RK, Yaffe SJ. Drugs in Pregnancy and Lactation, Fifth edition. Lippincott Williams & Wilkins, Philadelphia. 1998.

Canto-DeCetina TEC, Canto P, Luna MO. Effect of counseling to improve compliance in Mexican women receiving depot-medroxyprogesterone acetate. Contraception 63; 2001: 143-146. Cates W Jr., Steiner MJ. Dual protection against unintended pregnancy and sexually transmitted infections: What is the best contraceptive approach? Sex Transm Dis 2002;29:168-174.

Centers for Disease Control and Prevention. 1998 Guidelines for treatment of sexually transmitted diseases. MMWR 1998:47(No. RR-1).

Centers for Disease Control Cancer and Steroid Hormone Study. Long-term oral contraceptive use and the risk of breast cancer. JAMA. 1983; 249:1591-1595.

Cochrane Database of Systematic Reviews. Vander Wijden et al. Lactational amenorrhea for family planning. 2008.

Colditz GA, Rosner BA, et al. Risk factors for breast cancer according to family history of breast cancer. J Natl Cancer Inst. 1996;88:365-371.

Cole JA et al. VTE, MI and stroke among transdermal contraceptive system users. Ob & Gyn 2007; 109(2) 339-346.

Collaborative Group on Hormonal Factors in Breast Cancer. Breast cancer and hormonal contraceptives: collaborative reanalysis of individual data on 53,297 women with breast cancer and 100,239 women without breast cancer from epidemiological studies. Lancet 1996; 347:1713-1727.

Coutinho EM with Segal SJ. Is Menstruation Obsolete? Oxford University Press; Oxford; New York; 1999.

Cowman W.L. et al. Vaginal Misoprostol Aids in Difficult IUC Removal: a report of three cases. Contraception 2012;86:281-4.

Creinin MD, Burke AE. Methotrexate and misoprostol for early abortion: a multicenter trial. Acceptablity. Contraception 1996;54:19-22.

Creinin MD, Vittinghoff E, Schaff E, Klaisle C, Darney PD, Dean C. Medical abortion with oral methotrexate and vaginal misoprostol. Obstet Gynecol 1997;90:611-5.

Cromer BA, Lazebnik MD, Rome E et al. Double-blind controlled trial of estrogen supplementation in adolescent girls who receive depot medroxyprogesterone acetate for contraception. Am Jour Obstet Gynec 2005; 192:41-47.

Croxatto HB, Diaz S, Pavez M, et al. Plasma progesterone levels during long-term treatment with levonorgestrel silastic implants. Acta Endocrinol 1982;101:307-11.

Curtis et al. Contraception for Women in Selected Circumstances. Obstetrics and Gynecology, June 2002; 99 (6):1100-1112.

Cundy T, Evans M, Roberts H, Wattie D, Ames R, Reid IR. Bone density in women receiving depot medroxyprogesterone acetate for contraception. BMJ 1991; 303: 13-16.

Davis KR, Weller SC. The effectiveness of condoms in reducing heterosexual transmission of HIV. Fam Plann Perspect 1999;31(6):272-279.

Davis TC et al. Patient Understanding and use of OCPs in a Southern Public Health Family Planning Clinic. Southern Medical Jnl 99(7) 713-8. 2006 Jul.

de Abood M, de Castillo 2, Guerrero E, Espino M, Austin KL. Effect of Depo-Provera or Microgynon in the painful crises of sickle-cell anemia patients. Contraception 56; 1997:313.

Diaz J, Bahamondes L, Monteiro I, Peta C, Hildalgo MM, Arce XE. Acceptability and performance of the levonorgestrel-releasing intrauterine system (Mirena) in Campinas, Brazil. Contraception 2000; 62: 59-61.

Dieben T, Roumen F, Apter D. Efficacy, cycle control, and user acceptability of a novel combined contraceptive vaginal ring. Obstetrics and Gynecology. Sept 2002; 100:585-93.

Dinger JC et al. The safety of DRSP-containing OC: final results from the EURAS on OCs based on 142, 475 women-years of observation. Contraception 2007; 75:344.

Dragoman et al. Contraceptive Vaginal Ring Effectiveness is Maintained during 6 Weeks of Use: a prospective study of BMI and obese women. Contraception 2013;87:432-436.

Duke JM et al. Contraception 75 (2007) 27-31.

Dunson D, Sinai I, Colombo B. The relationship between cervical secretions and the daily probabilities of pregnancy. Effectiveness of the TwoDay algorithm. Hum Repro 2001; 16: 2278-2282.

Edwards, S.R. The role of men in contraceptive decision-making: Current knowledge and future implications. *Family Planning Perspectives* 1994; March/April.

Farley TM, Rosenberg MS, Rowe PJ, Chen SH, Meirck O. Intrauterine devices and pelvic inflammatory disease: an international perspective. Lancet 1992; 339: 785-88.

Feldblum PJ, Morrison CS, Roddy RE, Cates W Jr. The effectiveness of barrier methods of contraception in preventing the spread of HIV. AIDS 1995;9 (suppl A):585-93.

Fehring et al., Randomized comparison of two Internet supplied fertility-awareness-based methods of family planning. Contraception 2013; 88:24-30.

Fine PM et al. Safety and acceptability with the use of a contraceptive vaginal ring after surgical and medical abortion. Contraception 75 (2007) 367.

Finer LB, Henshaw SK. Abortion incidence and service in the United States in 2000. Perspectives on Sexual and Reproductive Health 2003; 35(1): 6-15.

Ford K, Labbok M. Contraceptive use during lactation in the United States: an update. American Institute of Public Health 1987; 77: 79-81.

Forrest JD. U.S. women's perceptions of and attitudes about the IUD. Obstet Gynecol Surv. 1996; 31:S30-34

Fraser SI, Affandi B, Croxatto HB, et al. Norplant consensus statement and background paper. Turku, Finland: Leiras Oy International, 1997.

Frezieres RG, Walsh TL, Nelson AL, Clark VA, Coulson AH: Breakage and acceptability of a polyurethane condom: A randomized controlled study. Fam Plann Perspect 1998;30;73-8.

Furlong LA. Ectopic Pregnancy risk when contraception fails. J Repro Med. 2002; Vol 47, No. 11.

Gallo I.D. et al. LNG-IUS Versus Oral Progestogen Treatment for Endometrial Hyperplasia: a long=term comperative cohort study. Hum Reprod 2013 Nov 28(11):2966-71.

Gallo MF, Grimes DA, Lopez LM et al. Non-latex versus latex male condoms for contraception. Cochrane Database Systematic reviews 2005.

Geere et al. Behind-the-counter status and availability of EC. AJOG 199(5): 478. 2008 Nov.

Glaser A. Can we identify women at risk of pregnancy despite using EC? Data from randomized trials of UPA and LNG. Contraception, 2011; 84(4):363

Glasier AF et al. Contraception 2003; 67:1-8.

Goldstein M, Girardi S. Vasectomy and vasectomy reversal. Curr Thera Endocrinol Metab 1997;6:371-80.

Goodman S. et al. Increasing intrauterine contracption use by reducing barriers to post-abortal and interval insertion. Contraception 78 (2008) 136-142.

Grabrick DH, Hartmann LC, Cerhan FR, Vierkant RA, Therneau TM, et al. Risk of Breast Cancer with Oral Contraceptive Use in Women With a Family History of Breast Cancer. JAMA; 284:1791-1798.

Gray RH, Campbell OM, Zacur H, Labbok MH, MacRae SL. Postpartum return of ovarian activity in non-breastfeeding women monitored by urinary assays. J Clin Endocrinol Metab 1987;64:645-50.

Grimes DA. Health benefits of oral contraception: update on endometrial cancer prevention. The Contraception Report 2001;12(3):4-7.

Grimes DA. Modern IUDs: an update. The Contraception Report; November, 1998.

Grimes DA. Should first-time OC users be screened for genetic thrombophilia? The Contraception Report; 10:1, p.p. 9-11; March 1999.

Grimes DA. Transdermal contraceptive patch awaiting US approval. The Contraception Report; 12(4):12-14.

Grimes DA. IN Hatcher. Contraceptive Technology, 18th Ed. Intrauterine Devices (IUDS).

Grimes DA, Gallo MF, Halpein V. Fertility awareness-based methods for contraception. Cochrone Database of Systematic Reviews.

Grimes DA, Lopez L, Raymond EG et al. Spermicide used alone for contraception. Cochrane Database of Systematic Reviews 2005.

Guillebaud J. Contraception, your questions answered, 3rd edition. London, Churchill Livingstone, 1999.

Guillebaud J. Personal communication; October 14, 2001.

Hafner DW, Schwartz P. What I've Learned about Sex. A Perigee Book: New York: The Berkeley Publishing Group, 1998.

Hakim-Elahi E, Tovell HMM, Burnhill MS. Complications of first-trimester abortion: a report of 170,000 cases. Obstet Gynecol 1990;76:129.

Hall KS et al. Progestin-only contraceptive pill

Hall PE. New once-a-month injectable contraceptives, with particular reference to Cyclofem/Cyclo-Provera. Int. J Gynaecol Obstet 1998; 62: S43-S56.

Hausknecht R. Mifepristone and misoprostol for early medical abortion: 18 months experience in the United States. Contraception 2003; 67:463-465.

Haws, J.M., et al. Clinical Practice of vasectomies in the United States in 1995. *Urology* 1998; October.

Henshaw SK. Unintended pregnancy in the United States. Fam Plann Perspect 1998;30:24-9, 46.

Harris Interactive Inc. prepared for The National Women's Health Resource Center. Menstrual Management Survey Report. Aug. 29, 2008. Accessed at www.healthywomen.org/Documents/MenstrualManagementReport.pdf

Hatcher RA, Trussell J, Stewart F, Cates W Jr, Stewart GK, Guest F, Kowal D. *Contraceptive Technology*, 17th ed. New York NY, Ardent Media, 1998

Hayes J et al. A pilot clinical trial of ultrasound-guided postplacental insertion of a levonorgestrel intrauterine device. Contraception 76(4): 292-6 2007 Oct.

Heinemann LA et al. Contraception 75 (2007) 328-336.

Heit et al. Ann Int Med 2005 143: 697-706.

Hennessy S., Berlin JA, Kinman JL et al. Risk of VTE from OCs containing desogestrel and gestodene versus levonorgestrel: a meta-analysis and formal sensitivity analysis. Contraception 64(2): 125-33, 2001 August.

Hilgers, T.W., Abraham, G.E., and Cavanagh, D. (1978), "Natural Family Planning. I. The Peak Symptom and Estimated Time of Ovulation", *Obstetrics and Gynecology* 52(5): 575-582.

Hogue CJR, Cates W Jr, Tietze C. The effects of induced abortion on subsequent reproduction. The Johns Hopkins University School of Hygiene and Public Health. Epidemiol Rev 1982;4:66

International Planned Parenthood Federation Handbook 1997.

Ito KE, Gizlice Z, Owen-O'Doud J. Parent opinion of sexuality education in a state mandated abstinence education: does policy match parental preference? J Adol Health. 39(5): 634, 2006 Nov.

Jain J, Jakimiuk AJ, Bode FR, Ross D, Kaunitz AM. Contraceptive efficacy and safety of DMPA-SC. Contraception 2004; 70:269-275.

Jamieson DJ, Costello C, Trussell J, Hillis SP, Marchbanks PA, Peterson HB. The risk of pregnancy after vasectomy. Obstetrics and Gynecology 2004; 103:848-850.

Jick S, et al. Further results on the risks of nonfatal VTE in users of the contraceptive transdermal patch compared to users of OCs containing norgestimate and 35 mcg of EE. Contraception 2007; 76: 4-7

Johnson JV. et al Contraception 75 (2007) 23-26.

Jones RK, Dorroch JE, Henshaw SK. Patterns with socioeconomic characterics of women obtaining abortions in 2000-2001. Perspectives in Sexual and Reproductive Health 2002,34:226-235.

Juliato CT et al. Usefulness of FSH measurements for determining menopause in long-term users of depot medroxyprogesterone acetate over 40 years of age. Contraception 76 (2007) 282-286.

Kaunitz AM. personal communications; December 28, 1998 and February 24, 1999.

Kaunitz AM, Garceau RJ, Cromie MA. Comparative safety, efficacy, and cycle control of Lunelle monthly contraceptive injection (medroxyprogesterone acetate and estradiol cypionate injectable suspension) and Ortho-Novum 7/7/7 oral contraceptive (norethindrone/ethinyl estradiol triphasic). Contraception 1999; 60(4):179-187.

Kennedy KI, Trussell J. Postpartum contraception and lactation. IN Hatcher RA, Trussell J, Stewart F et al: Contraceptive Technology, 17th ed.; New York: Ardent Media Inc; 1998: 592-4. [The same data are presented in the Family Health International Module for the teaching of Lactational Amenorrhea]

Kjos SL, Peters RK, Xiang A, Duncan T, Schaefer U, Buchanan TA. Contraception and the risk of type 2 diabetes mellitus in Latina women with prior gestational diabetes mellitus. JAMA 1998; 280: 533-38.

Klavon SL, Grubb G. Insertion site complications during the first year of Norplant use. Contraception 1990;41:27.

Krattenmacher R. Drospirenone: pharmacology and pharmacokinetics of a unique progestogen. Contraception 2000; 62:29-38.

Kuyoh MA, Toroitich-Ruto C, Grimes DA, et al. Sponge versus diaphragm for contraception: a Cochrane review. Contraception 2003; 67(1):15-18.

Kwiecien M et al. Contraception 2003; 67:9-13.

Lidegaard O et al. Hormonal contraception and risk of VTE: National follow-up study. BMJ 2009;339: b2890

Lipnick RJ, Buring JE, Hennekens CH, et al. Oral contraceptives and breast cancer: a prospective cohort study. JAMA. 1986; 255:58-61.

Lippes J (Guest Editor). Quinacrine sterilization: reports on 40,252 cases. Intl J of Gynec & Obstet Volume 83, supl 2, October 2003.

R. Lyus, et. al. Outcomes with same-day cervical preparation with Dilapan-S osmotic dilators and vaginal misoprostol before dilatation and evacuation at 18 to 21+6 weeks' gestation. Contraception vol 87(1):71-75

R. Lyus, et. al. Same day cervical preparation with misoprostol second trimester D-E: a case series. Contraception vol 88 (2013):116-121

Marcell, A.V., et al. Where Does Reproductive Health Fit Into the Lives of Adolescent Males? Perspectives of Sexual and Reproductive Health 2003; 35(4):180-186.

Marguilies R, Miller L. Increased depot medroxyprogesterone acetate use increases family planning program pharmaceutical supply costs. Contraception 2001 (63):147-149.

Michaelson, M.D., Oh, W.K. Epidemiology of and risk factors for testicular cancer. Available from http://www.utdol.com [Accessed 10 October 2004]

Miller L, Verhoeven CH, Hout J. Extended regimens of the contraceptive vaginal ring: a randomized trial. ObGyn. 106(3): 473-82, 2005 Sep.

Miller L, Grice J. Intradermal proximal field block: an innovative anesthetic technique for levonorgestrel implant removal. Obstet Gynecol 1998;91:294-297.

Miller L, Hughes J. Continuous combination oral contraceptive pills to eliminate withdrawal bleeding: a randomized trial. Obstet Gynecol 2003;101:653-61.

Moreau C & Trussell J. Results from Pooled Phase III Studies of VPA for Emergency Contraception. Contraception 2012;88:673-80.

Monteiro I, Bahamondes L, Diaz J, Perotti M, Petta C. Therapeutic use of levonorgestrel-releasing intra-uterine systems in women with menorrhagia: a pilot study. Contraception 65; 2002; 325-328.

Morroni C et al. The Impact of Oral Contraceptive Initiation on Young Women's Condom Use in 3 American Cities: Missed Opportunities for Intervention. PloSOne 2014 July 8; 9(7):e101804. doi:10.1371/jpurnal

Mosher WD et al. Use of contraception and use of family planning services in the U.S.: 1982-2000. Advance data from vital and health statistics, No. 350. 2004.

Mulders TMT, Dieben TOM. Use of the novel combined contraceptive vaginal ring NuvaRing for ovulation inhibition. Fertility and Sterility 2001; 75:865-870.

Mulders TMT, Dieben TOM, et al. Ovarian function with a novel combined contraceptive vaginal ring. Hum Reprod 2002;10:2594-2599.

Murray PP, Stadel BV, Schlesselman JJ. Oral contraceptive use in women with a family history of breast cancer. Obstet Gynecol. 1989; 73:977-983.

Narod ST. The Hereditary Ovarian Cancer Clinical Study Group. Oral contraceptives and the risk of hereditary ovarian cancer. N Engl J Med 1998;339;424-8.

Narod ST. et al. Lancet 357 [9267]: 1467-70, 2001.

Nelson AL. Recent use of condoms and EC by women who selected condoms as their contraceptive method. AJOG 194(6): 1710-5, 2006 Jun.

Ness RB, Grisso JA, Klapper J, et al. Risk of ovarian cancer in relation to estrogen and progestin dose and use characteristics of oral contraceptives. Am J Epidemiol 2000;152:233-241.

Ness, R.B., et al. Do men become infertile after having sexually transmitted urethritis? An epidemiologic examination. Fertility and Sterility 1997; 68(2):205-213.

Nilsson CG, Haukkamaa M, Vierok H, et al. Tissue concentrations of levonorgestrel in women using lng-releasing IUD. Clinical Endocrinology 17(6):529-36, 1982.

O'Hanley K, Huber DH. Postpartum IUDs: keys for success. Contraception 1992; 45: 351-361.

Peipert JF, Gutman J. Oral contraceptive risk assessment: a survey of 247 educated women. Obstet Gynecol 1993;82:112-7.

Pazol K, et al., Trnds in use of medical abortion in the US: reanalysis of surveillance data from the CDC and Prevention, 2001-2008. Contraception 2012; 86:746-751.

Penfield JA, The Filshie clip for female sterilzation: A review of world experience. AJOG 2000; 182:485-489.

Peterson HB, Jeng G, Folger SG et al for the U.S. Collaborative Review of Sterilization Working Group. N Engl J Med 2000; 343:1681-7.

Peterson HB, Pollack AE, Warshaw JS. Tubal sterilization. In: Rock JA, Thompson JD, eds. TeLinde's Operative Gynecology. 8th ed. Philadelphia: Lippincott-Raven, 1997:541-5.

Petta LA, Ferriani RA, Abrao RA et al. Randomized clinical trial of a levonorgestrel-releasing IUS and a depot GnRH analogue for the treatment of chronic pelvic pain in women with endometriosis. Human Reprod 2005; 20(7):1993-8.

Pinkerton SD, Abramson PR. Effectiveness of condoms in preventing HIV transmission. Soc Sci Med 1997 May; 44(9):1303-1312.

Plichta, S.B., et al. Partner-specific condom use among adolescent women clients of a family planning clinic. Journal of Adolescent Health 1992; 13(6):506-511.

Polaneczky M, Guarnaccia, Alon J, Wiley J. Early experience with the contraceptive use of depot medroxyprogesterone acetate in an inner-city clinic population. Family Planning Perspectives 1996; 28: 174-178.

Porter, L.E., Ku, L. Use of reproductive health services among young men, 1995. *Journal of Adolescent Health* 2000; 27(3):186-194.

Postlethwaite D et al. IUC: evaluation of clinician practice patterns in Kaiser Permanente Northern California. Contraception 75 (2007) 177-184.

Raudaskoski TH, Lahti EI, Kauppila AJ, Apaja-Sarkkinen MA, Laatikainen TJ. Transdermal estrogen with a levonorgestrel-releasing intrauterine device for climacteric complaints: clinical and endometrial responses. Am J Obstet Gynecol 1995;172:114-9.

Raymond EG nad Grimes DA. The comparative Safety of Legal Induced Abortion and Childbirth in the US Obstet Gynecol 2012; 119:215-9

Raymond EG, Trussel J, Polis C. Population effect of increased access to ECP: A systematic review. ObGyn 109(1): 181-8. 2007.

Redmond G, Godwin AJ, Olson W, Lippman JS. Use of placebo controls in an oral contraceptive trial: methodological issues and adverse event incidence. Contraception 1999;60:81-5.

Rocca CH, Schwart EB, Stewart FH et al. Beyond access: acceptability, use and non-use of EC among young women. AJOG 196(1):29e 1-6, 2007.

Ropes ASW. Menstrual suppression survey, 2002.

Rosenbaum JE. Patient Teenagers? A comparison of the sexual behavior of virginity pledgers and matched non-pledgers. Pediatrics 2009; 123: 110-120.

Roumen FJ, Apter D, Mulders TM, et al. Efficacy, tolerability and acceptability of a novel contraceptive vaginal ring releasing etonogestrel and ethinyl estradiol. Hum Reprod 2001;16:469-475.

Santelli J et al. Abstinence-only education policies and programs: A position paper of the society for adolescent medicine. J Adol Health 38(2006) 83-87.

Santelli JS, Abma J, Ventura S, et al. Can changes in sexual behaviors among high school students explain the decline in teen pregancy rates in the 1990's? Journal of Adolescent Health, 2004, 35(2); 80-90.

Schafer JE, Osborne LM, Davis AR et al. Acceptability and satisfaction using Quick Start with the contraceptive vaginal ring vs. an OC. Contraception 73(5): 488. 2006.

Schwallie PC, Assenzo JR. Contraceptive use-efficacy study initializing medroxy-progesterone acetate administered as an intramuscular injection once every 90 days. Fertil Steril 1973; 24(5):331-339.

Secura G., Madden T. et al. Provision of no cost, long-acting contraception and teen pregnancy NEJM Oct. 2 2014

Seeger JD et al. Risk of thromboembolism in women taking EE/DRSP and other OCs. Obstet/Gynecol 2007; 110:587.

Segal SJ. Is menstration obsolete? Lecture in Atlanta, Georgia. November 1, 2001.

Shelton JD. Repeat emergency contraception: facing our fears. Contraception 66;2002:15-17.

Schmidt JE, Millis SD, Marchbanks PA, Jerg G, Peterson HB. Fertil Steril 2000; 74(5):892-8.

Sidney et al. Recent Combined Hormonal Contraceptives and the Risk of Thromboembolism and Other Cardiovascular Events in Users. Contraception 2013;87:93-100.

Silvestre L, Dubois C, Renault M, Rezvani Y, Baulieu E, Ulmann A. Voluntary interruption of pregnancy with mifepristone (RU-486) and a prostaglandin analogue. N Engl J Med 1990; 322:645-8.

Sivin I, Stern J et al. Prolonged intrauterine contraception: a seven-year randomized study of the levonorgestrel 20 mcg/day (LNG 20) and the Copper T 380Ag IUDs. Contraception 1991; 44:473-80

Shulman LP, Oleen-Burkey M, Willke RJ. Patient acceptability and satisfaction with Lunelle monthly contraceptive injection (medroxyprogesterone acetate and estradiol cypionate injectable suspension). Contraception 1999;60(4):215-222.

Smith-McCune, Tvvesm JL, Rubin MM et al. Effect of Replens gel used with a diaphragm on tests for HPV and other lower genital tract infections. J of Lower Genital Tract Disease 10(4): 213-8, 2006 Oct.

Smith TW. Personal communication to James Trussell. December 13, 1993.

Sonfield, A. Looking at Men's Sexual and Reproductive Health Needs. *The Guttmacher Report on Public Policy* 2002; November.

Sonfield, A. Meeting the Sexual and Reproductive Health Needs of Men Worldwide. *The Guttmacher Report on Public Policy. 2004; March.*

Speroff L, Darney PD. A Clinical Guide for Contraception. Third Edition. Lippincott Williams & Wilkins; Philadelphia; 2001.

Speroff L, Glass RH, Kase NG. Clinical Gynecologic Endocrinology and Infertility. Sixth Edition. 1999; Lipincott Williams & Wilkins; Baltimore, Maryland.

Speroff L. The perimenospausal transition: maximizing preventive health care. In: Mooney B, Daughtery J, eds. Midlife Women's Health Sourcebook. Atlanta: American Health Consultants, 1995.

Steiner MJ. Cates W Jr, Warner L. The real problems with male condoms is nonuse. Sex Trans Dis 1999;26(8):459-61.

Steines M. et al. Decreased condom breakage and slippage rates after counseling men at a sexually transmitted infection clinic in Jamaica *Contraception 75 (2007) 289-293*

Stencheuer MA. Comprehensive Gynecology Fourth Edition. Mosby. 2001

Stewart FH, Harper CC, Ellertson CE, Grimes DA, Sawyer GF, Trussell J. Clinical breast and pelvic examination requirements for hormonal contraception: Current practice vs. evidence. JAMA 2001;285:2232-2239.

Strauss LT, Herndon J, Charg J et al. Abortion surveillance: U.S., 2002. In: CDC surveillance summaries, Nov 25, 2005 MMWR 2005; 54 no. 55-57.

Sulak PJ et al. Am J Obstet Gynecol 2002; 186:1142-1149.

Sulak PJ et al. Obstet Gynecol 2000; 95:261-266.

Swica et al. Acceptability of Home Use of Mifepristone for medical abortion. Contraception 2013; 88:122-127.

Task Force on Postovulatory Methods of Fertility Regulation. Randomized controlled trial of levonorgestrel versus the Yuzpe regimen of combined oral contraceptives for emergency contraception. Lancet 1998; 352:420-33.

The Alan Guttmacher Institute. Sex and America's Teenagers. New York and Washington: 1994.

The Hereditary Ovarian Cancer Clinical Study Group. Oral contraceptives and the risk of hereditary ovarian cancer. N Engl J Med 1998;339;424-8.

Truitt ST, Fraser AB, Grimes DA, Gallo MF, Schulz KF. Hormonal contraception during lactation: a systematic reivew of randomized controlled trials. Contraception 2003; 68:233-8.

Trussell J, Leveque JA, Koenig JD, London R, Borden S, Henneberry J, LaGuardia KD, Stewart F, Wilson TG, Wysocki S, Strauss M. The economic value of contraception: a comparison of 15 methods. Am J Public Health 1995;85:494-503.

Trussell J, Stewart F, Guest F, Hatcher RA. Emergency contraceptive pills: a simple proposal to reduce unintended pregnancies. Fam Plann Perspect 1992;24:269-73.

Tschugguel W, Berga SL. Treatment of functional hypothalamic amenorrhea with hypnotherapy. Fertil Steril. 2003; 80:982-985.

Use of at-home semi-quantitztive pregnancy tests serve as a replacement for clinical follow-up of medical abortion? A US study. Contraception 2012; 86:757-762.

Valle RF, Carignan CS, Wright TC, et al. Tissue response to STOP microcoil transcervical permanent contraceptive device: results from a prehysterectomy study. Fertil Steril 2001; 76:974.

Vander Wijden C, Kleijnen J, Vanden Berk T. Lactational amenorrhea for family planning. Cochrane Database Systematic Reviews 2005.

Vercellini P et al. Fertil Steril 2003; 80:560-63.

Vestergaard P, Rejnmark L., Mosekilde L. Oral contraceptive use and risk of fractures. Contraception 73; 2006: 571-576.

Von Hertzen H, Piaggio G, Ding J et al. Low dose Mifepristone and two regimens of levonorgestrel for emergency contraception: a WHO multicentre randomised trial. Lancet 2002; 360: 1803-10.

Walsh T, Grimes D, Frezieres R, Nelson A, Bernstein L, Coulson A, Bernstein G. Randomized controlled trial of prophylactic antibiotics before insertion of intrauterine devices. *Lancet* 1998:351;1005-1008.

Warner DL, Hatcher RA, Boles J, Goldsmith J. Practices and patterns of condom usage for prevention of infection and pregnancy among male university students (Session PS-12). Proceeding of the Eleventh Annual National Preventive Medicine Meeting. March 1994.

Warner L, Hatcher RA, Steiner MJ. Male Condoms. IN Hatcher RA et al. Contraceptive Technology 18th Edition. 2004.

Weidner, W., et al. Relevance of male accessory gland infection for subsequent fertility with special focus on prostatitis. *Human Reproduction Update* 1999; 5(5):421-432.

Westoff C, Kerns J, Morroni C, Cushman LF, Tiezzi L, Murphy PA. Quick Start: a novel contraceptive initiation method. Contraception 66; 2002:141-145.

Westhoff C et al. Changes in weight with depot medroxyprogesterone acetate subcutaneous injection 104 mg/0.65 ml Contraception 75 (2007) 261-267.

White MK, Ory HW, Rooks JB, Rochat RW. Intrauterine device termination rates and menstrual cycle day of insertion. Obstet Gynecol 1980; 55:220-4.

E. Wiebe, et. al., Can we safely avoid fasting before abortions with low dose procedural sedation? A retrospective cohort chart review of anesthesia-related complications in 47,748 abortions. Contraception 87(1) 2013:51-54.

Willett WC, Green A, Stampfer MJ, Speizer FE, Colditz GA, Rosner B, Monson RR, Stason W, Hennekens CH. Relative and absolute risks of coronary heart disease among women who smoke cigarettes. New Eng J Med 317:1303, 1987.

Winer RL, Hughes JP, Feng Q et al. Condom use and the risk of genital HPV infection in young women. NEJM 2006; 354:2645-54.

World Health Organization, Department of Reproductive Health and Research. Improving Access to Quality Care in Family Planning: Medical Eligibility Criteria for Contraceptive Use. Second Edition. Geneva. 2000.

World Health Organization. WHO Taskforce Postovulatory Methods of Fertility Regulation. Lancet Aug 8, 1998.

Writing Group for the Women's Health Initiative. Risks and benefits of estrogen plus progestin in healthy postmenopausal women. JAMA 2002; 288: 321-333.

Zhou et al. EC with Multiload Co-375 SL IUD: a multicenter clinical trial. Contraception 2001; 64:107-12.

Zieman M, Guillebaud J, Weisberg E, Shangold G, Fisher A, Creasy G. Integrated summary of contraceptive efficacy with the Ortho Evra transdermal system. Fertility and Sterility Supplement; Sept, 2001. S19

# IMPORTANT WEBSITES

| TOPIC | WEBSITE |
|---|---|
| Abortion | www.prochoice.org |
| | www.ipas.org |
| Adolescent Reproductive Health | www.teenpregnancy.org |
| | www.ama-assn.org/adolhlth/adolhlth.htm |
| | www.advocatesforyouth.org |
| Contraception | www.conrad.org |
| | www.who.int (World Health Organization Precautions) |
| | www.contraceptiononline.org/contrareport |
| | www.bestmethodforme.com |
| | www.managingcontraception.com |
| | www.ippfwhr.org |
| | www.plannedparenthood.org |
| | www.reproline.jhu.edu |
| | www.engenderhealth.org |
| Counseling | www.gmhc.org |
| Education | www.siecus.org |
| | www.cdc.gov |
| Emergency Contraception | www.not-2-late.com or princeton.edu |
| HIV/AIDS/STIs | www.CritPath.Org/aric |
| | www.cdc.gov/hiv |
| | www.cdc.gov/nchstp/dstd/dstdp.htm |
| Managing Contraception | www.managingcontraception.com |
| Menopause | www.menopause.org |
| | www.osteo.org |
| Natural Family Planning | www.canfp.org |
| (Fertility Awareness) | www.irh.org |
| | www.ccli.org |
| Population Organizations | www.popcouncil.org |
| | www.prb.org |
| | www.undp.org/popin/infoserv.htm |
| | www.population.org/homepage.htm |
| Professional Organizations | www.acog.org |
| | www.arhp.org |
| | www.fda.gov |
| | www.fhi.org |
| | www.jsi.com |
| | www.NPWH.org |
| | www.pathfind.org |
| | www.plannedparenthood.org |
| | www.societyfp.org |
| | www.who.int |
| Reproductive Health Research | www.guttmacher.org |
| | www.fhi.org |
| | www.ipm.microbicides.org |

# SPANISH/ENGLISH TRANSLATIONS

| SPANISH/ESPAÑOL | ENGLISH/INGLES |
| --- | --- |
| • Abstinencia | • Abstinence |
| • Amamantar a Su Bebe | • Breast-feeding |
| • Tapa Cervical | • Cervical Cap |
| • Retraer el pene antes de ejecular | • Coitus Interruptus (Withdrawal) |
| • Injecciones Combinadas | • Combined Injectables |
| • La Pildora | • Combined Oral Contraceptives (COCs) |
| • Condones parce hombres | • Condoms for Men |
| • Condones para Mujeres | • Condoms for Women |
| • La "T" o Dispositivo do Cobre | • Copper T 380-A |
| • Injecciones de Depo-Provera | • Depo-Provera |
| • El Diafragma | • Diaphragm |
| • Contraceptivo de Emergencia | • Emergency Contraception |
| • Consciente Sobre Metodos de Fertilidad | • Fertility Awareness Methods |
| • Espuma Contraceptiva | • Foam |
| • Metodos para el Futuro | • Future Methods |
| • Dispositivos | • IUDs |
| • Gelatina Anticonceptiva | • Jellies |
| • El Dispositivo de "Levo Norgestrel" | • Levonorgestrel IUD |
| • Implantes de NORPLANT | • Norplant Implant |
| • El Dispositivo de "Progestasert" | • Progestasert IUD |
| • Contraceptives de Progesterona Solamente | • Progestin-Only Contraceptives |
| • Pildoras de Progesterona Solamente | • Progestin-Only Pills (POPs) |
| • Mifepristone | • Mifepristone |
| • Espermicidas | • Spermicides |
| • Ligadura o Estirilizacion de las Trompas | • Tubal Sterilization |
| • Tela Anticonceptiva | • Vaginal contraceptive film |
| • Vasectomia | • Vasectomy |
| • Todos los dispositivos | • All other IUDs at this time |

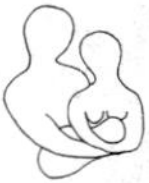

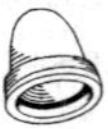

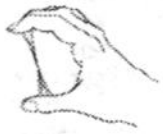

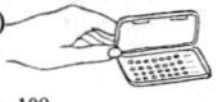

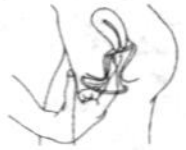

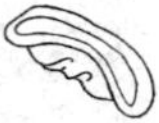

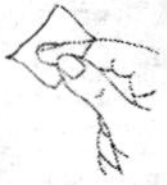

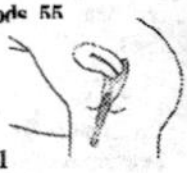

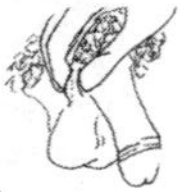

# Resources for Young Adults

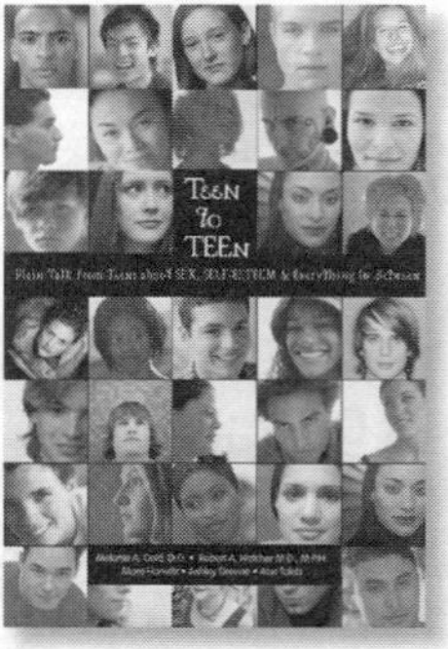


6" x 9" • 198 pages

## Teen to Teen

Teen to Teen is a book about living life as a young teenager! It was written specifically to educate today's teens and their parents in order to help them make responsible decisions. Some of the important areas covered in this book are: self esteem issues, creating a life plan, bullying, puberty, sexuality, and contraceptive choices. Written by teenagers under the direction of Dr. Melanie A. Gold, D.O., University of Pittsburgh School of Medicine, Children's Hospital of Pittsburgh and Robert A. Hatcher, M.D., Ph.D., Professor of Gynecology and Obstetrics, Emory University School of Medicine, Atlanta, GA.

**Code #5700**

**1-499 ($5.95 ea.)**
**500-1000 ($2.50 ea.)**

**NEWLY UPDATED**

---

## Sexual Etiquette 101 and More

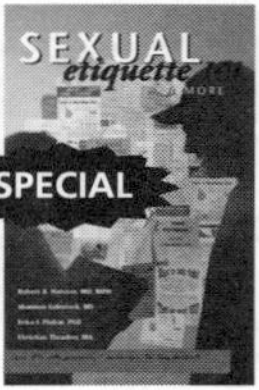


**SPECIAL**

**This book comes with a copy of Contraceptive Choices**
This book for college students contains stories, resources, ideas and other valuable tools to help you successfully navigate the often confusing world of relationships and sexuality.

**Code #4003**

**$2.50 ea. (min. 10)**

## The Quest for Excellence

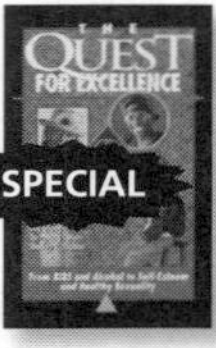


**SPECIAL**

This book for young adults contains stories, resources, ideas and other valuable tools to help you successfully navigate the often confusing world of relationships and sexuality.

**Code #4002**

**$2.00 ea. (min. 10)**

---

# Have your contraception questions answered by Dr. Hatcher at www.managingcontraception.com

---

**Order online: www.ManagingContraception.com**
**Order by Phone: (404) 875-5001 Fax: (404) 875-5030**

# Choices in Contraception
## Including Abstinence

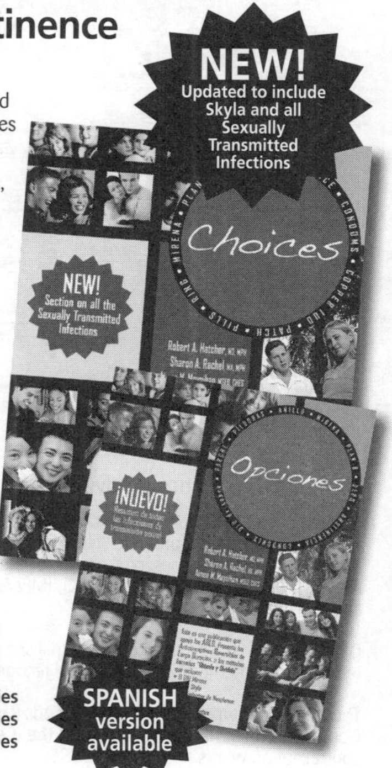


Choices includes 21 updated descriptions of contraceptives (birth control methods).

In writing these descriptions, we have tried to be brief, giving the most important information only, including the advantages and disadvantages of each one.

It is our desire that young people have a choice, including abstinence,when it comes to their sexual health.

Developed by
Dr. Robert A. Hatcher.

**Code #5100**

**$10.00 ea. • 1-10 copies**
**$9.00 ea. • 11-100 copies**
**$8.00 ea. • 101-300 copies**
**$7.50 ea. • 301-500 copies**
**$7.00 ea. • 501-999 copies**
**$4.00 ea. • 1000-2999 copies**
**$3.00 ea. • 3000-4999 copies**
**$2.50 ea. • 5000-9999 copies**
**$1.25 ea. • 10000+ copies**

BRIDGING THE GAP COMMUNICATIONS, INC.

**Order online: www.ManagingContraception.com**
**Order by Phone: (404) 875-5001 Fax: (404) 875-5030**

# ALL METHODS OF CO

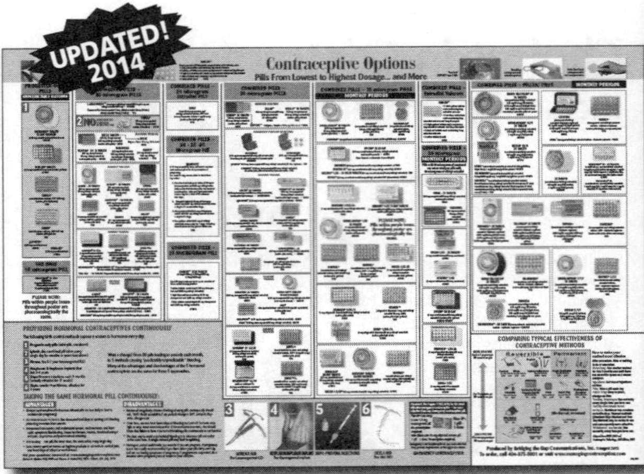


24" x 36" • Laminated with adhesive backing

## All Methods of Contraceptives Poster

All methods of CONTRACEPTIVE OPTIONS poster updated. NOW printed two sides with one side still showing all the pills from the lowest to the highest dosages, plus photos of the other methods including the COPPER T IUD, MIRENA, RING, IMPLANT, PATCH, SPONGE and CONDOMS.

GREAT for the patient to show which pill she is taking if she can't remember the name of the pill but will recognize the package.

The other side features the LARC methods (Long Acting Reversible Contraceptive). It has an illustration of the utertrus showing where contraception works and MUCH MORE!

BRIDGING THE GAP COMMUNICATIONS, INC.

**Order online: www.ManagingContraception.com**

# A Must Have for Every Exam Room!

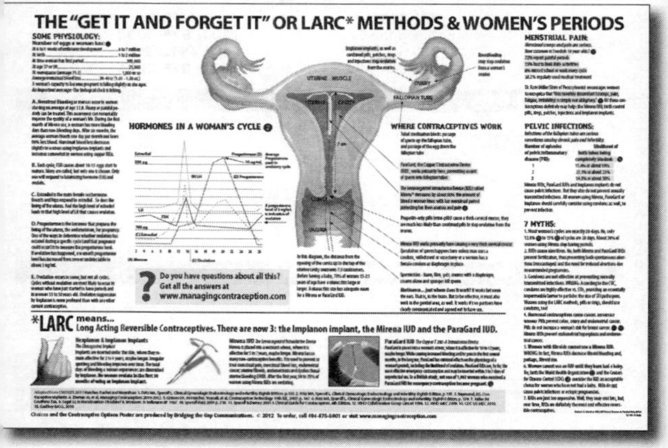


GREAT teaching tool!

The poster is 24"X36" and is laminated both sides safe and ready for display in the examination room or classroom!

**Code #6400 - 24"x36"**

**$25.00 ea. • 1 Copy**
**$20.00 ea. • 2 Copies**
**$18.00 ea. • 3-10 Copies**
**$15.00 ea. • 11-20 Copies**
**$12.00 ea. • 21+ Copies**

BRIDGING THE GAP COMMUNICATIONS, INC.

**Order online: www.ManagingContraception.com**
**Order by Phone: (404) 875-5001   Fax: (404) 875-5030**

# ORDER FORM

## To order, please see our website: www.ManagingContraception.com

**BY MAIL:**
Bridging the Gap
PO Box 79299
Atlanta, GA 30357

**BY FAX:**
(404) 875-5030
**BY PHONE:**
(404) 875-5001

**ORDERED BY**

Name ______________________ Title ______________________
Organization ______________________
Address ______________________
City ______________________ State __________ Zip __________
E-mail Address ______________________
Phone ______________________ Fax ______________________

**SHIP TO (Only if different from Ordered By)**

Name ______________________ Title ______________________
Organization ______________________
Address ______________________
City ______________________ State __________ Zip __________

| Item Code # | Description | Qty. | Price Ea. | Item Total |
|---|---|---|---|---|
| | | | | |
| | | | | |
| | | | | |
| | | | | |
| | | | | |
| | | | | |
| | | | | |

**Payment Method:**

☐ MasterCard ☐ VISA ☐ Discover
☐ American Express ☐ Personal Check
☐ Purchase Order #______________
(For Organizations Only)

Credit Card Number:
______________________

Valid through ______________________
Signature ______________________

Merchandise Subtotal: __________
GA Sales Tax (7%) __________
Subtotal __________
*Shipping (Add 18%) __________
Handling __________

TOTAL (US funds only) __________

Phone (required) ______________

**Thank You for Your Order!**

*International Shipping: Alaska, Hawaii, Puerto Rico, Canada and all others not in the 48 contiguous United States, call for shipping prices. Prices valid until superceded by subsequent publication.

# ORDER FORM

## To order, please see our website: www.ManagingContraception.com

**BY MAIL:**
Bridging the Gap
PO Box 79299
Atlanta, GA 30357

**BY FAX:**
(404) 875-5030

**BY PHONE:**
(404) 875-5001

**ORDERED BY**

Name ______________________ Title ______________________
Organization ______________________________________________
Address __________________________________________________
City ______________________ State __________ Zip __________
E-mail Address ____________________________________________
Phone ______________________ Fax ______________________

**SHIP TO (Only if different from Ordered By)**

Name ______________________ Title ______________________
Organization ______________________________________________
Address __________________________________________________
City ______________________ State __________ Zip __________

| Item Code # | Description | Qty. | Price Ea. | Item Total |
|---|---|---|---|---|
| | | | | |
| | | | | |
| | | | | |
| | | | | |
| | | | | |
| | | | | |
| | | | | |

**Payment Method:**

☐ MasterCard ☐ VISA ☐ Discover
☐ American Express ☐ Personal Check
☐ Purchase Order #______________
(For Organizations Only)

Credit Card Number:

________________________________

Valid through ______________________

Signature ______________________

Merchandise Subtotal: ____________
GA Sales Tax (7%) ____________
Subtotal ____________
*Shipping (Add 18%) ____________
Handling ____________

TOTAL (US funds only) ____________

Phone (required) ______________

**Thank You for Your Order!**

*International Shipping: Alaska, Hawaii, Puerto Rico, Canada and all others not in the 48 contiguous United States, call for shipping prices.
Prices valid until superceded by subsequent publication.

# PILLS AS EMERGENCY CONTRACEPTIVES:

3 Different Approaches:

Copper T IUD, Progestin-Only Pills OR Combined Pills

## COPPER T IUD

ParaGard, the Copper T IUD, is by the far the most effective emergency contraceptive — far more effective than any emergency contraceptive pill.

## PROGESTIN-ONLY PILLS

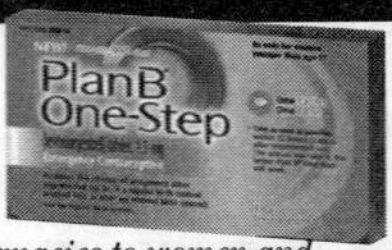


### Plan B®:

### 1 pill - 1 dose

Plan B® One-Step is one 1.5 mg levonogestrel pill.

*Plan B available without a prescription in pharmacies to women and men $\geq$ 17 years old. Plan B is NOT carried in all pharmacies. Check in advance. Ask your pharmacy to carry Plan B.*

## COMBINED ORAL CONTRACEPTIVES

*(Preven, Ogestrel and Ovral are NOT carried in all pharmacies. Check in advance.)*

### 2 + 2 pills 12 hours apart

Ogestrel *(white pills)*
Ovral *(white pills)*

### 4 + 4 pills 12 hours apart

Cryselle *(white pills)*
Enpresse *(orange pills)*
Jolessa *(pink pills)*
Low-Ogestrel *(white pills)*
Lo-Ovral *(white pills)*
Levora *(white pills)*
Levlen *(light orange pills)*
Nordette *(light orange pills)*
Portia *(pink pills)*
Quasense *(white pills)*
Seasonale *(pink pills)*
Seasonique *(light blue pills)*
Triphasil *(yellow pills)*
Tri-Levlen *(yellow pills)*
Trivora *(pink pills)*

**Have your patient take antinausea medication an hour before the first dose if using any of the combined oral contraceptives as emergency contraception. This is not necessary if using Plan B.**

### 5 + 5 pills 12 hours apart

Alesse *(pink pills)*
Levlite *(pink pills)*
Aviane *(orange pills)*
Lessina *(pink pills)*
Lutera *(white pills)*

# COLOR PHOTOS

## of Combined and Progestin-Only Oral Contraceptives

www.managingcontraception.com

**The thirteen color pages of pills are organized as follows:**



- Progestin-only pills with no estrogen: Micronor and NOR-QD
- Lowest estrogen pills with 20 micrograms of the estrogen, ethinyl estradiol: Alesse, Levlite, LoEstrin 1/20, and Mircette
- All of the 25-, 30- and 35-microgram pills (all ethinyl estradiol)
- All of the phasic pills
- Highest estrogen pills, with 50 micrograms of estrogen (ethinyl estradiol OR mestranol). Mestranol is converted in the body to ethinyl estradiol; 50 mcg of mestranol is equivalent to 35 mcg of ethinyl estradiol

**Pills which are pharmacologically exactly the same are grouped within boxes. The color and packaging of pills dispensed in clinics may differ from pills in pharmacies.*

**POSTERS** showing all pills can be ordered by calling 404-875-5001, on form at end of book, or on website: www.managingcontraception.com

## PROGESTIN - ONLY PILLS

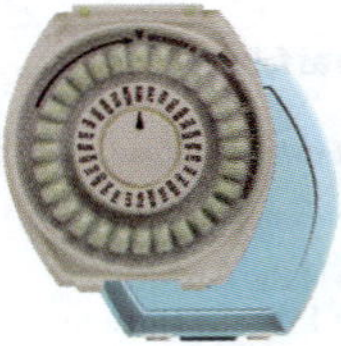

**MICRONOR® TABLETS 28-DAY REGIMEN**
(0.35 mg norethindrone)
(active pills lime green)
Janssen

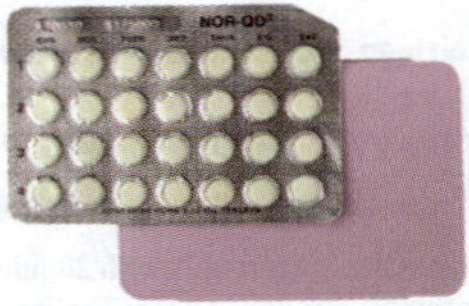


**NOR-QD® TABLETS**
(0.35 mg norethindrone)
(active pills yellow)
Actavis

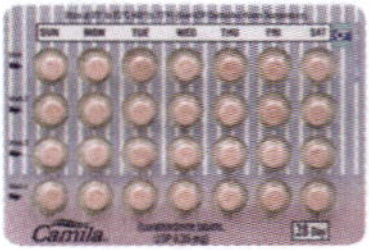


**CAMILA®**
(norethindrone tablets, USP 0.35 mg)
(active pills light pink)
Teva Pharmaceuticals USA

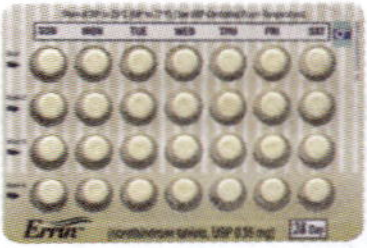


**ERRIN®**
(norethindrone tablets, USP 0.35 mg)
(active pills yellow)
Teva Pharmaceuticals USA

**JOLIVETTE®**
(0.35 mg norethindrone)
Actavis

**NORA-BE®**
(0.35 mg norethindrone)
Actavis

## THE ONLY 10 microgram PILL

→ **MINASTRINE® FE 1/10 CHEWABLE**
(1 mg norethindrone acetate/10 mcg ethinyl estradiol/75 mg ferrous fumarate [7d])
Actavis

## COMBINED PILLS - 20 microgram PILLS

**LoSEASONIQUE®**
**(levonorgestrel/ethinyl estradiol/0.10mg/ 20 mcg and ethinyl estridol 0.01 mg)**
Duramed

**CAMRESE®LO**
**(Levonorgestrel 0.1mg, ethinyl estradiol 20mcg (84 tabs)/ ethinyl estradiol 10mcg (7 tabs ))**
Teva Women's Health

## NO SCHEDULED PERIODS - No inactive pills

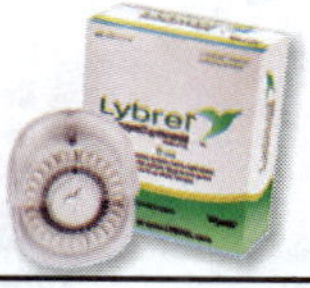


**LYBREL™**
**(90 mcg levonorgestrel/20 mcg ethinyl estradiol)**
(active pills pink)
Wyeth

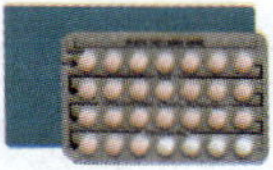

**YAZ® 28 TABLETS**
**(3.0 mg drospirenone/20 mcg ethinyl estradiol)**
(active pills pink)
Bayer

**GIANVI®**
**(3.0 mg drospirenone/20 mcg ethinyl estradiol)**
Teva Pharmaceuticals USA

**BEYAZ® 28 TABLETS**
**Beyaz = Yaz + 451mcg folic acid**
Bayer

**VESTURA® 3 X 28 TABLETS**
**(3.0 mg drospirenone/20 mcg ethinyl estradiol)**
(active pills pink)
ACTAVIS

**YASMINELLE**
**(3.0 mg drospirenone/0.02 mg ethinyl estradiol (as betadex clathrate))**
(active pills pink)
BAYER

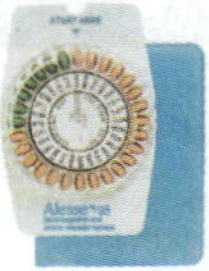

**ALESSE® - 28 TABLETS**
(0.1 mg levonorgestrel/20 mcg ethinyl estradiol)
(active pills pink)
Wyeth

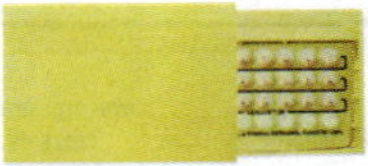

**LEVLITE™ - 28 TABLETS**
(0.1 mg levonorgestrel/20 mcg ethinyl estradiol)
(active pills pink)
Bayer

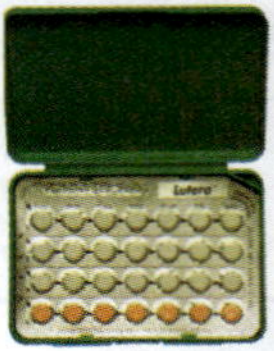

**LUTERA™**
(0.1 mg levonorgestrel/20 mcg ethinyl estradiol)
(active pills white)
Actavis

**AMETHYST® - 28 TABLETS**
(0.09 mg levonorgestrel/20 mcg ethinyl estradiol)
(active pills white)
ACTAVIS

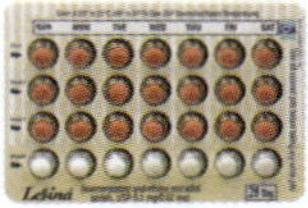

**LESSINA®**
(levonorgestrel/ethinyl estradiol tablets, USP 0.1 mg/20 mcg)
(active pills pink)
Teva Pharmaceuticals USA

**SRONYX®**
(0.1 mg levonorgestrel/ 20mcg ethinyl estradiol)
Actavis

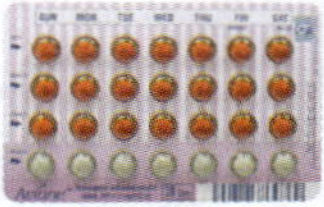

**AVIANE®**
(levonogestrel/ethinyl estradiol tablets, USP 0.10 mg/20 mcg)
(active pills orange)
Teva Pharmaceuticals USA

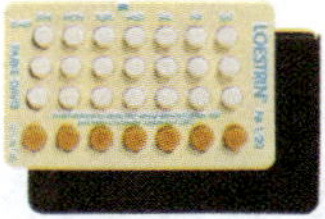

**LOESTRIN® FE 1/20**
(1 mg norethindrone acetate/ 20 mcg ethinyl estradiol/ 75 mg ferrous fumarate [7d])
(active pills white)
Teva Pharmaceuticals USA

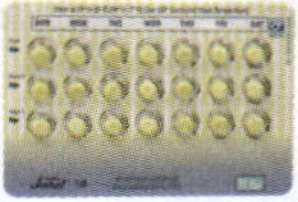

**JUNEL™**
(norethindrone acetate and ethinyl estradiol tablets, USP 1 mg/20 mcg)
(active pills light yellow)
Teva Pharmaceuticals USA

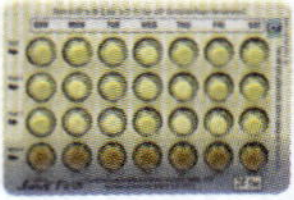

**JUNEL™ Fe**
(norethindrone acetate and ethinyl estradiol tablets, USP and ferrous fumarate tablets 1 mg/20 mcg)
(active pills light yellow)
Teva Pharmaceuticals USA

**MICROGESTIN® & MICROGESTIN FE®**
(1mg norethindrone acetate/ 20 mcg ethinyl estradiol FE also contains /75 mg ferrous fumarate
Actavis

**TILIA FE® - 28 TABLETS**
(1mg norethindrone acetate/ 20 mcg ethinyl estradiol FE)
Actavis

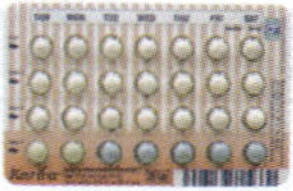

**KARIVA®**
(desogestrel/estradiol tablets 0.15 mg/
20 mcg and ethinyl estradiol tablets 0.01 mg)
(active pills white and light blue)
Teva Pharmaceuticals USA

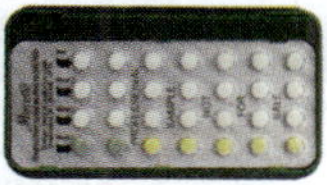

**MIRCETTE® - 28 TABLETS**
(0.15 mg desogestrel/ 20 mcg ethinyl estradiol X
21 (white)/placebo X 2 (green)/
10 mcg ethinyl estradiol X 5 (yellow)
Duramed

**MERCILON®**
(0.15 mg desogestrel/20 mcg ethinyl
estradiol/10mcg ethinyl estradiol)
Merck

**AZURETTE® - 28 TABLETS**
(0.15 mg desogestrel/ 20 mcg ethinyl estradiol X
21 (white)/placebo X 2 (green) 10 mcg ethinyl estradiol X 5 (blue)
ACTAVIS

## COMBINED PILLS - ESTRODIAL VALERATE

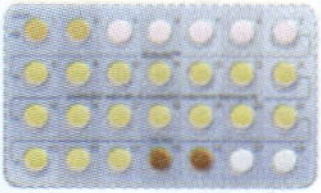

**NATAZIA™**

Natazia consists of 28 film-coated, unscored tablets in the following order:

- 2 dark yellow tablets each containing 3mg estradiol valerate
- 5 medium red tablets each containing 2mg estradiol valerate and 2mg dienogest
- 17 light yellow tablets each containing 2mg estradiol valerate and 3mg dienogest
- 2 dark red tablets each containing 1 mg estradiol valerate
- 2 white tablets (inert)

Bayer

## COMBINED PILLS - 20 microgram ESTRADIOL PILL

**ZOELY**
(norethindrone acetate and ethinyl estradiol tablets, USP and ferrous fumarate tablets 1 mg/20 mcg)
(active pills light yellow)
Teva Women's Health

## COMBINED PILLS - 20 - 25 -30 microgram PILL

**QUARTETTE**

A 91 day ascending-dose, extended-regimen oral contraceptive for the prevention of pregnancy.
For each 91-day course, take in the following order:

1. Start the first light pink tablet (0.15 mg of levonorgestrel and 0.02 mg ethinyl estradiol) on the first Sunday after the onset of menstruation. take one light pink tablet once a day for a total of 42 consecutive days.
2. One pink tablet (0.15 mg of levonorgestrel and 0.025 mg ethinyl estradiol) once a day for 21 consecutive days.
3. One purple tablet (0.15 mg of levonorgestrel and 0.03 mg ethinyl estradiol) once a day for 21 days.
4. One yellow tablet (0.01 mg of ethinyl estradiol) once a day for 7 days. Bleeding should occur during yellow tablet use.

Teva Women's Health

## COMBINED PILLS - 25 microgram PILL

**CAZIANT™ 3X28 TABLETS**
**(0.1mg/0.025mg, 0.125mg/0.025mg, 0.15mg/0.025mg)**

Each 28-day treatment cycle pack consists of three active dosing phases:

7 white tablets containing 0.100 mg desogestrel and 0.025 mg ethinyl estradiol;

7 light blue tablets containing 0.125 mg desogestrel and 0.025 mg ethinyl estradiol

7 blue tablets containing 0.150 mg desogestrel and 0.025 mg ethinyl estradiol.

ACTAVIS

## COMBINED PILLS - 30 microgram PILLS

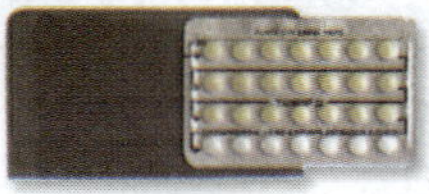

**YASMIN® 28 TABLETS**
**(3.0 mg drospirenone/30 mcg ethinyl estradiol)**
(active pills yellow)
BAYER

**SAFYRAL™**
Safyral = Yasmin + 451mcg Folic Acid
BAYER

**ZARAH™**
**(3.0 mg drospirenone/30 mcg ethinyl estradiol)**
(21 active pills)
Actavis

**OCELLA™ 28 TABLETS**
**(3.0 mg drospirenone/30 mcg ethinyl estradiol)**
(active pills yellow)
Teva Women's Health

## SCHEDULED PERIODS QUARTERLY

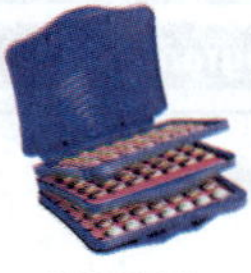

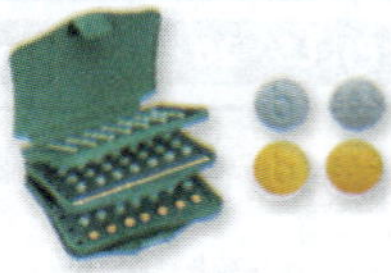

**SEASONALE®**
**(0.15 mg levonorgestrel/ 30 mcg ethinyl estradiol)**
84 active pink pills followed by 7 placebo pills
Duramed

**SEASONIQUE®**
**(0.15 mg levonorgestrel/ 30 mcg ethinyl estradiol)**
84 active pink pills followed by 7 pills with 10 mcg ethinyl estradiol
Teva Women's Health

**JOLESSA™**
**(0.15 mg levonorgestrel/ 30 mcg ethinyl estradiol)**
91 day regimen
Teva Women's Health

**CAMRESE™**
**(0.15 mg levonorgestrel/30 mcg ethinyl estradiol)**
84 active pink pills followed by 7 placebo pills
Teva Women's Health

**QUASENSE™**
(0.15 mg levonorgestrel/
30 mcg ethinyl estradiol)
Actavis

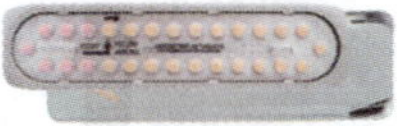

**NORDETTE®-28 TABLETS**
(0.15 mg levonorgestrel/30 mcg ethinyl estradiol)
(active pills light orange)
Wyeth

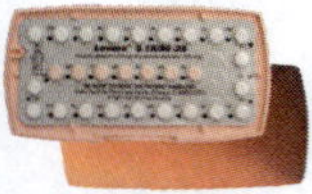

**LEVORA TABLETS**
(0.15 mg levonorgestrel/
30 mcg ethinyl estradiol)
(active pills white)
Actavis

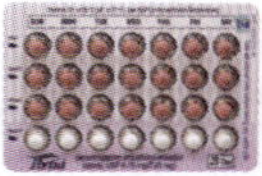

**PORTIA®**
(levonorgestrel and ethinyl estradiol
tablets, USP 0.15 mg/30 mcg)
(active pills pink)
Teva Pharmaceuticals USA

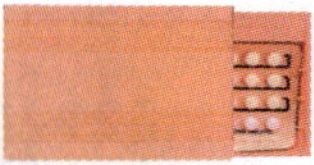

**LEVLEN® 28 TABLETS**
(0.15 mg levonorgestrel/
30 mcg ethinyl estradiol)
(active pills light orange)
MK Drughouse

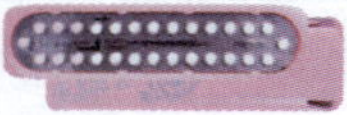

**LO/OVRAL®-28 TABLETS**
(0.3 mg norgestrel/
30 mcg ethinyl estradiol)
(active pills white)
Wyeth

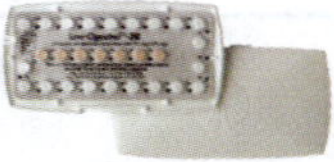

**LOW-OGESTREL® - 28**
(0.3 mg norgestrel/
30 mcg ethinyl estradiol)
(active pills white)
Actavis

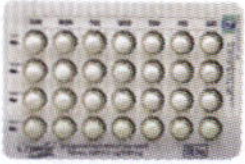

**CRYSELLE®**
(0.3 mg norgestrel/
30 mcg ethinyl estradiol)
(active pills white)
Teva Pharmaceuticals USA

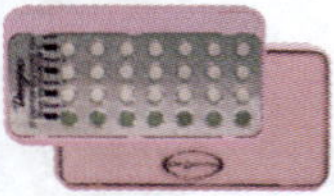

**DESOGEN® 28 TABLETS**
(0.15 mg desogestrel/
30 mcg ethinyl estradiol)
(active pills white)
Merck

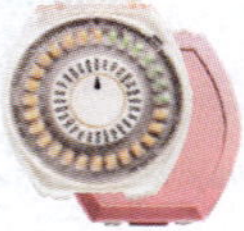

**ORTHO-CEPT® TABLETS
28-DAY REGIMEN**
(0.15 mg desogestrel/
30 mcg ethinyl estradiol)
(active pills orange)
Jannsen

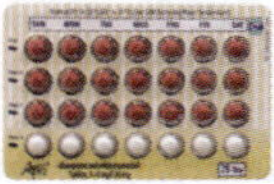

**APRI®**
(desogestrel/
ethinyl estradiol 0.15 mg/
0.03 mg tablets)
(active pills rose)
Teva Pharmaceuticals
USA

**RECLIPSEN™**
(0.15 mg desogestrel/30 mcg
ethinyl estradiol)
Actavis

**SOLIA™**
(0.15 mg levonorgestrel/30 mcg ethinyl estradiol)
Prasco

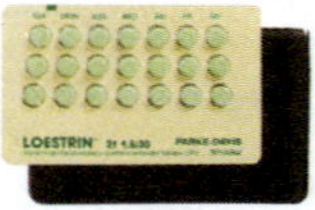

**LOESTRIN® 21 1.5/30**
(1.5 mg norethindrone acetate/30 mcg ethinyl estradiol)
(active pills green)
Teva Pharmaceuticals USA

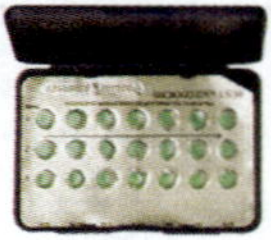

**MICROGESTIN® 1.5/30 with or without Fe**
(1.5 mg norethindrone acetate/
30 mcg ethinyl estradiol)
Actavis

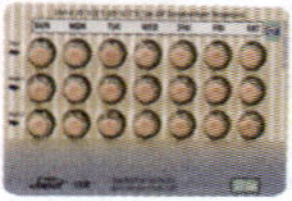

**JUNEL™**
(norethindrone acetate and ethinyl estradiol tablets, USP 1.5 mg./30 mcg.)
(active pills pink)
Teva Pharmaceuticals USA

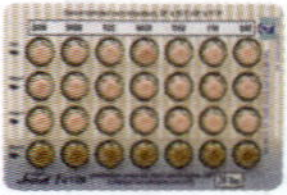

**JUNEL™ Fe**
(norethindrone acetate and ethinyl estradiol tablets, USP and ferrous fumarate tablets 1.5 mg/30 mcg)
(active pills pink)
Teva Pharmaceuticals USA

## COMBINED PILLS - 35 microgram PILLS

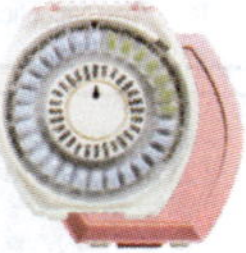

**ORTHO-CYCLEN® 28 TABLETS**
(0.25 mg norgestimate/
35 mcg ethinyl estradiol)
(active pills blue)
Jannsen

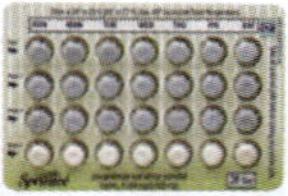

**SPRINTEC®**
(norgestimate and ethinyl estradiol tablets,
0.250 mg/35 mcg)
(active pills blue)
Teva Pharmaceuticals USA

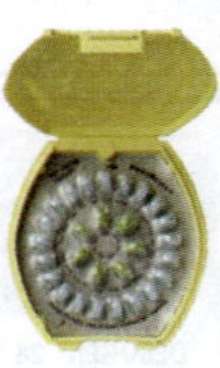

**MONONESESSA®**
(norgestimate and
ethinyl estradiol tablets,
0.250 mg/35 mcg)
Actavis

**PREVIFEM™**
(norgestimate and ethinyl estradiol tablets, 0.250 mg/35 mcg)
Qualitest

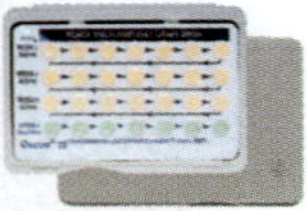

**OVCON® 35 28-DAY**
(0.4 mg norethindrone/
35 mcg ethinyl estradiol)
(active pills peach)
Actavis
Now there is a chewable
Ovcon-35 pill!

**ZENCHENT®**
(0.4 mg norethindrone/
35 mcg ethinyl estradiol)
Actavis

**FEMCON FE™**
(0.4 mg norethindrone/
35 mcg ethinyl estradiol)
Actavis

**BALZIVA™ 1/35**
**21 OR 28 TABLETS**
(0.4 mg norethindrone/
35 mcg ethinyl estradiol)
Teva Pharmaceuticals USA

**ZEOSA™**
(0.4 mg norethindrone/
35 mcg ethinyl estradiol)
(chewable)
Actavis

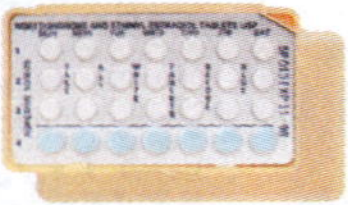

**NORETHIN 1/35E–28**
(1 mg norethindrone/35 mcg ethinyl estradiol)
(active pills white)
Shire

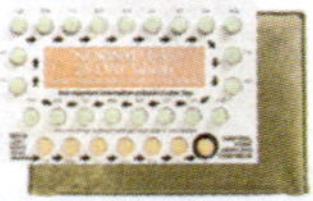

**NORINYL® 1+35 28-DAY TABLETS**
(1 mg norethindrone/35 mcg ethinyl estradiol)
(active pills yellow-green)
Actavis

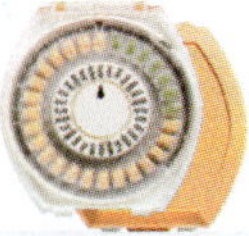

**ORTHO-NOVUM® 1/35 28 TABLETS**
(1 mg norethindrone/35 mcg ethinyl estradiol)
(active pills peach)
Jannsen

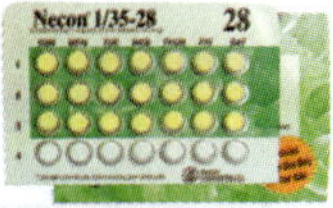


**NECON® 1/35-28**
(1 mg norethindrone/35 mcg ethinyl estradiol)
(active pills dark yellow)
Actavis

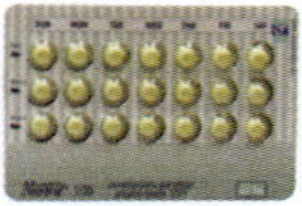

**NORTREL®**
(norethindrone and ethinyl estradiol tablets,
USP 1/35 mcg)
(active pills yellow)
Teva Pharmaceuticals USA

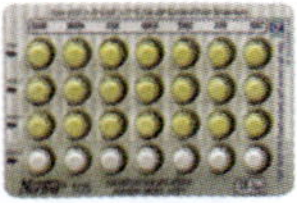

**NORTREL®**
(norethindrone and ethinyl estradiol tablets,
USP 1.0 mg/35 mcg 28-day regimen)
(active pills yellow)
Teva Pharmaceuticals USA

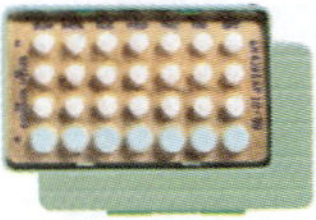

**DEMULEN® 1/35-28**
(1 mg ethynodiol diacetate/
35 mcg ethinyl estradiol)
(active pills white)
Pfizer

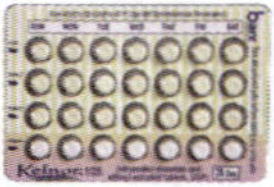

**KELNOR™**
(ethynodiol diacetate 1 mg. and
ethinyl estradiol 35 mcg, USP)
(active pills light yellow)
Teva Pharmaceuticals USA

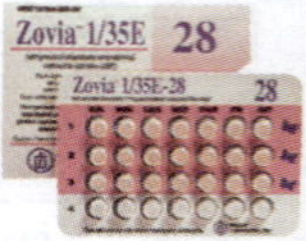


**ZOVIA® 1/35E–28**
(1 mg ethynodiol diacetate/
35 mcg ethinyl estradiol)
(active pills light pink)
Actavis

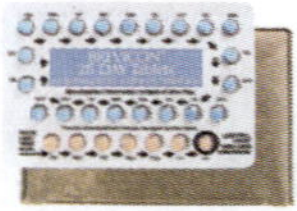

**BREVICON® 28-DAY TABLETS**
(0.5 mg norethindrone/35 mcg ethinyl estradiol)
(active pills blue)
Actavis

**NECON 0.5/35®**
(0.5 mg norethindrone/35 mcg ethinyl estradiol)
Actavis

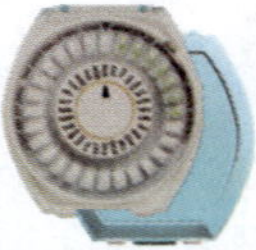

**MODICON® TABLETS**
**28-DAY REGIMEN**
(0.5 mg norethindrone/
35 mcg ethinyl estradiol)
(active pills white)
Jannsen

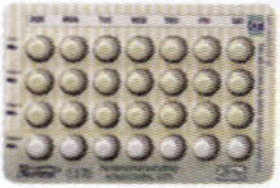

**NORTREL®**
(norethindrone and ethinyl estradiol
tablets, USP 0.5/35 mcg)
(active pills light yellow)
Teva Pharmaceuticals USA

# COMBINED PILLS - PHASIC PILLS

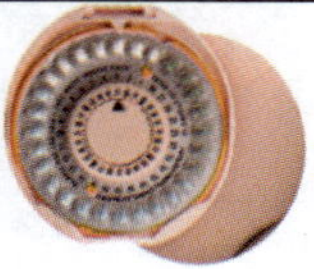

**ORTHO TRI-CYCLEN® LO - 28 TABLETS**
(norgestimate/ethinyl estradiol)
0.18 mg/25 mcg (7d) (white),
0.215 mg/25 mcg (7d) (light blue),
0.25 mg/25 mcg (7d) (dark blue)
remaining 7 placebo pills are green
Jannsen

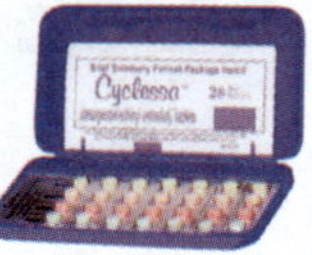


**CYCLESSA®**
(desogestrel/ethinyl estradiol - triphasic regimen)
0.1 mg/25 mcg (7d) (light yellow)
0.125 mg/25 mcg (7d) (orange)
0.150 mg/25 mcg (7d) (red)
Merck

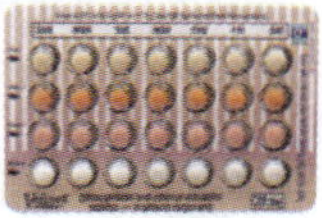

**VELIVET™**
(desogestrel/ethinyl estradiol tablets - triphasic regimen)
(active pills beige, orange and pink)
Teva Pharmaceuticals USA

**CESIA™**
(desogestrel/ethinyl estradiol tablets - triphasic regimen)
Prasco

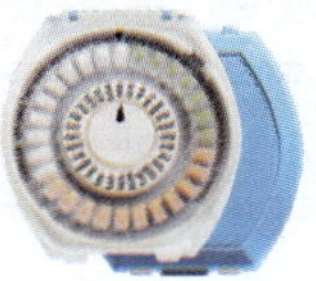

**ORTHO-NOVUM® 10/11 - 28 TABLETS**
(norethindrone/ethinyl estradiol)
0.5 mg/35 mcg (10d) (white),
1 mg/35 mcg (11d) (peach)
Jannsen

**ARANELLE™**
(norethindrone/ethinyl estradiol tablets)
Norethindrone 0.5mg, ethinyl estradiol 35micrograms (7 tabs); norethindrone 1mg, ethinyl estradiol 35micrograms (9 tabs); norethindrone 0.5mg, ethinyl estradiol 35micrograms (5 tabs); inert (7 tabs)
Teva Pharmaceuticals USA

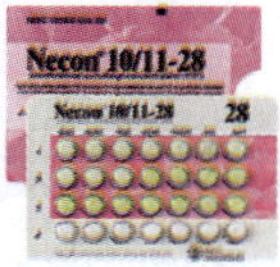


**NECON® 10/11 - 28 TABLETS**
(norethindrone/ethinyl estradiol)
0.5 mg/35 mcg (10d) (white),
1 mg/35 mcg (11d) (peach)
Actavis

**LEENA®**
(norenthindrone/ethinyl estradiol) 0.5mg/35 mcg (light blue), 1 mg/35 mcg (yellow-green)
Actavis

**TRI-NORINYL®**
(norenthindrone/ethinyl estradiol) 0.5mg/35 mcg (blue), 1 mg/35 mcg (yellow-green)
Actavis

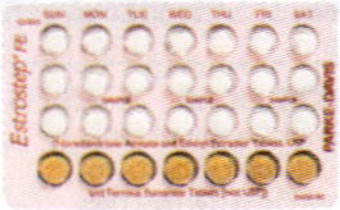

**ESTROSTEP® FE - 28 TABLETS**
(norethindrone acetate/ethinyl estradiol)
1 mg/20 mcg (5d) (white triangular),
1 mg/30 mcg (7d) (white square),
1 mg/35 mcg (9d), 75 mg ferrous
fumarate (7d) (white round)
Actavis

**TRI-LEGEST® FE**
(norethindrone acetate/ethinyl estradiol)
1 mg/20 mcg (5d) , 1 mg/30 mcg (7d)
1 mg/35 mcg (9d), 75 mg ferrous fumarate (7d)
Teva Pharmaceuticals USA

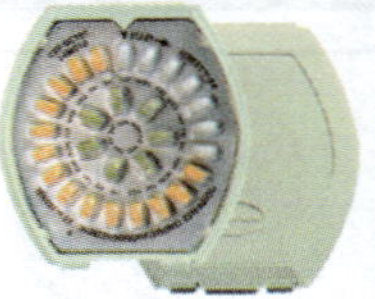

**JENEST® 28 TABLETS**
(norethindrone/ethinyl estradiol)
0.5 mg/35 mcg (7d) (white),
1 mg/35 mcg (14d) (peach)
Organon

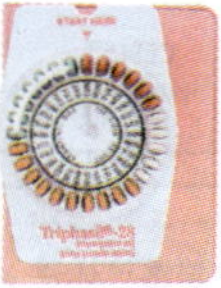

**TRIPHASIL®- 28 TABLETS**
(levonorgestrel/ethinyl estradiol—triphasic regimen)
0.050 mg/30 mcg (6d) (brown),
0.075 mg/40 mcg (5d) (white),
0.125 mg/30 mcg (10d) (light yellow)
Wyeth

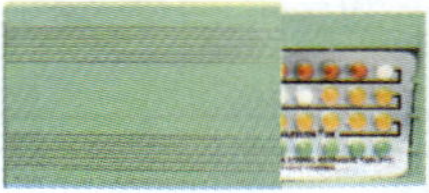

**TRI-LEVLEN® 28 TABLETS**
(levonorgestrel/ethinyl estradiol—triphasic regimen)
0.050 mg/30 mcg (6d) (brown),
0.075 mg/40 mcg (5d) (white),
0.125 mg/30 mcg (10d) (light yellow)
MK Drughouse

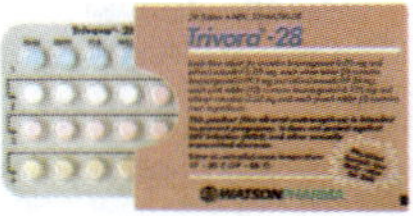

**TRIVORA®**
(levonorgestrel/ethinyl estradiol—triphasic regimen)
0.050 mg/30 mcg (6d), 0.075 mg/
40 mcg (5d), 0.125 mg/30 mcg (10d) (pink)
Actavis

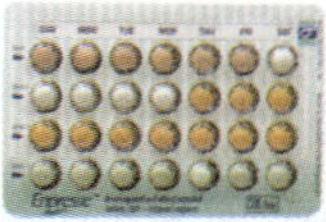

**ENPRESSE®**
(levonorgestrel and ethinyl estradiol tablets,
USP - triphasic regimen)
(active pills pink, white and orange)
Teva Pharmaceuticals USA

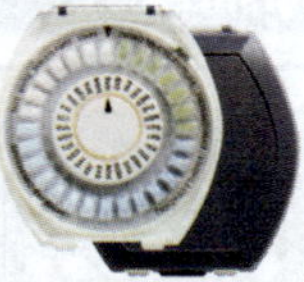

**ORTHO TRI-CYCLEN® - 28 TABLETS**
(norgestimate/ethinyl estradiol)
0.18 mg/35 mcg (7d) (white),
0.215 mg/35 mcg (7d) (light blue),
0.25 mg/35 mcg (7d) (blue)
Jannsen

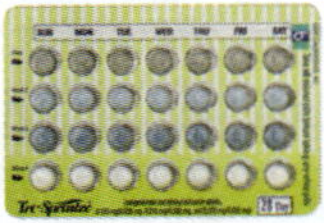

**TRI-SPRINTEC®**
(norgestimate and ethinyl estradiol tablets - triphasic regimen)
(active pills gray, light blue and blue)
Teva Pharmaceuticals USA

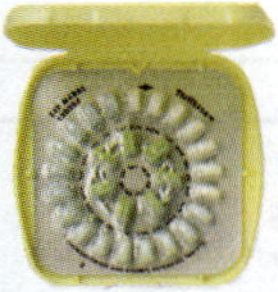

**TRINESSA®**
(norgestimate/ethinyl estradiol)
0.18 mg/35 mcg (7d) (white),
0.215 mg/35 mcg (7d) (light blue),
0.25 mg/35 mcg (7d) (dark blue)
remaining 7 placebo pills are green
Actavis

**TRI-PREVIFEM™ - 28 TABLETS**
(norgestimate and ethinyl estradiol tablets - triphasic regimen)
Qualitest

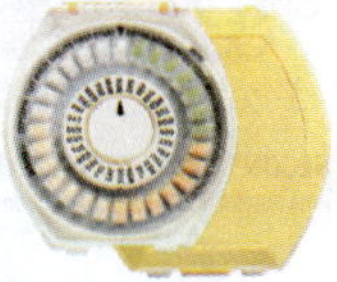

**ORTHO-NOVUM® 7/7/7 - 28 TABLETS**
(norethindrone/ethinyl estradiol)
0.5 mg/35 mcg (7d) (white),
0.75 mg/35 mcg (7d) (light peach),
1 mg/35 mcg (7d) (peach)
Jannsen

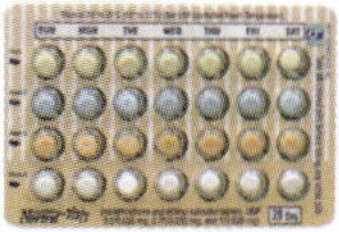

**NORTREL® 7/7/7**
(norethindrone and ethinyl estradiol tablets, USP - triphasic regimen)
(active pills light yellow, blue and peach)
Teva Pharmaceuticals USA

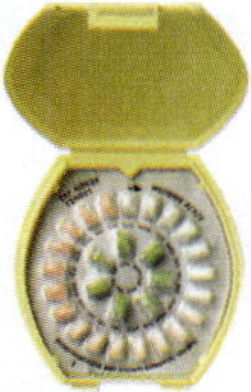

**NECON® 7/7/7**
0.5 mg/35 mcg (7d) (yellow),
0.75 mg/35 mcg (7d) (blue),
1 mg/35 mcg (7d) (peach)
Actavis

# COMBINED PILLS - 50 microgram PILLS

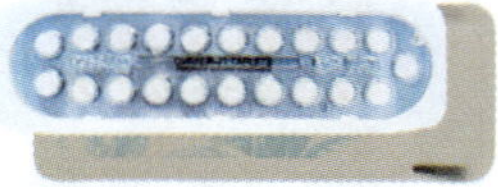

**OVRAL® - 21 TABLETS**
(0.5 mg norgestrel/50 mcg ethinyl estradiol)
(active pills white)
Wyeth

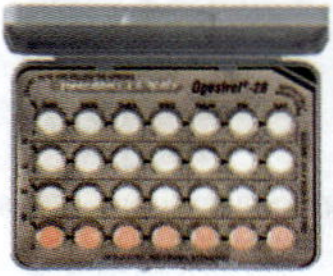

**OGESTREL®**
(0.5 mg norgestrel/50 mcg ethinyl estradiol)
(active pills white)
Actavis

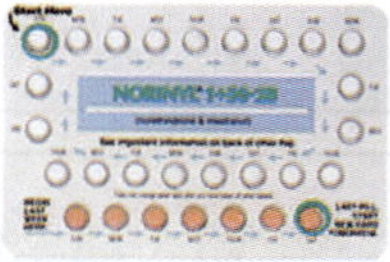

**NORINYL® 1/50**
(1 mg norethindrone/50 mcg mestranol)
Actavis

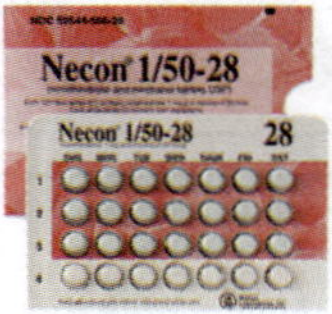


**NECON® 1/50 - 28 TABLETS**
(1 mg norethindrone/50 mcg mestranol)
Actavis

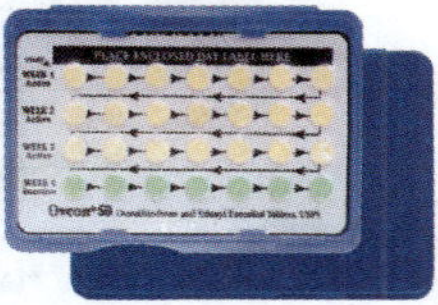

**OVCON® 50 28-DAY**
**(1 mg norethindrone/50 mcg ethinyl estradiol)**
(active pills yellow)
Warner-Chilcott

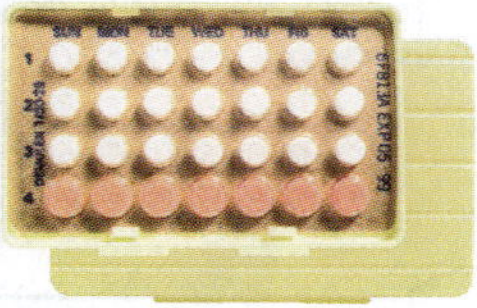

**DEMULEN® 1/50-28**
**(1 mg ethynodiol diacetate/50 mcg ethinyl estradiol)**
(active pills white)
Pfizer

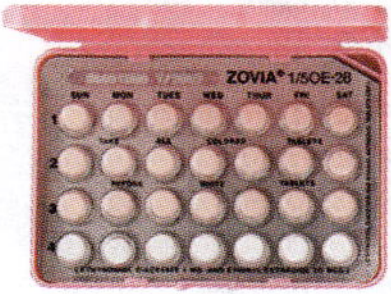

**ZOVIA® 1/50**
**(1 mg ethynodiol diacetate/50 mcg ethinyl estradiol)**
Actavis

# PILLS AS EMERGENCY CONTRACEPTIVES:

2 Different Approaches: Progestin-Only Pills OR Combined Pills

## PROGESTIN-ONLY PILLS

### Plan B

**1 + 1 pill** 12 hours apart OR
2 Plan B Pills *(white)* ASAP after unprotected sex

*Plan B available without a prescription in pharmacies to women and men ≥ 18 years old. Plan B is NOT carried in all pharmacies. Check in advance. Ask your pharmacy to carry Plan B.*

Barr Laboratories

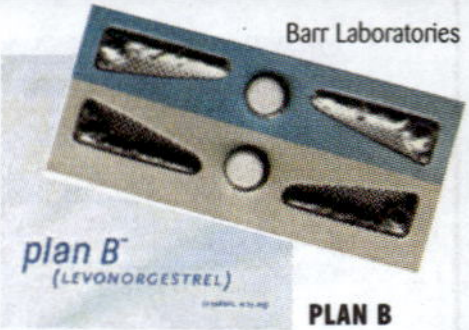


PLAN B

**Antinausea meds not necessary**

## COMBINED ORAL CONTRACEPTIVES

**2 + 2 pills** 12 hours apart
Ogestrel *(white pills)*
Ovral *(white pills)*

*(Ogestrel and Ovral are NOT carried in all pharmacies. Check in advance.)*

**4 + 4 pills** 12 hours apart
Cryselle *(white pills)*
Enpresse *(orange pills)*
Jolessa *(pink pills)*
Low-Ogestrel *(white pills)*
Lo-Ovral *(white pills)*
Levora *(white pills)*
Levlen *(light orange pills)*
Nordette *(light orange pills)*
Portia *(pink pills)*
Quasense *(white pills)*
Seasonale *(pink pills)*
Seasonique *(light blue pills)*
Triphasil *(yellow pills)*
Tri-Levlen *(yellow pills)*
Trivora *(pink pills)*

**Have your patient take antinausea medication an hour before the first dose if using any of the combined oral contraceptives as emergency contraception. This is not necessary if using Plan B.**

**5 + 5 pills** 12 hours apart
Alesse *(pink pills)*
Levlite *(pink pills)*
Aviane *(orange pills)*
Lessina *(pink pills)*
Lutera *(white pills)*